Alcohol: A Dangerous and Unnecessary Medicine, How and Why

by Martha M. Allen

I0429759

CONTENTS.

CHAPTER IV.

TEMPERANCE HOSPITALS.

CHAPTER V.

THE EFFECTS OF ALCOHOL UPON THE HUMAN BODY.

CHAPTER VI.

ALCOHOL AS MEDICINE.

CHAPTER VII.

ALCOHOL IN PHARMACY.

and acetic acid to preserve drugs--Non-alcohol tinctures in use at London Temperance Hospital--Sale of liquor in drug-stores condemned by pharmacists 131

CHAPTER VIII.

DISEASES, AND THEIR TREATMENT WITHOUT ALCOHOL.

CHAPTER IX.

ALCOHOL AND NURSING MOTHERS.

CHAPTER X.

COMPARATIVE DEATH-RATES WITH AND WITHOUT THE USE OF ALCOHOL.

CHAPTER XI.

REASONS WHY ALCOHOL IS DANGEROUS AS MEDICINE.

CHAPTER XII.

WHY DOCTORS STILL PRESCRIBE ALCOHOLICS.

CHAPTER XIII.

ALCOHOLIC PROPRIETARY OR "PATENT" MEDICINES.

CHAPTER XVII.

MISCELLANEOUS.

INTRODUCTION.

This book is the outcome of many years of study. With the exception of a few quotations, none of the material has ever before appeared in any book. The writer has been indebted for years past to many of the physicians mentioned in the following pages for copies of pamphlets and magazines, and for newspaper articles, bearing upon the medical study of alcohol. Indeed, had it not been for the kindly counsels and hearty co-operation of physicians, she could never have accomplished all that was laid upon her to do as a state and national superintendent of Medical Temperance for the Woman's Christian Temperance Union. She is also under obligation for helps received from the secretaries of several State Boards of Health, and from eminent chemists and pharmacists.

The object of the book is to put into the hands of the people a statement of the views regarding the medical properties of alcohol held by those physicians who make little, or no use of this drug. In most cases their views are given in their own language, so that the book is, of necessity, largely a compilation.

It is hoped that while the laity may be glad to peruse these pages because of the very useful and interesting information to be obtained from them, the medical profession, also, may be pleased to find, in brief form, the teachings of some of their most distinguished brethren upon a question now frequently up for discussion in society meetings.

The writer does not presume to set forth her own opinions upon a question which is still a subject of dispute among the members of a learned profession; she simply culls from the writings of those members of that profession who, having made thorough examination of the claims of alcohol, have decided that this drug, as ordinarily used, is more harmful than beneficial, and that medical practice would be upon a higher plane, were it driven entirely from the pharmacopoeia.

PREFACE TO SECOND EDITION.

When the first edition of this book was published in 1900, there were only a few leading physicians either in Europe or America who were ready to condemn the medical use of alcohol. Sir Benjamin Ward Richardson, Sims Woodhead, and a few others in England; Forel, Kassowitz and one or two more on the Continent, and Nathan S. Davis, T. D. Crothers and J. H. Kellogg, in America, were about all that could be quoted largely as opposed to alcoholic liquors as remedies in disease. Whisky was then looked upon as necessary in the treatment of consumption and diphtheria. Ten years have brought about a great change. There are many American physicians now willing to admit that they have very little or no use for alcoholic liquors as remedial agents, and now, instead of recommending whisky for consumption anti-tuberculosis literature almost everywhere warns against the use of intoxicating drinks. The use of anti-toxin in diphtheria has driven out whisky treatment in that disease with markedly favorable results. Under the whisky treatment death-rates ran up to fifty-five and sixty per cent.; now the diphtheria death-rate is very low. Ten years ago many good authorities still ranked alcohol as a stimulant; now, almost all rank it as a depressant. In England, leading physicians and surgeons have spoken so strongly against alcohol in the last few years that the London Times, England's leading newspaper, said: "According to recent developments of scientific opinion, it is not impossible that a belief in the strengthening and supporting qualities of alcohol will eventually become as obsolete as a belief in witchcraft."

So far as the writer can learn from replies sent to her inquiries by teachers of medicine, and by study of text-books on medicine, and articles in good medical journals, alcohol now has only a very limited use in medicine with the great majority of successful physicians. Some recommend wine in diabetes mellitus, saying that it acts less like a poison and more like a food in that disease than in any other. Some use alcoholic liquors in fevers as a food "to save the burning of tissue," but an article on "Therapeutics" in the

Journal of the American Medical Association, for November 6, 1909, page 1564, says that sugar would probably have equal value in such case. The same article says that hot baths, with hot lemonade, and a quickly acting cathartic, will abort a cold without any need of recourse to alcohol.

The writer wishes here to make grateful acknowledgment of courtesies received from busy physicians who have aided materially in her work by answering personal letters of inquiry, also letters published in the Journal of the American Medical Association, by kindness of the editor. Especially would she thank those professors of medicine and superintendents of large hospitals, who so courteously aided her in preparing a paper for the International Congress on Alcoholism, held in London, July, 1909, to which she was a delegate, representing the United States government. A few of the replies received at that time are given in this book. There was not room for all.

She wishes also to acknowledge kindness and much help received from pharmacists and druggists in the fight against dangerous patent medicines and drug drinks sold at soda fountains. The Druggists' Circular, of New York, deserves special mention in this connection.

It has been necessary to make many changes in this edition because of the changing views on alcohol and the publicity on patent medicines. Physicians will find Chapter XVI entirely new, and of great interest.

M. M. A.

* * * *

ALCOHOL.

CHAPTER I.

HISTORY OF THE STUDY OF ALCOHOL.

The only intoxicating drinks known to the ancients were wines and beers. That these were used for medicinal as well as beverage purposes is evident from sacred and secular history. About the tenth century of the Christian era, an Arabian alchemist discovered the art of distillation, by which the active principle of fermented liquors could be drawn off and separated. To the spirit thus produced the name alcohol was given. A plausible reason cited for this name is that the Arabian for evil spirit is Al ghole, and the effects of the mysterious liquid upon men suggested demoniacal possession.

Medical knowledge at this time was very limited: there was no accurate way of determining the real nature of the new substance, nor its action upon the human system. It could be judged only by its seeming effects. As these were pleasing, it was supposed that a great medical discovery had been made. The alchemists had been seeking a panacea for all the ills to which flesh is heir, indeed for something which would enable men even to defy Death, and the subtle new spirit was eagerly proclaimed as the long-looked-for cure-all, if not the very aqua vit?itself. Physicians introduced it to their patients, and were lavish in their praises of its curative powers. The following is quoted from the writings of Theoricus, a prominent German of the sixteenth century, as an example of medical opinion of alcohol in his day:--

"It sloweth age, it strengtheneth youth, it helpeth digestion, it cutteth phlegme, it cureth the hydropsia, it healeth the strangurie, it pounces the stone, it expelleth gravel, it keepeth the head from whirling, the teeth from chattering, and the throat from rattling; it keepeth the weasen from stiffling, the stomach from wambling, and the heart from swelling; it keepeth the hands from shivering, the sinews from shrinking, the veins from crumbling, the bones from aching, and the marrow from soaking."

Being a medicine, which very rapidly creates a craving for itself, the demand for it became enormous, and, as time advanced, people began prescribing it for themselves, until its use both as medicine and beverage became almost general.

If the medical profession is responsible for the wide-spread belief that alcoholics are of service to mankind both as food and medicine, it should not be forgotten that it is to members of the same profession the world is indebted for the correction of these errors. All down through the centuries there have been physicians who doubted and opposed its claims to merit. It remained for the medical science of the latter half of the nineteenth century to clearly demonstrate with nicely adjusted chemical apparatus and appliances the wisdom of these doubts.

The scientific study of the effects of alcohol upon the human body began about sixty years ago. The first American investigator was Dr. Nathan S. Davis, of Chicago, who was the founder of the American Medical Association. During the months of May, June, July, September and October, 1848, Dr. Davis published in the Annalist, a monthly medical journal of New York City, a series of articles controverting the universal opinion that alcoholic drinks are warming, strengthening and nourishing. In 1850 he executed an extensive series of experiments to determine the effects of a diet exclusively carbonaceous (starch), one exclusively nitrogenous (albumen), and alcohol (brandy and wine), on the temperature of the living body; on the quantity of carbonic acid exhaled; and on the circulation of the blood. The results of these investigations were embodied in a paper read before the American Medical Association in May, 1851. They showed that alcohol, instead of increasing animal heat, and promoting nutrition and strength, actually produced directly opposite effects, reducing temperature, the amount of carbonic acid exhaled, and the muscular strength. So opposed were these conclusions to the generally accepted teachings of the day that the Association did not refer the paper to the committee of publication. It was published later in the Northwestern Medical and Surgical Journal.

In 1854 Dr. Davis published one of the most remarkable of the numerous works which have come from his prolific pen; it was entitled, "A Lecture on the Effects of Alcoholic Drinks on the Human System, and the Duty of Medical Men in Relation Thereto." This lecture was delivered in Rush Medical College, Chicago, on Christmas, 1854. An appendix to the work contained a full account of the series of original experiments which the author had been conducting in relation to the effect of alcohol upon respiration and animal heat, and gave the same conclusions as those presented before the A. M. A. several years previously. These experiments laid the foundation for the scientific study of the physiological effects of alcohol; and their bearing upon the study of the temperance question can even yet scarcely be appreciated. They were the first experiments which showed conclusively that the effect of alcohol is not that of a stimulant, but the opposite.

In 1855 Prof. R. D. Mussey, of Vermont, read an able paper before the American Medical Association upon "The Effects of Alcohol in Health and Disease," in which he said, "So long as alcohol retains its place among sick patients, so long will there be drunkards."

In England as early as 1802, Dr. Beddoes pointed out the dangers attendant upon the social and medical use of intoxicating drinks, laying stress upon "The enfeebling power of small portions of wine regularly drunk." In 1829 Dr. John Cheyne, Physician General to the forces in Ireland said:--

"The benefits which have been supposed from their liberal use in medicine, and especially in those diseases which are vulgarly supposed to depend upon mere weakness, have invested these agents with attributes to which they have no claim, and hence, as we physicians no longer employ them as we were wont to do, we ought not to rest satisfied with the mere acknowledgment of error, but we ought also to make every retribution in our power for having so long upheld one of the most fatal delusions that ever took possession of the human mind."

Dr. Higginbotham, F. R. S., of Nottingham, a keen and able clinical practitioner, abandoned the prescription of alcohol in 1832, saying:--

"I have amply tried both ways. I gave alcohol in my practice for twenty years, and have now practiced without it for the last thirty years or more. My experience is, that acute disease is more readily cured without it, and chronic diseases much more manageable. I have not found a single patient injured by the disuse of alcohol, or a constitution requiring it; indeed, to find either, although I am in my seventy-seventh year, I would walk fifty miles to see such an unnatural phenomenon. If I ordered or allowed alcohol in any form, either as food or as medicine, to a patient, I should certainly do it with a felonious intent."--Ipswich Tracts. No. 346.

In 1839 Dr. Julius Jeffreys drew up a medical declaration which was signed by seventy-eight leaders of medicine and surgery. This document declared the opinion to be erroneous that wine, beer or spirit was beneficial to health; that even in the most moderate doses, alcoholic drinks did no good. This, of course, dealt only with the beverage use of alcoholics. In 1847 a second declaration was originated, signed by over two thousand of the most eminent physicians and surgeons. This also referred only to liquor as a beverage. In 1871 a third declaration, signed by two hundred and sixty-nine of the leading members of the medical profession was published in the London Times.

This declaration was in part as follows:--

"As it is believed that the inconsiderate prescription of large quantities of alcoholic liquids by medical men for their patients has given rise, in many instances, to the formation of intemperate habits, the undersigned, while unable to abandon the use of alcohol in the treatment of certain cases of disease, are yet of opinion that no medical practitioner should prescribe it without a sense of grave responsibility.

"They are also of opinion that many people immensely exaggerate the value of alcohol as an article of diet, and they hold that every medical practitioner is bound to exert his utmost influence to inculcate habits of great moderation in the use of alcoholic liquids."

In the same year the American Medical Association passed a resolution that "alcohol should be classed with other powerful drugs, and when prescribed medically, it should be done with conscientious caution, and a sense of great responsibility."

The physicians of New York, Brooklyn and vicinity not long afterward published a declaration practically the same as that of the A. M. A., adding: "We are of opinion that the use of alcoholic liquor as a beverage is productive of a large amount of physical disease."

The publication of these later declarations was the beginning of a marked change in the medical use of alcohol.

In England the scientific temperance movement began with Dr. B. W. Richardson, afterwards knighted by Queen Victoria for his great services to humanity as a medical philanthropist. Dr. Richardson's success in bringing before physicians the remarkable medicinal agent known as nitrite of amyl, led to a request from the British Association for the Advancement of Science that he investigate other chemical substances. The result was that several years of study, beginning with 1863, were given to the physiological effects of various alcohols, ethylic alcohol, which is the active principle in wines, beers and other intoxicating drinks, receiving special attention.

The following is taken from his "Results of Researches on Alcohol":--

"In my hands ethylic alcohol and other bodies of the same group; viz. methylic, propylic, butylic, and amylic alcohols were tested purely from the physiological point of view. They were tested exclusively as chemical substances apart from any question as to their general use and employment, and free from all bias for or against their influence on mankind for good or for evil.

"The method of research that was pursued was the same that had been followed in respect to nitrite of amyl, chloroform, ether, and other chemical substances, and it was in the following order: First, the mode in which living bodies would take up or absorb the substance was considered. This settled, the quantity necessary to produce a decided physiological change was ascertained, and was estimated in relation to the weight of the living body on which the observation was made. After these facts were ascertained the special action of the agent was investigated on the blood, on the motion of the heart, on the respiration, on the minute circulation of the blood, on the digestive organs, on the secreting and excreting organs, on the nervous system and brain, on the animal temperature and on the muscular activity. By these processes of inquiry, each specially carried out, I was enabled to test fairly the action of the different chemical agents that came before me. * * * * *

"The results of these researches were that I learned purely by experimental observation that, in its action on the living body, alcohol deranges the constitution of the blood; unduly excites the heart and respiration; paralyzes the minute blood-vessels; disturbs the regularity of nervous action; lowers the animal temperature, and lessens the muscular power.

"Such, independent of any prejudice of party or influence of sentiment, are the unanswerable teachings of the sternest of all evidences, the evidences of experiment, of natural fact revealed to man by testing of natural phenomena."

When Dr. Richardson reported to the Association for the Advancement of Science the results of his researches so at variance with commonly accepted ideas, the Association was as incredulous as the American Medical Association had been in 1851 when Dr. Davis gave a similar report, and Dr. Richardson's paper was returned to him for correction.

It should be stated here that Dr. Richardson was not a total abstainer when he began his study of the effects of alcohol, but became an ardent and enthusiastic advocate of total abstinence, and later of non-alcoholic medication, because of what he learned by his experiments with this drug. He was the first to suggest that scientific temperance be taught in the public schools, and he prepared the first text-book ever published for this purpose. In 1874 he delivered his famous "Cantor Lectures on Alcohol," by request of the Society of Arts. This series of lectures created a sensation, being attended by crowds of people, as it was the first time that any physician of eminence had spoken from experimental evidence in favor of total abstinence.

The agitation begotten in medical circles by the discussion of Dr. Richardson's researches upon alcohol led to extensive experimenting upon the same line by scientists of England, Continental Europe and America. The efforts of the National Woman's Christian Temperance Union of the United States, led by that intrepid woman, Mrs. Mary H. Hunt, to introduce scientific temperance instruction into public schools gave impetus to the study in this country. The call for text-books caused publishers to request professors in medical colleges to make minute research into the nature and effects of alcohol, that the demands of the new educational law might be met. The bitter opposition to these temperance education laws was a great stimulant to the scientific study of alcohol, for it was hoped by many that the teachings regarding the deleterious effects of alcohol might be proved incorrect. Unfortunately for the lovers of the bibulous, the proof was all the other way; great medical men could not be bought by distillers or brewers to tell anything but the truth, and the truth of experimental research was all against alcohol. The text-books endorsed by Mrs. Hunt and her advisory committee being assailed again and again as containing erroneous teaching, were finally, in 1897, submitted to an examining committee of medical experts, nearly all of whom were connected with medical colleges. This committee consisted of Dr. N. S. Davis, Sr., of Chicago, Ill.; Dr. Leartus Connor, of Detroit, Michigan; Dr. Henry Q. Marcy, of Boston, Mass.; Dr. E. E. Montgomery, of Philadelphia, Pa.; Dr. Henry D. Holton, of Brattleboro, Vt.; and Dr. George F. Shrady, of New York City. From their reports upon the books the following is culled:--

"I find no errors in the teaching of any of them on this subject."

"No statement was found at variance with the most reliable studies of especially competent investigators."

"I was asked to point out any errors in these books which need correcting. I find no such errors."

"I find their teaching completely in accordance with the facts determined through scientific experimentation and investigation."

"I find them to be in substantial accord with the results of the latest scientific investigations."

Dr. Baer, of Berlin, Germany, the foremost European specialist on the subject treated in these text-books, has recently subjected the books to rigid examination. He says in his report upon them:--

"On the basis of the examination I have made I can assert that the above mentioned school text-books, (the endorsed physiologies), in respect to their statements regarding alcoholic drinks contain no teachings which are not in harmony with the attitude of strict science."

Still the opposers of the text-books were not satisfied, and a self constituted Committee of Fifty undertook an investigation. Men of unquestioned ability were chosen to make researches, but the result of their investigations was so different from what was looked for, that, with the exception of Professor Atwater's contention for the food value of alcohol, the report of the Committee of Fifty did not stir up much controversy.

The school text-books deal exclusively with the effects of alcohol used as a beverage; for obvious reasons this is all they can do. But as intoxicating drinks have been generally supposed to contain great virtue as remedial agents, this phase of their nature and effects has not been overlooked by those pursuing inquiries concerning them. While full agreement has not yet been reached by experts as to the value of alcoholic liquids as medicines, it is noteworthy that some of the most eminent investigators were led to drop alcohol from their pharmaceutical outfit, and the remainder to admit that its sphere of usefulness is extremely limited.

There are now medical colleges of high standing where students are advised against the use of alcohol as a remedy; hospitals are gradually using it less and less, some entirely discarding it; and many progressive physicians, while saying nothing as to their position upon the alcohol question, yet show their lack of faith in this drug by ignoring it unless patients or their friends desire it.

CHAPTER II.

THE WOMAN'S CHRISTIAN TEMPERANCE UNION IN OPPOSITION TO ALCOHOL AS MEDICINE.

When the W. C. T. U. was first organized there was no thought among its members of antagonizing the use of alcohol in medicine. One almost immediate result of the organization, however, was that the women began to study the causes of inebriety, and prominent among the prevailing influences leading to drunkenness they found the medical use of alcoholics. The early efforts of these women were chiefly in rescue work through Gospel temperance meetings, and visitations of jails and poor-houses. By reason of this contact with the effects of inebriety they learned many sad tales of ruined lives, blighted homes and lost souls, through the appetite for strong drink created, or aroused, by alcoholic prescription. They saw, as time passed, that some of the drunkards reclaimed through their influence lapsed again into their evil habits because a little beer, or wine, "for the stomach's sake," or some other sake, had been advised them. Some of the workers had this trouble in their own homes, husband, son or other relative enslaved to alcohol through prescription in disease. Is it any wonder that women of the spirit of the Crusaders, having once had their attention thoroughly aroused to the danger of alcohol in medicine, should begin to examine this stronghold of the enemy to discover, if possible, whether or not, his fortress, the medicine-chest, was impregnable? Greatly to their joy they found that the medical profession was not a unit in commending alcoholics as remedial agencies, that all along since alcohol came into common use there have been physicians who distrusted, and opposed it. They learned, too, that some of the most distinguished physicians of America and of England were using little or no alcohol in their practice, and that a hospital had been established in London, England, which was clearly demonstrating the superiority of non-alcoholic medication by its small death-rate in comparison with hospitals using alcohol.

This knowledge encouraged those possessing it so that they began to refuse alcoholics as remedies in their own households, and rarely did they find physicians unwilling or unable to supply another agent when asked to do so, and thousands of women can now testify to the fact of having recovered from ill health without the wine, beer or brandy they were advised to take. So the W. C. T. U. discovered several good reasons for opposing alcohol in medicine.

1. Its liability to create or revive an uncontrollable appetite.

2. A considerable number of the leading physicians of America and of Great Britain discard it from their list of remedies, considering it harmful rather than helpful.

3. The lessened mortality consequent upon its entire disuse demonstrated by the London Temperance Hospital.

4. By their own experience they knew that alcohol is not necessary to the restoration of health, nor to the upbuilding of strength.

The first active work touching the medical use of alcohol was a memorial from the National W. C. T. U. to the International Medical Congress of 1876, which met in Washington, D. C. This memorial was suggested by Miss Frances E. Willard, and co-operated in by the National Temperance Society. It asked for a deliverance from the Congress upon alcohol as a food and as a medicine.

The Congress was divided into sections for the more thorough discussion of the various topics. Upon the program was a paper on "The Therapeutic Value of Alcohol as Food, and as a Medicine," by Ezra M. Hunt, M. D., delegate from the New Jersey Medical Society. This paper was read before the "Section on Medicine," and, after earnest discussion, the conclusions of the author were adopted "quite unanimously" as the sentiments of the Section on Medicine. As such they were reported for acceptance to the General Congress, and by it ordered to be transmitted as a reply to the memorialists.

The report was published in full by the National Temperance Society, and may be obtained from it in paper binding for twenty-five cents. As it makes a book of 137 pages the conclusions only will be quoted here. They are as follows:--

1. "Alcohol is not shown to have a definite food value by any of the usual methods of chemical analysis or physiological investigation.

2. "Its use as a medicine is chiefly that of a cardiac stimulant, and often admits of substitution.

3. "As a medicine it is not well fitted for self-prescription by the laity, and the medical profession is not accountable for such administration, or for the enormous evil arising therefrom.

4. "The purity of alcoholic liquors is in general not as well assured as that of articles used for medicine should be. The various mixtures when used as medicine should have definite and known composition, and should not be interchanged promiscuously."

It is matter for sincere regret that this deliverance was not, in some way, brought prominently before every physician in the land. There are, doubtless, thousands of physicians who never heard of it, and, consequently have never been influenced by it to doubt the utility of the popular brandy bottle.

In 1883 Mrs. Mary Towne Burt, President of New York State W. C. T. U., in her annual address, suggested that a department of work be created to endeavor to induce physicians to not prescribe alcohol, unless in such cases as allowed of the use of no other agent. Mrs. (Rev.) J. Butler, of Fairport, was the first superintendent of this department, which was named, "Influencing Physicians to not Prescribe Alcoholics as Medicines." The National W. C. T. U. adopted the department in 1883, but soon dropped it. In 1895 it was reinstated and Mrs. Martha M. Allen, New York's superintendent, was made national superintendent. In 1905 the name of the department was changed from Non-Alcoholic Medication, which it had borne for fifteen years, to Medical Temperance.

The objects of this department of work are:

1. To inform the public of the objections to the medical use of alcoholic drinks now held by many successful physicians.

2. To show the dangers in the home-prescription of alcohol and other powerful drugs.

3. To expose fraudulent and dangerous proprietary and "patent" medicines and liquid "foods," the main ingredients of which are alcohol and morphine.

4. To use persuasion with publishers of newspapers and magazines against fraudulent medical advertising. Also to seek legislation which shall hinder such advertising.

5. To endeavor to win the attention of physicians who prescribe alcoholic

liquors to the teachings of great leaders in their profession who have abandoned such practice.

6. To bring to the attention of nurses the same teachings, and to seek their co-operation in education against the self-prescription of alcohol.

7. To work for legislation which shall correct the evils of the whisky drug-store, the whisky-prescribing doctor, and the dangerous "patent" medicine.

8. To gather the opinions upon alcohol of well-known physicians who do not use it, and publish them.

This department originated the public agitation against injurious and fraudulent "patent" medicines which later was so ably carried on by Collier's Weekly, and the Ladies' Home Journal. That its early work in this direction was not better known to the general public was due to the fact that religious as well as secular papers were reaping large revenues from the advertising of these nostrums, and consequently refused to publish anything which might injure the trade. Indeed, in accepting some of this advertising, newspaper managers had to sign a contract that they would not publish any reading matter opposed to the nostrum business.

The Christian Advocate of New York city deserves special mention for having published in 1898 two articles written by Mrs. Allen under the caption, "The Danger and Harmfulness of Patent Medicines." These were in the fall of that year published in pamphlet form, and a copy sent to every local W. C. T. U. in the United States for study. Tens of thousands of copies of this and other leaflets on that theme were distributed within a few years, some local unions placing them in every home in their community. Medical journals took note of this work and commended it highly. When Mr. Bok began his campaign of education in the Ladies' Home Journal, for which he deserves lasting gratitude, the American Druggist said he was "bowing to the clamor of the W. C. T. U."

This department which began in weakness, and was for years regarded as fanatical even by many members of the W. C. T. U. has entered upon an era of victories. The National Pure Food Law requires the percentage of alcohol in patent medicines, and the presence of different dangerous drugs, to be stated upon the label. The prohibition law of Georgia forbids physicians to prescribe alcoholic beverages, absolute alcohol only being permitted. Kansas has amended her law so that whisky drug-stores are eliminated. If physicians prescribe alcohol the law forbids charge for it. Alabama forbids the sale of liquor for everything but the communion. The Internal Revenue Department has examined a large number of "patent" medicines and has listed them as intoxicating beverages. Two state medical societies and some county societies in 1908 passed resolutions to discourage the medical use of alcoholic liquors. Two national societies of druggists and pharmacists in 1908 passed resolutions against whiskey drug-stores.

These are some of the results of Medical Temperance agitation. Much more may be expected in the next decade if the work is as faithfully and fearlessly carried on as in the past.

This book contains much of the teachings of the department of Medical Temperance. When these views are generally accepted the liquor-problem will be well-nigh solved.

CHAPTER III.

ALCOHOL AS A PRODUCER OF DISEASE.

That alcohol is a poison is attested by all chemists and other scientific men; taken undiluted it destroys the vitality of the tissues of the body with which it comes in contact as readily as creosote, or pure carbolic acid. The term intoxicating applied to beverages containing it refers to its poisonous nature, the word being derived from the Greek toxicon, which signifies a bow or an arrow; the barbarians poisoned their arrows, hence, toxicum in Latin was used to signify poison; from this comes the English term toxicology, which is the science treating of poisons. Druggists in selling proof spirits usually label the bottle, "Poison." Apart from the testimony of science in regard to its poisonous nature, it is commonly known that large doses of brandy or whisky will speedily cause death, particularly in those unaccustomed to their use. The newspapers frequently contain items regarding the death of children who have had access to whisky, and drunk freely of it. Cases are reported, too, of men, habituated to drink, who after tossing off several glasses of brandy at the bar of a saloon have suddenly dropped dead.

Dr. Mussey says:--

"A poison is that substance, in whatever form it may be, which, when applied to a living surface, disconcerts and disturbs life's healthy movements. It is altogether distinct from substances which are in their nature nutritious. It is not capable of being converted into food, and becoming a part of the living organs. We all know that proper food is wrought into our bodies; the action of animal life occasions a constant waste, and new matter has to be taken in, which, after digestion, is carried into the blood, and then changed; but poison is incapable of this. It may indeed be mixed with nutritious substances, but if it goes into the blood, it is thrown off as soon as the system can accomplish its deliverance, if it has not been too far enfeebled by the influence of the poison. Such a poison is alcohol--such in all its forms mix it with what you may."

Dr. Nathan S. Davis said in an address given in 1891:--

"When largely diluted with water, as it is in all the varieties of fermented and distilled liquids, and taken into the stomach, it is rapidly imbibed, or taken up by the capillary vessels and carried into the venous blood, without having undergone any digestion or change in the stomach. With the blood it is carried to every part, and made to penetrate every tissue of the living body, where it has been detected by proper chemical tests as unchanged alcohol, until it has been removed through the natural process of elimination, or lost its identity by molecular combination with the albuminous elements of the blood and tissues, for which it has a strong affinity.

"The most varied and painstaking experiments of chemists and physiologists, both in this country and Europe, have shown conclusively that the presence of alcohol in the blood diminishes the amount of oxygen taken up through the air-cells of the lungs; retards the molecular and metabolic changes of both nutrition and waste throughout the system and diminishes the sensibility and action of the nervous structures in direct proportion to the quantity of alcohol present. By its stronger affinity for water and albumen, with which it readily unites in all proportions, it so alters the hemaglobin of the blood as to lessen its power to take the oxygen from the air-cells of the lungs and carry it as oxyhemaglobia to all the tissues of the body; and by the same affinity it retards all atomic or molecular changes in the muscular, secretory and nervous structures; and in the same ratio it diminishes the elimination of carbon-dioxide, phosphates, heat and nerve force. In other words, its presence diminishes all the physical phenomena of life.

"I say, then, that from the facts hitherto adduced, whether from accurate experimental investigations in different countries, from the pathological results developed in the most scientific societies, from the most reliable statistics of sickness and mortality, as influenced by occupations and social habits, or from the life insurance records kept on a uniform basis through periods of ten, twenty, thirty or even forty years, it is clearly shown that alcohol when taken into the human system not only acts upon the nervous system, perverting its sensibility, and, if increased in quantity, causing intoxication or insensibility, but it also, even in small quantities, lessens the oxygenation and decarbonization of the blood and retards the molecular changes in the structures of the body. When these effects are continued through months and years, as in the most temperate class of drinkers, they lead to permanent structural changes, most prominently in the liver, kidneys, stomach, heart, blood-vessels and nerve structures, and lessen the natural duration of life in the aggregate from ten to fifteen years. Consequently there is no greater, nor more destructive error existing in the public mind than the belief that the use of fermented and distilled drinks does no harm so long as they do not intoxicate.

"Another popular error is the opinion that the substitution of the different varieties of beer and wine in the place of distilled liquors promotes temperance, and lessens the evil effects of alcohol on the health and morals of those who use them. Accurate investigations show that beer and wine drinkers generally consume more alcohol per man than the spirit drinkers; and while they are not as often intoxicated, they suffer fully as much from diseases and premature death as do those who use distilled spirits. Again, the beer drinker drinks more nearly every day, and thereby keeps some alcohol in his blood more constantly; while a large percentage of spirit drinkers drink only periodically, leaving considerable intervals of abstinence, during which the tissues regain nearly their natural condition. The more constant and persistent is the presence of alcohol in the blood and the tissues, even in moderate quantity, the more certainly does it lead to perverted and degenerative changes in the tissues, ending in renal (kidney) and hepatic (liver) dropsies, cardiac (heart) failures, gout, apoplexy and paralysis."

Sir B. W. Richardson says:--

"Alcohol produces many diseases; and it constantly happens that persons die of diseases which have their origin solely in the drinking of alcohol, while the cause itself is never for a moment suspected. A man may say quite truthfully that he never was tipsy in the whole course of his life; and yet it is quite possible that such a man may die of disease caused by the alcohol he has taken, and by no other cause whatever. This is one of the most dreadful evils of alcohol, that it kills insidiously, as if it were doing no harm, or as if it were doing good, while it is destroying life. Another great evil of it is that it assails so many different parts of the body. It hardly seems credible at first sight that the same agent can give rise to the many different kinds of diseases it does give rise to. In fact, the universality of its action has blinded even learned men as to its potency for destruction.

"Step by step, however, we have now discovered that its modes of action are all very simple, and are all the same in character; and that the differences that have been and are seen in different persons under its influence are due mainly to the organs, or organ, which first give way under it. Thus, if the stomach gives way first, we say that the person has indigestion or dyspepsia, or failure of the stomach; if the brain gives way first, we say the person has paralysis, or apoplexy, or brain disease; if the liver gives way first, we say the man has liver disease, and so on.

"All persons who indulge much in any form of alcoholic drink are troubled with indigestion. When they wake in the morning they find their mouth dry, their tongue coated, and their appetite bad. In course of time they become confirmed 'dyspeptics,' and as many of them find a temporary relief from the distress at the stomach, and the deficient appetite from which they suffer by taking more liquor, they increase the quantity taken, and so make matters much worse. * * * * *

"There are a great number of diseases caused by alcohol, some of which are known by terms that do not convey to the mind what really has been the cause of the diseases." They are:

(a) Diseases of the brain and nervous system: indicated by such names as apoplexy, epilepsy, paralysis, vertigo, softening of the brain, delirium tremens, loss of memory and that general failure of the mental power called dementia. (b) Diseases of the lungs: one form of consumption, congestion and subsequent bronchitis. (c) Diseases of the heart: irregular beat, feebleness of the musculcar walls, dilation, disease of the valves. (d) Diseases of the blood: scurvy, dropsy, separation of fibrine. (e) Diseases of the stomach: feebleness of the stomach and indigestion, flatulency, irritation and sometimes inflammation. (f) Diseases of the bowels: relaxation or purging, irritation. (g) Diseases of the liver: congestion, hardening and shrinking cirrhosis. (h) Diseases of the kidneys: change of structure into fatty or waxy-like condition and other changes leading to dropsy. (i) Diseases of the muscles: fatty changes in the muscles, by which they lose their power for proper active contraction. (j) Diseases of the membranes of the body:

thickening and loss of elasticity, by which the parts wrapped up in the membrane are impaired for use, and premature decay is induced.

But it constantly happens that when deaths from these diseases are recorded and alcohol has been the primary cause, some other cause is believed to have been at work.

While drinking parents by virtue of a strong constitution sometimes escape the penalty of their bibulous habit, it is not uncommon to see their children suffering from some disease or nervous weakness such as is caused by alcohol, "the sins of the father being visited upon the children."

Erasmus Darwin says upon this point:--

"It is remarkable that all the diseases from drinking spirituous or fermented liquors are liable to become hereditary, even to the third generation, gradually increasing, if the cause be continued, till the family become extinct."

Prof. Christison, of Edinburgh, in answer to inquiries from the Massachusetts State Board of Health, says of general diseases due to alcohol:--

"I recognize certain diseases which originate in the vice of drunkenness alone, which are delirium tremens, cirrhosis of the liver, many cases of Bright's disease of the kidneys, and dipsomania, or insane drunkenness.

"Then I recognize many other diseases in regard to which excess in alcoholics acts as a powerful predisposing cause, such as gout, gravel, aneurism, paralysis, apoplexy, epilepsy, cystitis, premature incontinence of urine, erysipelas, spreading cellular inflammation, tendency of wounds and sores to gangrene, inability of the constitution to resist the attacks of epidemics. I have had a fearful amount of experience of continued fever in our infirmary during many epidemics, and in all my experience I have only once known an intemperate man of forty and upwards to recover."

Professor Christison also claims that three-fourths, or even four-fifths, of Bright's disease in Scotland is produced by alcohol.

Dr. C. Murchison, in speaking of alcohol as a preventive of disease, says:--

"There is no greater error than to imagine that a liberal allowance of alcoholic liquids fortifies the system against contagious diseases."

In a paper read before the Royal Medical and Chirurgical Society, Oct. 22, 1872, Dr. W. Dickinson gave the following conclusions:--

"Alcohol causes fatty infiltration and fibrous encroachments; it engenders tubercles; encourages suppuration, and retards healing; it produces untimely atheroma (a form of fatty degeneration of the inner coats of the arteries), invites hemorrhage, and anticipates old age. The most constant fatty changes, replacement by oil of the material of epithelial cells and muscular fibres, though probably nearly universal, is most noticeable in the liver, the heart and the kidneys. Drink causes tuberculosis, which is evident not only in the lungs, but in every amenable organ."

Dr. William Hargreaves says:--

"Brandy is not a prophylactic. To the temperate it is an active, exciting cause. It is well known that a single act of intemperance during the prevalence of cholera, will often produce a fatal attack. The sense of warmth and irritation (called stimulation) produced by alcoholic liquors, has led to the erroneous notion that they may prevent cholera. But the contrary we have seen is the truth, for the effects of alcoholics are to reduce the temperature of the body, and instead of stimulating, they narcotize, and reduce the life-forces, and predispose the system to all kinds of disease."

The following testimonies are culled from the writings of eminent physicians:--

Sir Andrew Clark, M. D., F. R. C. P., London, Physician in Ordinary to the Queen, Senior Physician at the London Hospital: "As I looked at the hospital wards to-day, and saw that seven out of ten owed their diseases to alcohol, I could but lament that the teaching about this question is not more direct, more decisive and more home-thrusting. * * * * * Can I say to you any words stronger than these of the terrible effects of alcohol? When I think of this I am disposed to give up my profession, and go forth upon a holy crusade, preaching to all men--Beware of this enemy of the race."

Sir William Gull, F. R. S. (late Physician to her Majesty): "I should say, from my experience, that alcohol is the most destructive agent that we are aware of in this country. I would like to say that a very large number of people in society are dying day by day, poisoned by alcohol, but not supposed to be poisoned by it."

Dr. Abernethy: "If people will leave off drinking alcohol, live plainly, and take very little medicine they will find that many disorders will be relieved by this treatment alone."

Dr. Forel, of the University of Zurich, Switzerland: "Life is considerably shortened by the use of alcohol in large quantities. But a moderate consumption of the same also shortens life by an average of five to six years. This is consistently and unequivocally seen in the statistics kept for thirty years by English insurance companies, with special sections for abstainers. They give a large discount, and still make more profit, as not nearly so many deaths occur as might be expected under the usual calculations. According to federal statistics in the fifteen largest towns of Switzerland, over ten per cent. of the men over twenty years of age die solely, or partly of alcoholism."

Dr. J. H. Kellogg, Battle Creek, Mich.: "Every organ feels the effect of the abuse through indulgence in alcohol, and no function is left undisturbed. By degrees, disordered function, through long continuance of the disturbance, induces tissue change. The most common form of organic or structural disease due to alcohol is fatty degeneration, which may effect almost every organ in the body. * * * * * No class of persons are so subject to nervous diseases due to degeneration of nerves and nerve-centres as drinkers. Partial or general paralysis, locomotor ataxia, epilepsy and a host of other nervous disorders, are directly traceable to the use of alcohol."

One of the visiting physicians of Bellevue Hospital, New York, states that at least two-thirds of all the diseases treated there originated in drink.

Dr. W. A. Hammond: "It is of all causes most prolific in exciting derangements of the brain, the spinal cord, and the nerves."

CHAPTER IV.

TEMPERANCE HOSPITALS.

THE LONDON TEMPERANCE HOSPITAL.

In 1865 Dr. S. Nicholls, medical officer of the Longford Poor-law Union, published a report of the results of non-alcoholic treatment of disease as practiced by him for sixteen years in the institutions under his control. The figures for 1865 were:--

ADMITTED. RECOVERED. DIED.

Fever, 142 135 7 Scarlatina, 33 30 3 Small-pox, 48 47 1 Measles, 8 8 0 --- --- --- 231 220 11

The treatment was altogether without wines, spirits or alcohol in any form.

The death-rate reported by Dr. Nicholls was so small that some of the more observing and progressive physicians were led by it to begin similar experiments in the disuse of alcohol in other hospitals. Among these was Dr.

James Edmunds, senior physician at the Lying-In Hospital, London. The experiments continued a year with a reduced death-rate among both mothers and children. But the great brewers of London, who contributed largely to the support of this hospital raised such a storm of opposition to the discontinuance of alcoholic liquors that the experiments had to be abandoned.

The establishment of a temperance hospital was now suggested, and in October, 1873, a temporary institution was opened in Gower Street, accommodating only seventeen in-patients at one time. Later a fine site was secured on Hampstead Road, and in 1881 the east wing and centre were opened by the Lord Mayor of London. In 1885 the west wing was finished, and the opening ceremonies conducted by the Bishop of London.

At the time of the launching of this enterprise, wine and spirits were literally "poured into" sick persons, with frightful results. Death-rates were enormous. The success of the Temperance Hospital has no doubt had much to do in modifying this abuse. Its death-rate, on an average, has been only 6 per cent. throughout the years since its beginning. This is lower than that of any other general hospital in London, and certainly proves conclusively that alcohol is not necessary in the treatment of disease. The physicians connected with it have been men of eminence in the profession, such as Dr. James Edmunds, Dr. J. J. Ridge and Sir B. W. Richardson.

The visiting staff is not compelled to pledge disuse of alcohol, but is required to report if it is used. During all these years it has been given only seventeen times, then almost entirely in surgical cases, and in nearly all of these a fatal result proved it to be useless. The patients who are restored to health leave without having had aroused or implanted in them a desire for alcoholic liquors, neither have they been taught to regard them as valuable aids to the recovery of health and strength. On the contrary, there have been many who have come in, suffering from this delusion, who have had it thoroughly dispelled, both by their own experience and the experience of their fellow patients.

Sir B. W. Richardson took charge of this hospital from 1892 until his death in 1897. In his report in 1893 he said:--

"I remember quite well when according to custom, I should have prescribed alcohol in all those cases that were not actually inflammatory (speaking of diseases of the alimentary system); but I never remember having seen such quick and sound recoveries as those which have followed the non-alcoholic method."

The following selection showing points of practice in this hospital is taken from the same report:

"For medicinal purposes, we are as free as possible from all complexity. We use glycerine for making what may be called our tinctures, and in my clinique I am introducing a series of 'waters'--aqua ferri, aqua chloroformi, aqua opii, aqua quin? and so on--to form the menstruums of other active drugs when they are called for. I also follow the plan of having the medicines administered with a free quantity of water, and with as accurate a dosage as can be obtained, for I agree with Mr. Spender's original proposition that the administration of medicines in comparatively small and frequent doses is more effective and useful than the more common plan of large doses given at long intervals.

"I treat many cases by inhalation, and for this end I use oxygen in a new and, I hope, efficient manner. I make oxygen gas a medium for carrying other volatile substances that admit of being inhaled with it. The mode is very simple. * * * * * In the pneumonic and bronchial cases the treatment has been of the simple and sustaining kind. The medicines that have been given during the acute febrile stages have been chiefly liquor ammoni?acetatis and carbonate of ammonia in small and frequently repeated doses. The patients have all been well and carefully fed on the milk and middle diet until convalescence was declared. In some of the more extreme instances, where there was fear of collapse from separation of fibrine in the heart or pulmonary artery, ammonia has been given freely according to the method I have for so many years inculcated. I have also in cases of depression under which fibrinous separation is so easily developed, lighted on a mode of administering ammonia which combines feeding with the medicine. I direct that a three or five-grain tabloid of bicarbonate of ammonia shall be dissolved in a cup of coffee or of coffee with milk, and be taken by the patient in that manner. The coffee can be sweetened with sugar if that is desired by the patient, and the ammonia can be so administered without any objectionable taste to the beverage. After what is called the crisis in acute pneumonia, I administer very little medicine of any kind; I trust rather to careful feeding with an occasional alterative or expectorant, as may be required. * * * * * I am satisfied that no aid I could have derived from alcoholic stimulants, as they are called, could have bettered my results. I feel sure any candid medical brother who will have the steady courage to put aside many old and unproven, though much-practiced, methods, based only on unquestioning and unquestioned experience, and to move into these new fields of observation and experience, will, in the end, find no fault with me for leaving a track which, though it be beaten very firmly and be very wide and smooth to traverse, may not, after all, be the surest and soundest path to the golden gate of cure."

THE FRANCES E. WILLARD NATIONAL TEMPERANCE HOSPITAL.

This hospital is situated at 343-349 South Lincoln Street, Chicago, in a handsome and well-equipped building. It is connected with a medical school. The history of its origin is best told in the words of the woman to whom the conception of such an institution first came, Dr. Mary Weeks Burnett, for several years the physician in charge:--

"In the fall of 1883 there came to a few of us the thought that there was a point of weakness in the temperance pledge. It reads, 'We promise to abstain from all liquors--as a beverage.' We had found in many instances in reform work that pledging to abstain from liquor 'as a beverage,' and leaving the victim to the unlimited use of it in physicians' prescriptions, was simply a skirmish with the devil's outposts, that the conflict, based upon these grounds, was short, and defeat almost sure; and the great fact remained that the innermost recesses of evil force and power were by this pledge still left unassailed. We found that this power of evil had largely entered the homes of our land through the family physicians, and that willingly or not, the physicians were being used to bring in even our innocent children as recruits to this unrighteous warfare.

"Now, how could we hope to eliminate those three little words 'as a beverage' from our pledge?

"In some way we must bring about an arrest of thought in the minds of 100,000 men and women physicians whose medical education warranted them in supposing that they knew that of alcohol which justified them in its full and free use in medical practice. Nothing short of a great national object lesson could ever convict and convert this broad constituency through which the power of darkness is doing his deadliest work.

"In January, 1884, four of us met and organized under the name of the National Temperance Hospital. To have our sick properly cared for in our hospital we found that we should be obliged to train our own nurses. The nurse who has always been accustomed to administering alcohol under the physician's prescription at all times and under all circumstances, and to administering it herself at her own discretion if the physician is not at hand, is a terror to the temperance physician. So we included in our charter a Training School for Nurses. It is now open, and we expect, as the years go by, to send out armed with our training school diplomas, grand, noble women and men thoroughly trained in true temperance methods for relieving the sick.

"Our organization lived on paper, and was sustained in purpose by prayer and planning for two years. In September, 1885, Mr. R. G. Peters, of Manistee, Michigan, signified to us his intention to give $50,000 toward our buildings whenever we had satisfactorily materialized. About the same time a good old gentleman in Michigan placed in his will for us $2,500. The dear man is still living, and we hope will live many years. Even the money when it comes can never be of greater service to us than was the knowledge at that time that the Lord was our leader and was raising up helpers in the work.

"In January, 1886, we found, according to the law under which our charter was obtained, that we must commence active operations at once, or obtain a new charter. After a blessed season of prayer and counseling together in the board meeting held January 29, there being present only the members of the board at that time, Mrs. Plumb offered to advance $3,500, if necessary, toward the expenses for the first year. We accepted it with great thankfulness, rented a building the 15th of March, 1886, and formally opened the National Temperance Hospital on the 4th of May, 1886.

"In April, 1886, we took a firm stand upon the alcohol question, and decided to eliminate it entirely from our list of therapeutics, as we had become convinced that there were better and more reliable remedies as stimulants and tonics.

"In September, 1886, at our annual meeting, we reaffirmed this decision, and we now have the following as one of the articles of our constitution: 'All medicines used in the hospital must be prepared without alcohol, and all physicians accepting positions on the medical staff of the hospital or dispensary must pledge themselves not to administer alcohol in any form to any patient in hospital or dispensary, nor to call in counsel for such patients any physician who will advise the use of alcohol.

"Any physician of pure character, and in good standing, who is a total abstainer from liquor and tobacco can, by subscribing to this pledge, become a member of our physicians' association, and if so desired, be placed upon the visiting and consulting staff of the hospital.

"The cases treated in the hospital include many of the serious medical and surgical maladies. In no case has any particle of alcohol been used, and the usual inflammatory secondary symptoms resulting when alcohol is used have been entirely avoided.

"Our course of building-up treatment is, we believe, unique in hospital practice. It consists of treatment by massage, heat, rest, passive exercise, etc., together with proper medication and a thoroughly nutritious diet adapted to the individual needs of the patient.

"To alleviate, and, if possible, cure disease, is the design of all hospital treatment. In our hospital we seek to gain this result by means which the highest science of the day approves, and in addition to this we have especially at heart the advancement of the temperance reform. There are, we believe, thousands of temperance adherents, who do not yet fully apprehend the importance of this hospital to the permanent extension and progress of temperance principles. Although prohibition as a principle has been accepted by many, yet in its practical application in the home in serious illness, it is still feared by the immense majority of even our strongest prohibitionists. We are organized upon the basis no alcohol in medicine, and we are preparing to demonstrate fully and scientifically, so he who runs may read, that as in health, so in disease and accident, alcohol in any form works to the hindrance and injury of the vital forces, and prevents the establishment and advancement of health processes in the system."

At the opening of the hospital, May 4, 1886, Miss Frances E. Willard, the president of the National W. C. T. U., gave the following address:

"Nothing is changeless except change. The conservatives of one epoch are the madmen of the next, even as the radicals of to-day would have been the lunatics of yesterday. To prove this, just imagine the founders of this hospital declaring to my great-grandfather that because he had taken a cold was no reason why he should take a toddy; and per contra, imagine my great-grandfather's doctor marching into our presence here and now, with saddle-bags on arm, and after treating us each to a glass of grog for our stomach's sake, giving us a scientific disquisition on the sovereign virtues of the blue pill, and informing us that bleeding, cupping and starvation were the surest methods of cure!

"That the story of Evolution is true I am by no means certain, but that 'We, Us, and Company,' are 'evoluting' with electric speed ourselves it is useless to deny. This very hospital is the latest mile-stone on the highway of progress in the American temperance reform. The conditions that have made its existence possible have developed in this country within about twelve years.

"Public opinion, that mightiest of magicians, has within that time been educated up to this level and has said in its omnipotence: 'Hospital, be!' and, behold, the hospital is.

"When I joined the ranks of temperance workers in 1874, a thought so adventurous as that alcoholics in relation to medicine were a curse and not a blessing had never lodged within my cranium. But, as in duty bound, I studied the subject from the practical, which is the nineteenth century standpoint.

"I investigated the cause of inebriety, and found the medical use of alcoholic stimulants a prominent factor in this horrible result; I sought for expert testimony, and found Dr. N. S. Davis, ex-President American Medical Association, saying 'that in his ample clinical practice he had for over thirty years tested the medical uses of alcoholics, and had found no case of disease and no emergency arising from accident that he could not treat more successfully without any form of fermented or distilled liquors than with'; found Dr. James R. Nichols, of Boston, so long editor of The Journal of Chemistry, declaring as his deliberate scientific opinion that the entire banishment of these liquors 'would not deprive us of a single one of the indispensable agents which modern civilization demands'; found Dr. Green, of Boston, saying before the physicians of that city that it is upon the members of the medical profession and the exceptional laws which it has always demanded, that the whole liquor fraternity depends more than upon anything else to screen it from opprobrium and just punishment for the evils it entails, and that after thirty years of professional experience he felt assured that alcoholic stimulants are not required as medicines, and that many, if not a majority of the best physicians, now believe them to be worse than useless. Meanwhile I learned that across the sea such great physicians as Dr. Benjamin Ward Richardson, Sir Andrew Clark, Sir Henry Thompson and Sir William Gull held views which for their latitude were almost equally radical; and Dr. James Edmunds, founder of the London Temperance Hospital had demonstrated publicly and on a grand scale the more excellent way, his hospital having 4-1/2 per cent. fewer deaths than any other in London, taking the same run of cases, and that the Royal Infirmary at Manchester reported the medicinal use of alcohol fallen off 87 per cent. in recent years, with a decrease in its death-rate of over one-third. Besides all this, and independent of any such investigation, the 'intuitions' of our most earnest women were leading them out of the wilderness. As is their custom, they determined to put this matter to the test of that 'experience which one experiences when he experiences his own experience,' and a whole body of divinity upon the advantages of non-alcoholic treatment could be furnished from their evidence. I was not able personally to pursue this method, my own condition of good health having become chronic. Away back in 1875, in executive committee, one of our leading officers was stricken with angina pectoris. A physician was promptly summoned. 'Give her brandy,' he said, and insisted so stoutly upon it as vital to her recovery that we should probably have sent for it, but the dear woman gasped out faintly, 'I can die, but I can't touch brandy.' She is alive and flourishing to-day. Another national officer absolutely refused whisky for a violent attack of a very different character, the physician telling her that she could not live through the night without it; but she is still an active worker--a living witness that doctors are not infallible. Instances like these have multiplied by hundreds and thousands in our Woman's Christian Unions and Bands of Hope. 'No, mamma I can't touch liquor; I've signed the pledge,' is a protest 'familiar as household words.' Meanwhile, I beg you to contemplate something else that has happened. Behold, our own beloved beverage itself,

'Sparkling and bright, In its liquid light,'

has come grandly to our rescue in this crusade against alcohol in the sick room. Water has become a favorite--nay, even a fashionable--medicine! The most conservative physicians freely prescribe it in the very cases where some form of alcohol was the specific so long. To be sure, they give it hot, but we do not object to that, since 'water hot ne'er made a sot,' and it cures dyspepsia and all forms of indigestion as whisky never did, but only made believe to; while its external use as a fomentation is banishing alcohol even for old folks' 'rheumatiz' where, as a remedy, it would be likely to make its final stand.

"Farewell, thou cloven-foot, Alcohol! Thou canst no longer hide away in the home-like old camphor bottle, paregoric bottle, peppermint bottle or Jamaica-ginger bottle; and a tender good-by, Mrs. Winslow's Soothing Syrup, for be it known to you that the wonderful discovery stumbled over for six thousand years has in our day been made, namely, that hot water will soothe the baby's stomach-aches and the grown people's pains, and drive out a cold when all else fails. Jubilate! Clear out the cupboard and top shelf of the closet now that the sideboard has gone. Let great Nature have a glance to 'mother up' humanity with the medicine, as well as the beverage, brewed in Heaven."

THE RED CROSS HOSPITAL.

A philanthropic young woman, Miss Bettina A. Hofker, entered Mount Sinai Training School for Nurses in 1891. Her desire was to fit herself as a nurse for the poor. After her graduation in 1893, she met Mrs. Charles A. Raymond, a benevolent lady, who offered her pecuniary assistance in her work. Miss Hofker suggested that she would like to institute a Red Cross Hospital and Training School for Nurses. Mrs. Raymond succeeded in interesting others in the proposition. The name of Red Cross however could not be used without permission of the officers of the society bearing that name, but after consultation with Miss Barton, permission was granted.

Several years previous to this, Dr. A. Mon?Lesser, Dr. Thomas McNicholl and Dr. Gottlieb Steger had opened a small hospital under the name of St. John's Institute. This was now amalgamated with the Red Cross, and Dr. George F. Shrady and Dr. T. Gaillard Thomas, two of New York's leading physicians, were requested to act as consulting physicians.

The hospital does not confine itself to service in its building alone, but sends its workers wherever called, to mansion or tenement. The "Sisters" are trained for field service or for any national calamity such as floods, earthquakes, forest fires, epidemics, etc. When neither war nor calamities require their presence, they devote themselves to the service of the needy poor, or wait upon the rich, if called. The heroic service rendered by the surgeons and nurses from this hospital in the Cuban War, brought their work into great prominence.

At the suggestion of Miss Barton, the medical department of the hospital was commissioned to treat diseases without the use of alcoholic liquids.

Dr. Lesser, the executive surgeon, is a German, and of German education, having received his medical education in the Universities of Berlin and Leipsic. In a conversation with a press representative, Dr. Lesser said some time ago:--

"We have been convinced that the use of alcohol can be entirely eliminated from our medical practice, and this has been practically accomplished at the Red Cross Hospital. We find that where stimulants are required, such remedies as caffeine, nitro-glycerine and kolafra take the place of alcohol, and are even more satisfactory. The main use of alcohol is to stimulate the action of the heart in various ailments. The blood is thus forced to the remote parts of the system, and poisonous substances carried away. But, besides serving this good purpose, the drug tears down and ultimately destroys the cellular tissues of the body. A relapse is certain to follow the application. The drugs that I have mentioned serve exactly the same purpose without the disastrous results. We are proving this every day at the Red Cross Hospital.

"Only a few days ago a boy was brought in, apparently at the point of death. He was put into bed and watched by the nurse. After a little ammonia had been given to him as a stimulant, he unconsciously expressed himself to the effect that it was not the same as they gave him in another place, and gradually when it dawned upon him that no alcohol was administered by the Red Cross, he said, 'Gin has allers made me better.' The doctor in charge, who already suspected that the boy was pretending illness for the sake of the drink, was not surprised an hour or two afterwards to learn that he had demanded his clothes, dressed himself, and left the hospital most ungratefully, but apparently quite well."

Dr. George F. Shrady, one of the consulting physicians, is famous as having been in attendance upon both President Garfield and President Grant. He is the editor of the Medical Record, one of the most important medical journals published in America. While not a non-alcoholic physician, he says of the medical use of intoxicants:--

"There is altogether too much looseness among physicians in prescribing alcohol. It is a dangerous drug. There is much more alcohol used by physicians than is necessary, and it does great harm. Whisky is not a preventive; it prevents no disease whatever, contrary to a current notion. Another thing, we physicians get blamed wrongfully in many cases. People who want to drink, and do drink, often lay it on to the physician who prescribed it. * * * * * I think that in most cases where alcohol is now used, other drugs with which we are familiar could be used with far better effect, and with no harmful results."

Dr. Steger, another physician of the staff, says:--

"I don't use alcohol at all in my practice. I used to use it, but my observation has been that other drugs do the same work without the harmful results. Alcohol over-stimulates the heart, and tears down the cellular tissues of the system, besides causing other deleterious effects. The use of alcohol is simply a superstition among physicians. They have used it so long that they think they always must. I am not a total abstainer, but that only shows that I take better care of my patients than I do of myself. It is not good for a healthy man to drink, but sometimes folks like myself do things which had better be left undone. I have seen patients in hospitals made absolutely drunk by their physicians."

The following interesting items in regard to practice in this hospital are culled from the report of 1897:--

"Temperature was never reduced by active drugs known as antipyretics.

"Water was allowed freely after all kinds of surgical operations and in fevers.

"Alcohol was never used as an internal medicine.

"The free use of water in saline solutions directly injected into the tissues was found of great service. Quarts have been injected that way with most satisfactory results.

"Antipyretics were altogether discarded as it is well known that their action diminishes the tone of the heart. Artificial reduction of temperature only deludes one into the belief that the drug has improved the condition of the patient, while in reality, it has no beneficial influence on the disease, and has reduced the vital resistance of the patient. In no case has high temperature harmed a patient and there was every evidence that in some instances a high temperature was preferable to a low one.

"Special attention has been given to the use of alcohol in disease, not with any desire to approve or disapprove it, but solely for the purpose of discovering the truth, for nothing seems of greater public interest from a medical standpoint than the truth regarding a subject for which so many virtues are claimed on the one hand, and so many destructive elements proven on the other. * * * * *

"We criticise the treatment of no institution, antagonize no school of medicine, claim no unusual or peculiar scientific virtue, but what we do maintain and insist upon is this: that the human body may be ever so afflicted, ever so reduced, the heart ever so feeble, and the spark of life ever so dim, the conscientious student of medicine can secure as good results without as with administration of antipyretics, sparkling wines, beers or liquors.

"Experience teaches that true science does not antagonize nature. In surgical cases, in septic 鎚 ia, in pneumonia, or in any of the fevers, water freely administered has proven to be a real source of comfort, and an aid to recovery. It is amazing how favorably diseases terminate under this beneficent beverage. The withholding of food does not retard, but rather hastens convalescence.

"In the conduct of our Red Cross patients, irrespective of their condition when admitted, it can be truly said that after treatment began, delirium has not been witnessed in a single instance, and as our hospital reports indicate, our mortality has been unusually small.

"Alcohol has not figured as a life-saver in our institution. Cases of extreme collapse following major operations, cases of pneumonia, where the pulse ranged from 160 to 220, patients suffering from pernicious an 鎚 ia, septic 鎚 ia, py 鎚 ia, cholera infantum and typhoid fever, some of whom when first seen were in the worst stages of delirium and collapse have without alcohol regained consciousness, overcome delirium and made excellent recoveries.

"The following cases very forcibly illustrate the results of non-alcoholic treatment:--

"Case No. 1. A child, aged nine months, under treatment for six days for pneumonia, came under our notice on the seventh day. The temperature was 106 5-10; pulse was 220; respirations 90. Whisky, which had been given previously to the extent of two ounces daily, was stopped. Carbonate of ammonia, caffeine salicylate, nitro-glycerine and 1-10 of a drop of aconite were given internally; camphorated lard applied externally; with the result that on the ninth day temperature stood 99; pulse 100; respiration 20. The child made a complete recovery.

"Case No. 2. L. was a child aged eight months, suffering from a very violent attack of entero-colitis. For three weeks previous to coming under our notice the patient received brandy, stimulating foods and alkaline mixtures. Fearfully emaciated, temperature 106, feeble pulse 182, frequent bloody discharges from the bowels, numbering as much as thirty in a day and constant vomiting, the child was considered beyond hope. Under these circumstances, and at this time we first saw her. Brandy and all foods were stopped; bowel flushings were given, 1-12 of a drop of tincture of aconite was administered every half hour and salicylate of caffeine every two hours. In twenty-four hours the temperature was 105 and the pulse 160. In two days, temperature was 102 and the pulse 140. In one week, temperature was 99 5-10, pulse 110. In three weeks, the patient was discharged cured.

"Case No. 3. Mrs. C., aged forty-three, who had been under treatment for seven weeks for metrorrhagia, nietortes and peritonitis came under our notice. Brandy which had been previously given in large quantities had proved of no avail and the patient was considered beyond recovery. We found her completely prostrated, temperature 102, pulse 170, and unconscious. The heart very weak and irregular. The brandy was discontinued, salicylate of caffeine and nitrate of strychnia were given with the result that in a short time the patient was convalescent and finally recovered.

"Each case in our hospital is an additional proof that whether found in wines, spirits or beers, alcohol can claim no right as an indispensable medicine."

Dr. Lesser, who was Surgeon-General of the American Red Cross in the Cuban War said after his return from his first visit to Cuba that four out of six of his patients, to whom he allowed liquor to be given as a concession to the popular idea that it was necessary, died; while subsequently in treating absolutely without alcohol sixty-three similar cases, only one died, and he upon the day on which he was received at the hospital.

ALCOHOL IN OTHER HOSPITALS.

In the spring of 1909 a circular letter was sent to some of the best known hospitals throughout the country asking if the use of alcoholic liquors had decreased in those institutions during the past ten years. From the replies received the following statements are taken:

Cook County Hospital, Chicago, sent figures for two years only, 1907, and 1908. With 28,932 patients treated in 1907, the bill for wines and liquors amounted to only $719.40. In 1908 with 31,202 patients the bill for liquors amounted to $970.65. This makes a per capita expenditure for liquors for 1907 of .024 cents, and for 1908 a per capita expenditure of .031 cents. The per capita expenditure for liquors during the same years in Bellevue and Allied Hospitals of New York city, with from 30,000 to 40,000 patients treated was .0246 and .029. Two or three cents as the yearly per capita expenditure for alcoholic liquors in the two largest hospitals in America is striking evidence that the physicians practicing there have not large faith in whisky, or other alcoholic liquors as remedial agents.

Long Island, N. Y., State Hospital:--"We are not using more than half the amount of alcohol we used ten years ago."

Manhattan State Hospital, Ward's Island, New York City:--"Our patient population has averaged nearly 4,500 the last four years, and we have had about 750 employees, many of whom are prescribed for by institution physicians. The per capita cost of distilled liquors for the last fiscal year was

.0273 at this hospital."

Milwaukee City Hospital:--"No alcoholic liquors are used to any extent in this hospital, or prescribed by the staff. I know of no move against such use of liquors, but venture the assertion that the physicians believe they have more reliable agents at their command for most cases."

Pennsylvania Hospital, Philadelphia:--"We are now using about one-third the amount of liquor that was used in the Pennsylvania Hospital ten years ago."

The Presbyterian Hospital of Philadelphia sent figures for the years from 1900 to 1908. Those for 1900 show the cost of liquors to be $774.20 and for 1908 only $331.48. The number of patients was not given.

Grady Hospital, Atlanta, Georgia:--"That less liquor is now used than formerly is a fact well known to all connected with the institution."

Garfield Memorial, Washington, D. C., sent figures for ten years. For 1899 the cost of liquors was $490.08, with a steady decrease to 1908 when the cost was $274.58. Number of patients in 1899 was 1,171; in 1908, 1,898 patients. The per capita for 1908 was .144 cents.

University Hospital, Ann Arbor, Michigan:--"Very little alcohol is prescribed in this hospital."

Maine General Hospital, Portland:--"Comparatively speaking, we use but little alcohol for the reason that we now have many remedies which, especially for continued use, are superior to alcohol, which twenty years ago we did not have. For the conditions or emergencies in which we think alcohol has a value it is used when required or deemed best."

Buffalo, New York, State Hospital sent figures for six years which include cost of alcohol used in the manufacture of pharmaceutical preparations, which, of course, makes a very decided difference. Per capita for 1903 was 22 cents; for 1908 it was 18 cents.

Buffalo, New York, General Hospital:--"The use of alcohol as a drug in this hospital has diminished about one-third in the past ten years, but I wish to add in this connection that the use of all drugs has diminished in this hospital, and to the best of my knowledge in other institutions of a like character. The use of the microscope, and other studies have advanced the science of medicine the same as all other branches of learning, and other methods are coming to be used beside the use of drugs."

Mount Sinai, New York City:--"The use of alcoholic beverages here for medical purposes is the exception rather than the rule. The majority of our cases are surgical cases, and in these alcoholic liquors are rarely prescribed for any purpose whatsoever."

Massachusetts Homeopathic Hospital, Boston, sent figures for five years. For 1904 the cost of alcoholic liquors was $197.69 with 3,720 patients; for 1908, the cost was $69.82 with 4,543 patients. The per capita cost for the five years is as follows: 1904, cost .0531 cents; 1905, cost .0474; 1906, cost .034; 1907, cost .0171; 1908, cost .0153.

In the Boston Medical and Surgical Journal of April 15, 1909, Dr. Richard C. Cabot gave a table showing the decrease in the use of alcoholic liquors, and of other drugs in Massachusetts General Hospital, Boston.

The following is his table:

1898 1899 1900 1901

Ale and Beer $759.00 $793.90 $1,062.00 $723.00 Wines and liquors, 1,563.00 2,209.00 1,348.00 1,063.00 --------- --------- --------- --------- Total for alcoholic drinks, $2,321.00 $3,002.00 $2,410.00 $1,786.00

Total for other medicines, $8,424.00 $10,013.00 $10,132.00 $9,168.00

Number of patients, 5,005 5,203 5,012 5,495 Cost of alcohol per patient, $0.46 $0.57 $0.48 $0.32 Cost of medicine per patient, 1.68 1.92 2.02 1.66

1902 1903 1904 1905

Ale and beer, $605.00 $338.00 $431.00 $301.00 Wines and liquors, 799.00 688.00 904.00 144.00 --------- --------- --------- ------- Total for alcoholic drinks, $1,404.00 $1,026.00 $1,335.00 $445.00

Total for other medicines, $9,772.00 $7,815.00 $9,162.00 $7,018.00

Number of patients, 5,342 5,429 5,709 5,531 Cost of alcohol per patient, $0.26 $0.19 $0.23 $0.09 Cost of medicine per patient, 1.88 1.43 1.60 1.26

1906 1907

Ale and beer, $192.00 $203.00 Wines and liquors, 546.00 610.00 --------- -- ------- Total for alcoholic drinks, $738.00 $813.00

Total for other medicines, $5,981.00 $5,492.00

Number of patients, 5,513 5,966 Cost of alcohol per patient, $0.13 $0.13 Cost of medicine per patient, 1.00 0.92

Dr. Cabot says:--

"Since there has been no fall in the price of stimulants or medicine, the diminished expenditure corresponds to a diminution in the number of doses of medicine and stimulants, and indicates a rapid and striking change of view among the members of the staff of the hospital, especially in the past five years, when it has become generally known that alcohol is not a stimulant but a narcotic and that drugs can cure only about half a dozen of the diseases against which we are contending.

"There has been during this period no increase in the proportion of surgical cases among the whole number treated, so that the decreased use of medicines and alcoholic beverages has not resulted from an increased resort to surgical remedies. On the other hand, there has been a great increase in the utilization of baths (hydrotherapeutics), of massage, of mechanical treatment and of psychical treatment, all of which accounts no doubt for part of the falling off in the use of alcohol and drugs."

CHAPTER V.

THE EFFECTS OF ALCOHOL UPON THE HUMAN BODY.

The body is made up mainly of cells, fibres and fluids. The cell is the most important structure in the living body. Life resides in the cell, and every animal may be considered a mass of cells, each of which is alive, and each of which has its own work to accomplish in the building up of the body.

The matter which forms the mass of a cell is called protoplasm, or bioplasm. It resembles somewhat the white of a raw egg, which is almost pure albumen. Cells make up the body, and do its work. Some are employed to construct the skeleton, others are used to form the organs which move the body; liver-cells secrete bile, and the cells in the kidneys separate poisonous matters from the blood in order that they may be expelled from the system.

These cells, composing the mass of the body, being very delicate, are easily acted upon by substances coming into contact with them. If substances other than natural foods or drinks are introduced into the body, the cells are injuriously affected. Alcohol is especially injurious to cells, "retarding the changes in their interior, hindering their appropriation of food, and elimination of waste matters, and therefore preventing their proper development and growth."

"Bioplasm is living matter; it is structureless, semi-fluid, transparent and colorless. It is the only matter that can grow, move, divide itself and multiply, the only matter that can take up pabulum (food) and convert it into its own substance; and is the only matter that can be nourished. The bioplasm in the cell gets its nourishment by drawing in of the pabulum through the cell wall, and in that way building up the formed material while it is being disintegrated on the outer surface. This process is continually being carried on, and is what is meant by nutrition. Disintegration of the formed material is as essential as the building up of it. All organic structure is the result of change taking place in bioplasm. These small cell-like bioplasts are the workmen of the organism. All wounds are repaired by them, all fractures are united, and all diseased tissues brought back to their normal and healthy condition, unless there is not vitality enough to overcome disease, or they have been injured or killed by poisonous material. The body is kept in repair by this living matter, and all the functions of the body are but the result of its action. We may examine, watch and study bioplasm under the microscope; we see it take up pabulum and convert that which is adapted to itself into its own substance, while all other substances are rejected. We take a solution of what we call a stimulant and immerse the bioplasm in it, and we find that it increases its activity, moves faster, takes up more pabulum, and divides more rapidly than in the unstimulated condition. We next add an astringent, and it begins to move more slowly, and soon contracts into a spherical shape and remains contracted, or may move slowly to a limited extent, depending on the strength of the solution. We next take a relaxant, and gradually the living matter begins to spread in all directions, in a laxy-like manner, and becomes so thin as to be almost undiscernible, and takes up very little, if any, pabulum. If sufficiently relaxed or astringed, the movements may entirely cease so as to appear lifeless, but when a stimulant is again added the same result is obtained as before--it begins to move, and acts as vigorous as ever, which shows that it was not injured in the least by the agents used. Alcohol is called a stimulant. We take a weak solution of alcohol and try it in the same way; but we find that almost instantly the living matter contracts into a ball-like mass. Now, we may through ignorance suppose that alcohol acts as an astringent, and so we try to stimulate it with the same harmless agent before used, but no impression is made on it; it does not move; it is dead matter. These are demonstrable facts, and lie at the foundation of physiology, pathology and the practice of medicine. Alcohol destroys the very life force that alone keeps the body in repair. For a more simple experiment as to the action of alcohol, take the white of an egg (which consists of albumen, and is very similar to bioplasm), put it into alcohol, and notice it turn white, coagulate and harden. The same experiment can be made with blood with the same result--killing the blood bioplasts. Raw meat will turn white and harden in alcohol. Alcohol acts the same on food in the stomach as it does on the same substances before introduced into the stomach, and acts just the same on blood and all the living tissues in the system as out of it; and this alone is enough to condemn its use as a medicine." From Alcohol, Is It a Medicine? by W. F. Pechuman, M. D., of Detroit, Michigan.

ALCOHOL AND STOMACH DIGESTION.

The nitrogenous portions of the food are the only ones digested in the stomach. The oily and fatty, as well as the starchy portions, are digested in the small intestines.

Very little was known about digestion until 1833, when Dr. Beaumont published the results of his investigations upon the stomach of Alexis St. Martin. St. Martin received a severe wound in the left side from a shot-gun. The wound in healing left an opening into the stomach about 4/5 of an inch in diameter, closed on the inside by a flap of mucous membrane. Through this opening the interior of the stomach could be thoroughly examined. Dr. Beaumont made hundreds of observations upon this young man, who was in his home several years. He says:--

"In a feverish condition, from whatever cause, obstructed perspiration, excitement by alcoholic liquors, overloading the stomach with food, fear, anger or whatever depresses or disturbs the nervous system, the lining of the stomach becomes somewhat red and dry, at other times pale and moist, and loses its smooth and healthy appearance, the secretions become vitiated, greatly diminished or entirely suppressed."

One day after giving St. Martin a good wholesome dinner, digestion of which was going on in regular order, Dr. Beaumont gave him a glass of gin. The digestive process was at once arrested, and did not begin again until after the absorption of the spirit, after which it was slowly renewed, and tardily finished.

Gluzinski made some conclusive experiments with a syphon. He drew off the contents of the stomach at various times with and without liquor. He concluded that alcohol entirely suspends the transformation of food while it remains in the stomach.

Dr. Figg, of Edinburgh, fed two dogs with roast mutton; to one of them he gave 1-1/2 ounces of spirit. Three hours later he killed both dogs. The dog without liquor had digested the mutton; the other had not digested his at all. Similar experiments have been made repeatedly with like result.

The elements of our food which the stomach can digest depend upon the pepsin of the gastric juice for their transformation. Alcohol diminishes the secretions of the gastric juice, unless given in very minute quantities, and kills and precipitates its pepsin. It also coagulates both albumen and fibrine, converting them into a solid substance, thus rendering them unfit for the action of the solvent principles of the gastric juice. Hence, any considerable quantity of alcohol taken into the stomach must for the time retard the function of digestion.

Many experiments have been made with gastric juice in vials, one, having alcohol added, the other, not having alcohol. The meat in the vials without alcohol, in time dissolved till it bore the appearance of soup; in the vials to which alcohol was added the meat remained practically unchanged. In the latter a deposit of pepsin was found at the bottom, the alcohol having precipitated it. Dr. Henry Munroe, of England, one of the experimenters in this line of research, says:--

"Alcohol, even in a diluted form, has the peculiar power of interfering with the ordinary process of digestion.

"As long as alcohol remains in the stomach in any degree of concentration, the process of digestion is arrested, and is not continued until enough gastric juice is thrown out to overcome its effects."--Tracy's Physiology, page 90.

In The Human Body, Dr. Newell Martin says:--

"A vast number of persons suffer from alcoholic dyspepsia without knowing its cause; people who were never drunk in their lives and consider themselves very temperate. Abstinence from alcohol, the cause of the trouble, is the true remedy."

Sir B. W. Richardson:--

"The common idea that alcohol acts as an aid to digestion is without foundation. Experiments on the artificial digestion of food, in which the natural process is closely imitated, show that the presence of alcohol in the solvents employed interferes with and weakens the efficacy of the solvents. It is also one of the most definite of facts that persons who indulge even in what is called the moderate use of alcohol suffer often from dyspepsia from this cause alone. In fact, it leads to the symptoms which, under the varied names of biliousness, nervousness, lassitude and indigestion, are so well and extensively known.

"From the paralysis of the minute blood-vessels which is induced by alcohol, there occurs, when alcohol is introduced into the stomach, injection of the vessels and redness of the mucous lining of the stomach. This is attended by the subjective feeling of a warmth or glow within the body, and according to some, with an increased secretion of the gastric fluids. It is urged by the advocates of alcohol that this action of alcohol on the stomach is a reason for its employment as an aid to digestion, especially when the digestive powers are feeble. At best this argument suggests only an artificial aid, which it cannot be sound practice to make permanent in place of the natural process of digestion. In truth, the artificial stimulation, if it be resorted to even moderately, is in time deleterious. It excites a morbid habitual craving, and in the end leads to weakened contractile power of the vessels of the stomach, to consequent deficiency of control of those vessels over the current of blood, to organic impairment of function, and to confirmed indigestion. Lastly, it is a matter of experience with me, that in nine cases out of ten, the sense of the necessity, on which so much is urged, is removed in the readiest manner, by the simple plan of total abstinence, without any other remedy or method."

In Medicinal Drinking, by John Kirk, M. D., this passage occurs:--

"Especially in the matter of support, it is essential to our inquiry to examine fully into alcoholic influence on the change by which food introduced into the stomach becomes capable of passing into the circulation and constituent elements of the living frame. It may be best to suppose a case for illustration. Here, then, is a child of, say, six or seven years of age. This child is of the slenderer sex and has been brought into a state of extreme weakness as the consequence of fever. The fury of the disease is expended, but it has, as nearly as may be, extinguished life. The medical man's one hope for saving this child is now concentrated in what he fancies to be 'support.' Beef-tea, arrowroot and port wine are prescribed. Let it be kept in mind that the pure wine of the grape is discarded in favor of alcoholic wine. Our question is, What effect will the alcohol in this wine have on that process by which the food is to prove really nourishing, and so to be that support which is the only hope for this child? Will it help her? or will it so hinder the necessary change in the food as to kill her, unless she has sufficient strength left to get above its influence? These are surely important questions. Neither of them can be set at rest by the fact that she recovers; for she may have strength enough, as many have had, to survive even a serious error in her treatment.

"What light, then, does true science throw on these important questions? All who know anything on the subject are aware that alcohol, instead of dissolving food, or aiding in its dissolution, is one of the most powerful agents in preventing that dissolution. On what principle, then, is it possible that its being mixed with the materials of food, in this case, can aid in their dissolution, so that they may more easily be changed into the fresh blood required to sustain and recover life in this child?"

He then refers to the experiments with gastric juice in vials, and proceeds:--

"Here, then, is indisputable evidence that alcohol effectually prevents that process which is known as digestion, and which is essential to food's being of any use to support life in man. On what principle can the physician explain his introduction of it into the stomach of a child whose thread of life is attenuated to the slenderest hair?

"We urge the chemical truth that the alcohol, given to promote support, is of such a nature as to prevent that which would nourish, from effecting the end so much to be desired, and for which true food is adapted."

The pure, unfermented juice of the grape, free from chemical preservatives, is now used by many physicians where the miserable concoction of drugs and alcohol, known as port wine, was once considered essential. Unfermented grape juice contains all the nutriment of the grape, without any of the poison, alcohol. After being opened it should be kept in a cool place, or it will ferment and produce alcohol. Fruit juices are very grateful to a fever patient, and should not be withheld as they are in so many cases. Dr. J. H. Kellogg, and other non-alcoholic physicians, recommend them highly. They are better than milk, as milk frequently produces "feverishness," while fruit juices allay it.

For those who think beer or ale an incentive to appetite, Dr. N. S. Davis, and others, recommend an infusion of hops, made fresh each day. It is the bitter which promotes appetite, not the alcohol. For the sake of the little bitter in beer, it is not wise to vitiate the tone of the stomach with the alcohol it contains, and which is its active principle. Many mothers have become drunkards, secret drunkards, possibly, through the use of beer as a fancied aid to digestion. Multitudes of men suffer untold horrors from dyspepsia, caused by the beer which they mistakenly suppose to be a friend to their stomach.

EFFECTS OF ALCOHOL UPON THE BLOOD.

"The blood is a thick, opaque fluid, varying in color in different parts of the body from a bright scarlet to a dark purple, or even almost black." If a drop of blood be placed under a microscope, immense numbers of small bodies will be seen. These are called blood-globules, or corpuscles, or discs. There are both red, and white or colorless, corpuscles. Each red corpuscle is soft and jelly-like. Its chief constituent, besides water, is a substance called hemoglobin, which has the power of combining with oxygen when in a place where that gas is plentiful, and of giving it off again in a region where oxygen is absent, or present only in small quantity. Hence, as the blood flows through the lungs, which are constantly supplied with fresh air, its corpuscles take up oxygen, which, as it flows on, is carried by them to distant parts of the body where oxygen is deficient, and there given up to the tissues. This oxygen-carrying is the function of the red corpuscles.

Hemoglobin, as the coloring-matter of the blood is called, is dark purplish-red in color; combined with oxygen it is bright "scarlet red." Accordingly, the blood which flows to the lungs after giving up its oxygen is dark red in color, its dark color being due to the impurities it contains; and that which, having received a fresh supply of oxygen, flows away from the lungs is bright scarlet--having been cleansed of its impurities. The bright red blood is called arterial, and the dark red venous.

The work assigned to the blood in the economy of the human system is: first, to pick up nutriment in its course through the walls of the alimentary canal, and oxygen, as it flows through the lungs, and convey these to all other parts of the body. Second, to act as a sort of sewage stream that drains off waste matter, and to carry this to the organs of excretion by which waste is expelled from the body.

"The blood is the great circulating market of the body, in which all the things that are wanted by all parts, by the muscles, the brain, the skin, the lungs, liver and kidneys, are bought and sold. What the muscles want they buy from the blood; what they have done with, they sell back to the blood; and so with every other organ and part. As long as life lasts this buying and selling is forever going on, and this is why the blood is forever on the move, sweeping restlessly from place to place, bringing to each part the thing it wants, and carrying away those with which it has done. When the blood ceases to move, the market is blocked, the buying and selling cease, and all the organs die, starved for lack of the things they want, choked by the abundance of things for which they have no longer any need."--FOSTER.

This is one way of saying that the processes of repair and waste are constantly going on in the body. Every action of the body, every impulse of the mind uses up some cell-matter, which must then be passed from the body as waste. This is called tissue disintegration. New cells to repair tissue waste are built up from the nutriment which the blood carries from the alimentary canal after the process of food digestion is accomplished. This is called tissue construction, or the process of assimilation. Technically, these are the metabolic, or destructive and constructive processes. Both are essential to health and life. Any substance taken into the body, which will interfere with these processes of nutrition and waste is inimical to health, and in time of disease, dangerous to life.

Alcohol is such a substance.

The cells and tissues of the body which are touched by alcohol are more or less hardened and injured by it, hence are less perfectly nourished than they are when alcohol is not present in the blood. Even a teaspoonful of alcohol to a 1/2 gallon of water hinders natural growth. If liquor is given to puppies it keeps them small. Young growing-cells are most affected by it, because they are most tender. There are growing-cells in adults as well as in children, for people are growing and changing all through their lives.

Hence, when alcohol is administered in sickness the cells are hindered in the full performance of their function of taking up food for the building up of tissue, and as a consequence, the patient's body is really robbed of nutriment by the agent which is supposed to be "keeping up his strength." Truly, "Wine is a mocker, strong drink is raging, and whosoever is deceived thereby is not wise."

That alcohol interferes with the passage of waste matter from the body is generally conceded. Indeed this is claimed by the advocates of its medicinal use as one of its virtues: the fact that less waste passes from the body being urged as evidence that there is less waste, that in some way alcohol preserves tissue from being used up in the natural way. Those who speak thus seem to think that they know better than the Creator how the body should be treated. He made the body so that in health, work, waste and repair should be equal to one another.

Dr. Ezra M. Hunt says in Alcohol as a Food and as a Medicine:--

"We believe that any one who will candidly review the claims put forth for alcohol, in that it delays in any of these hypothetical ways, tissue-change, will conclude that it has no such power in a salutary sense, and that it is unwarrantably assumed that to retard tissue metamorphosis (change) is equivalent to tissue nutrition."

Dr. N. S. Davis says:--

"It seems hardly possible that men of eminent attainments in the profession should so far forget one of the most fundamental and universally recognized laws of organic life as to promulgate the fallacy here stated. The fundamental law to which we refer is, that all vital phenomena are accompanied by, and dependent upon, molecular or atomic changes; and whatever retards these retards the phenomena of life; whatever suspends these suspends life. Hence, to say that an agent which retards tissue metamorphosis is in any sense a food, is simply to pervert and misapply terms."

Non-alcoholic physicians unite in declaring that the retention of waste matter in the system, caused by alcohol, invites disease, and tends to inflammatory action; and in illness retards, and frequently prevents, recovery, for the germs of disease remain longer in the body than they would were it not for the delay in the passage of effete matter.

Alcohol not only hinders the blood in its work of tissue nutrition; it also prevents the full oxidation of the blood in the lungs.

"In order that a steam engine may work and keep warm it is not merely necessary that it have plenty of coal, but it must also have a draft of air through its furnace. Chemistry teaches us that the burning in this case consists in the combination of a gas called oxygen, taken from the air, with other things in the coals; when this combination takes place a great deal of heat is given off. The same thing is true of our bodies; in order that food matters may be burnt in them and enable us to work and keep warm, they must be supplied with oxygen; this they get from the air by breathing. We all know that if his supply of air be cut off a man will die in a few minutes. His food is no use to him unless he gets oxygen from the air to combine with it; while he usually has stored up in his body an excess of food matters which will keep him alive for some time if he gets a supply of oxygen, he has not stored up in him any reserve, or, if any, but a very small one, of oxygen, and so he dies very rapidly if his breathing be prevented. In ordinary language we do not call oxygen a food, but restrict that name to the solids and liquids which we swallow; but inasmuch as it is a material which we must take from the external universe into our bodies in order to keep us alive, oxygen is really a food as much as any of the other substances which we take into our bodies from outside, in order to keep them alive and at work. Suffocation, as death from deficient air supply is named, is really death from oxygen-starvation."--Martin's Human Body.

Much of the food taken into the body is burned to supply energy and heat. This burning is called oxidation. When food is burned, or oxidized, either in the body, or out of it, three things are produced, carbon dioxide (carbonic acid gas), water and ashes. These are waste matters, and must be expelled from the body, or they will clog up the various organs, as the ashes and smoke of an engine would soon put its fire out if they were allowed to accumulate in the furnace. It is the duty of the lungs to pass the carbon dioxide out to the air. With every breath exhaled, this poison gas, generated in the body through the oxidation of food, passes from the system. With every breath inhaled the life-giving oxygen is taken into the body; providing that the person is not in a close room from which the fresh air is excluded.

Any substance taken into the body which interferes with the reception of oxygen into the blood, and with the giving off of carbon dioxide from the same is a dangerous substance.

Alcohol is such a substance.

It has already been stated that it is the duty of the little red corpuscles in the blood to take up oxygen in the lungs, and carry it to every part of the body, and upon the return passage to the lungs to convey the d 閣 ris, or used-up material, from the tissues, called carbon dioxide gas. A little vapor and ammonia accompany this gas. The action of alcohol upon these little corpuscles, or carriers of the blood, is to somewhat harden and shrivel them, so that they are unable to take up and carry as much oxygen as they can when no injurious substance is present in the blood. In consequence of this, the blood can never be so pure when alcohol is present, as it may be in the absence of this agent.

The following is taken from The Temperance Lesson Book, by B. W. Richardson, M. D.:--

"When the blood in the veins is floating toward the right side of the heart, which communicates with the lungs, it carries with it the carbonic acid (carbon dioxide), and, as I have found by experiment, a great part of this gas is condensed in these little bodies, the corpuscles. Arrived at the lungs, the blood comes into such contact with the air we breathe, that the oxygen gas in the air is freely absorbed by the little corpuscles, while the carbonic acid is given up into the air-passages of the lungs, and is thrown off with every breath we throw out. In this process the blood changes in color. It comes into the lungs of a dark color; it goes out of them a bright red. * * * * * The parts of the blood on which alcohol acts injuriously are the corpuscles and the fibrine. The red corpuscles are most distinctly affected. They undergo a peculiar process of shrinking from extraction of water from them. They also lose some of their power to absorb oxygen from the air. In confirmed spirit-drinkers the face and hands are often seen of dark mottled color, and in very bad specimens of the kind, the face is sometimes seen to be quite dark. This is because the blood cannot take up the vital air in the natural degree. * * * * *

"If anything whatever interferes with the proper reception of oxygen by the blood, the blood is not properly oxidized, the animal warmth is not sufficiently maintained, and life is reduced in activity. If for a brief interval of time the process of breathing is stopped in a living person, we see quickly developed the signs of difficulty, and we say the person is being suffocated. We observe that the face becomes dark, the lips blue, the surface cold. Should the process of arrest or stoppage of the breathing be long continued the person will become unconscious, will stagger and fall, and should relief not be at hand, he will in a very few minutes die.

"I found by experiment that in presence of alcohol in blood the process of absorption of oxygen was directly checked, and that even so minute a quantity as one part of alcohol in five hundred of blood proved an obstacle to the perfect reception of oxygen by the blood. The corpuscles are reduced in size, when large quantities of alcohol are taken, and become irregular in shape."

Dr. J. J. Ridge says in Addresses on the Physiological Action of Alcohol:--

"It has been found by experiment that, when alcohol is taken, less carbonic acid comes away in the breath than when it is not. This is partly because the blood-corpuscles cannot carry so much, and partly because so much is not produced, because there is less oxygen to join with the food and produce it. Just as burning paper smokes when it does not get enough oxygen, so other things are formed and get into the blood when there is not enough oxygen to make carbonic acid. These things make the blood impure, and cause extra work and trouble to get rid of them. This is why persons who drink alcohol are more liable to have gout and other diseases, than total abstainers."

Dr. Alfred Carpenter, formerly president of the Council of the British Medical Association, says in Alcoholic Drinks:--

"A blood corpuscle cannot come into direct contact with an atom of alcohol, without the function of the former being spoiled, and not only is it spoiled, but the effete matter which it has within its capsule cannot be exchanged for the necessary oxygen. The breath of the drunken man does not give out the quantity of carbonic acid which that of the healthy man does, and the ammoniacal compounds are in a great measure absent. Some of the carbon and effete nitrogenous matter is kept back. The retention of these poisonous matters within the body is highly injurious. Let the drinker suffer from any wound or injury and this effete matter in his blood is ready at a moment's notice to prepare and set up actions called inflammatory or erysipelatous, or some other kind; by means of which too often the drinker is hurried into eternity, although, perhaps, he may have been regarded as a perfectly sober man, and have never been drunk in his life."

In the light of these scientific facts, what can appear more utterly foolish than the swallowing of alcoholic patent medicines which are widely advertised as "Blood Purifiers"? That they will render the blood impure is only too evident in the light of scientific truth.

Dr. Nathan S. Davis has written much in disapproval of the use of alcohol in fevers, pneumonia and diphtheria, putting stress upon the fact that these diseases, of themselves, interfere with the reception of oxygen into the blood, and hence the use of all remedies that notably diminish the internal distribution of oxygen, or impair the corpuscles of the blood, should be avoided. Not only is alcohol of such a nature, but all the coal-tar series of antipyretics also. Since the internal distribution of oxygen, and the processes of tissue change are essential to the repair of the body, and alcohol hinders the blood in the full performance of its duties in these respects, it certainly seems clear that those physicians, who are extremely cautious in the use of this drug, or who do not use it at all, are more likely to be successful in saving their patients than are those who use it freely. Death-rates, with and without alcohol, show conclusively the superiority of the latter treatment.

ALCOHOL AND THE HEART.

The organs of circulation are the heart and the blood-vessels. The blood-vessels are of three kinds, arteries, capillaries and veins. The arteries carry blood from the heart to the capillaries; the veins collect it from the capillaries and return it to the heart. There are two distinct sets of blood-vessels in the body, both connected with the heart; one set carries blood to, through and from the lungs, the other guides its flow through all the remaining organs; the former are known as the pulmonary, the latter as the systemic blood-vessels.

The smallest arteries pass into the capillaries, which have very thin walls, and form very close networks in nearly all parts of the body; their immense number compensating for their small size. It is while flowing in these delicate tubes that the blood does its nutritive work, the arteries being merely supply-tubes for the capillaries, through whose delicate walls liquid containing nourishment exudes from the blood to bathe the various tissues.

The quantity of blood in any part of the body at any given time is dependent upon certain relations which exist between the blood-vessels and the nervous system. The walls of the arteries are abundantly supplied with involuntary muscular fibres, which have the power of contraction and relaxation. This power of contraction and relaxation is controlled by certain nerves called vasomotor nerves, because they cause or control motion in the vessels to which they are attached. When arteries supplying blood to any particular part of the body contract, the supply of blood to that part will be diminished in proportion to the amount of contraction. If the nervous control be altogether withdrawn, the arterial walls will completely relax, and the amount of blood in the part affected will be increased correspondingly.

Alcohol, even in moderate doses, paralyzes the vasomotor nerves which control the minute blood-vessels, thus allowing these vessels to become dilated with the flowing blood.

"With the disturbance of power in the extreme vessels, more disturbance is set up in other organs, and the first organ that shares in it is the heart. With each beat of the heart a certain degree of resistance is offered by the vessels when their nervous supply is perfect, and the stroke of the heart is moderate in respect both to tension and to time. But when the vessels are rendered relaxed, the resistance is removed, the heart begins to run quicker like a clock from which the pendulum has been removed, and the heart-stroke is greatly increased in frequency. It is easy to account in this manner for the quickened heart and pulse which accompany the first stage of deranged action from alcohol."--RICHARDSON.

Dr. Parkes of England, assisted by Count Wollowicz, conducted inquiries upon the effects of alcohol upon the heart, with a young and healthy man. At first they made accurate count of the heart beats during periods when the young man drank water only; then of the beats during successive periods in which alcohol was taken in increasing quantities. Thus step by step they measured the precise action of alcohol on the heart, and thereby the precise primary influence induced by alcohol. Their results are stated by themselves as follows:--

"The average number of beats of the heart in 24 hours (as calculated from eight observations made in 14 hours), during the first, or water period, was 106,000; in the earlier alcoholic period it was 127,000, or about 21,000 more; and in the later period it was 131,000, or 25,000 more.

"The highest of the daily means of the pulse observed during the first, or water period, was 77.5; but on this day two observations are deficient. The next highest daily mean was 77 beats.

"If, instead of the mean of the eight days, or 73.57, we compare the mean of this one day; viz. 77 beats per minute, with the alcoholic days, so as to be sure not to over-estimate the action of the alcohol, we find:--

"On the 9th day, with one fluid ounce of alcohol, the heart beat 4,300 times more.

On the 10th day, with two fluid ounces, 8,172 times more.

On the 11th day, with four fluid ounces, 12,960 times more.

On the 12th day, with six fluid ounces, 20,672 times more.

On the 13th day, with eight fluid ounces, 23,904 times more.

On the 14th day, with eight fluid ounces, 25,488 times more.

But as there was ephemeral fever on the 12th day, it is right to make a deduction, and to estimate the number of beats in that day as midway between the 11th and 13th days, or 18,432. Adopting this, the mean daily excess of beats during the alcoholic days was 14,492, or an increase of rather more than 13 per cent.

The first day of alcohol gave an excess of 4 per cent., and the last of 23 per cent.; and the mean of these two gives almost the same percentage of excess as the mean of the six days.

Admitting that each beat of the heart was as strong during the alcoholic period as in the water period (and it was really more powerful), the heart on the last two days of alcohol was doing one-fifth more work.

"Adopting the lowest estimate which has been given of the daily work of the heart; viz. as equal to 12.2 tons lifted one foot, the heart during the alcoholic period, did daily work excess equal to lifting 15.8 tons one foot, and in the last two days did extra work to the amount of 24 tons lifted as far.

"The period of rest for the heart was shortened, though, perhaps, not to such an extent as would be inferred from the number of beats, for each contraction was sooner over. The heart, on the fifth and sixth days after alcohol was left off, and, apparently at the time when the last traces of alcohol were eliminated, showed in the sphygmographic tracing signs of unusual feebleness; and, perhaps, in consequence of this, when the brandy quickened the heart again, the tracings showed a more rapid contraction of the ventricles, but less power than in the alcoholic period. The brandy acted, in fact, on a heart whose nutrition had not been perfectly restored."

Richardson quotes these experiments of Parkes and Wollowicz as if he agrees with them that increased heart-beat must of necessity mean increased work done by the heart. Dr. Nathan S. Davis, Dr. Newell Martin, Dr. A. B. Palmer, and some other investigators, show conclusively that mere increased frequency of beat above the natural standard is no evidence of increased force or efficiency in the circulation.

"The more frequent beats under the influence of alcohol constitute no exception to the general rule, for while the heart beats more frequently, its influence on the vasomotor nerves causes dilatation of the peripheral and systemic blood-vessels, as proved by the pulse-line written by the sphygmograph, which more than counterbalances the supposed increased action of the heart. The truth is, that under the influence of alcohol in the blood the systolic action of the heart loses in sustained force in direct proportion to its increase in frequency, until, by simply increasing the proportion of alcohol, the heart stops in diastole, as perfectly paralyzed as are the coats of the smaller vessels throughout the system. This was clearly demonstrated by the experiments of Professor Martin of Johns Hopkins University, to determine the effects of different proportions of alcohol on the action of the heart of the dog; and those of Drs. Sidney Ringer and H. Sainsbury, to determine the relative strength of different alcohols as indicated by their influence on the heart of the frog. Professor Martin states that blood containing 1/4 per cent. by volume of absolute alcohol, almost invariably diminishes, within a minute, the work done by the heart."

(This estimate would equal in an adult man an amount equal to the absolute alcohol in two or three ounces of whisky or brandy.)

"These investigations of Professor Martin, being directly corroborated by those of Drs. Ringer and Sainsbury, complete the series of demonstrations needed to show the actual effects of alcohol on the cardiac, as well as on the vasomotor, and also on the direct contractability of the muscular structure, when supplied with blood containing all gradations in the relative proportion of alcohol, leaving no longer any basis for the idea, popular both in and out of the profession, that alcohol in any of its forms is capable of increasing, even temporarily the force or efficiency of the heart's action."--Dr. N. S. Davis in Influence of Alcohol On the Human System.

The following letter will be of great interest to all students of the physiological effects of alcohol:--

"CHICAGO, ILL., March 3, 1899.

"To MRS. MARTHA M. ALLEN, "Syracuse, N. Y.,

"MADAM: Your letter asking my attention to the apparent contradiction of authorities concerning the work done by the heart when influenced by alcohol was received yesterday.

"The explanation is not difficult. It depends entirely on the different views of what constitutes the work of the heart.

"One class of investigators, led by the original and valuable experiments of Parkes and Wollowicz base their estimate of the heart's work entirely on the number of times it contracts or beats per minute. Thus Dr. Parkes, finding that moderate doses of alcohol increased the number of contractions of the heart from three to six beats per minute more than natural, readily estimated the number of additional contractions that would occur in twenty-four hours, and thereby demonstrated a large amount of increased work done by the heart under the influence of alcohol. All writers who speak of 'stimulating' or increasing the action of the heart by alcohol follow this method of measuring the amount of work done. They generally add that it is like applying 'the whip to a tired horse.'

"The other class of investigators who claim that alcohol diminishes the actual work done by the heart base their estimates on the amount of blood the heart passes through its cavities into the arteries in a given time. This is the physiological function of the heart; i.e. to aid in circulating the blood. Professor Martin's experiments were admirably contrived to determine, not how frequently the heart beat, but the amount of blood it delivered per minute under the influence of alcohol and without alcohol.

"He, and all others who take this basis of work, found that alcohol in any dose diminished the efficiency of the heart in circulating the blood in direct ratio to the quantity taken.

"My own original experiments, made fifty years ago, uniformly showed that alcohol quickly increased the number of heart beats per minute, but at the same time diminished the efficiency of the circulation generally. Every experienced practitioner knows that the weaker the heart becomes, the faster it beats. Consequently, the number of times the heart contracts per minute is no measure of the efficiency of its work in circulating the blood. Indeed the mechanism of the heart is such that there must be sufficient time between each of its contractions for its cavities to fill, or it is made to contract on an insufficient supply, and the efficiency of the circulation is diminished.

"Yours respectfully, "N. S. DAVIS."

The International Medical Congress of 1876 adopted as its reply to the Memorial of the National Temperance Society, and of the National Woman's Christian Temperance Union respecting "Alcohol as a Food and as a Medicine," the paper by Dr. Ezra M. Hunt, one conclusion of which was, "Its use as a medicine is chiefly that of a cardiac stimulant."

As experiments conducted since that time show that it is not a cardiac stimulant, but a direct cardiac paralyzant, what excuse is there for using it as a medicine now?

"Whenever the heart is compelled to more rapid contraction than is natural, it has less time to rest. Although it seems to be constantly at work, it really rests more than half the time, so that, although the periods of relaxation are very short, they are so numerous that the aggregate amount of rest in a day is very great. Now, if the rapidity of the contractions is increased materially and continuously, although the aggregate amount of time for rest may be the same as before, yet the waste caused by the contractions is greater, while the time for rest after each one is shorter. This lack of rest produces exhaustion of the heart-muscle, ending in partial change of the muscular tissue into fat. The heart then becomes flabby and weak and its walls become thinner, a condition known to physicians as a 'fatty heart,' often resulting in sudden death."--Tracy's Physiology, page 158.

Dr. T. D. Crothers, of Hartford, Conn., has made many observations with the sphygmograph to learn the effects of alcohol upon the heart. He says:--

"On general principles, and clinically, the increased activity and subsequent diminution of the heart's action brings no medicinal aid or strength to combat disease. This is simply a reckless waste of force for which there is no compensation. Without any question or doubt the increased heart's action, extending over a long period, is dangerous.

"The medicinal damage done by alcohol does not fall exclusively upon the heart, although this organ may show it more permanently than others."-- Transactions of Second Annual Meeting of A. M. T. A.

Dr. I. N. Quimby, of Jersey City, N. J., in an address before the American Medical Temperance Association, after describing two clinical cases which ended in death, made the following statement:

"There was nothing so strange about the death of these two patients, although they both died unexpectedly to the physician and their friends, but the declaration I am about to make may be somewhat new and startling, namely: That neither of these patients, in my candid judgment, died from the effect of disease, but rather from vasomotor paralysis of the heart, superinduced by the administration of the alcohol, which brought on a sudden and unexpected collapse and death."

Alcohol causes fatty degeneration of the heart and other muscular structures. Old age also causes these degenerations, hence alcohol is said to produce premature aging of the body.

"In fatty degeneration the cells and fibres of the body become more or less changed into fat. If a muscular fibre undergoes fatty degeneration, the particles of which it is made disappear one by one, and particles of oil or fatty matter take their place, so that the degree or amount of degeneration varies according to the extent to which this change has gone on. When the fibres of which a muscle is composed have become thus altered by fatty degeneration they become softer according to the amount of it; they are more easily torn and may even tear across when the muscle is being used during life. The more a muscle is thus degenerated the weaker it is, because it contains less muscular substance and more fat. Not only do the heart and other voluntary muscles thus degenerate, but those of the arteries also.

"Fatty degeneration is promoted by alcohol because alcohol prevents the proper removal of fat, which has been seen to accumulate in the blood; alcohol prevents the proper oxidation or burning up of waste matters; growing cells which are affected by the chemical influence of alcohol are not quite natural or healthy, so are more liable to degeneration; alcohol hinders the proper removal of waste matter from individual cells and tissues."--DR. J. J. RIDGE, London.

Dr. Newell Martin says in The Human Body:--

"Although fatty degeneration of the heart may occur from other causes, alcoholic indulgence is the most frequent one. Fatty liver or fatty heart is rarely if ever curable; either will ultimately cause death."

Dr. Ridge says these degenerations occur in the tissues of thin people as well as in those of stout persons. In thin people they are usually in the fibres only, not between them.

It is because of this degeneration of the heart and other muscles caused by alcohol that athletes in training need to be so very careful to avoid the use of beer and other intoxicating drinks.

Diseases such as fevers, diphtheria, and pneumonia which interfere with the reception, and internal distribution of oxygen, favor granular and fatty degeneration of the heart and other structures of the body. Hence non-alcoholic physicians urge that alcohol and such other drugs, as have like action in hindering full oxidation of the blood, and causing fatty degenerations should be studiously avoided. These physicians attribute many of the deaths from heart-failure in such diseases to the combined action of the disease and the alcohol in exhausting the heart, and weakening its structure.

Comparative death-rates with and without alcohol show conclusively the superiority of the latter treatment.

EFFECTS OF ALCOHOL UPON THE LIVER.

The liver is a very large organ, the largest and heaviest in the body, weighing in a healthy adult from three to four pounds. It secretes the bile. Its cells also store up, "in the form of a kind of animal starch called glycogen," excess of starchy or sugary food absorbed from the intestine during the digestion of a meal. This it gradually doles out to the blood for general use by the organs of the body until the next meal is eaten.

Dr. William Hargreaves says:--

"The office of the liver is to take up new substances having not yet become blood, as well as the portions of integrated matter that can be worked over, and brought again into use. It is in fact the economist of the system. It excretes bile, and liver-sugar, and renews the blood. When the liver is disordered the whole body is more or less deranged and the proper nutrition of its parts arrested."

Dr. Alfred Carpenter says:--

"The liver has to do several things; a considerable part of its duty is to purify the blood from d 閜 ris (waste matter), to filter out some things, to break up and alter others, and to expel them from the body in the form of bile. There are certain diseases in which the liver suddenly declines to do any more work. Acute atrophy of the liver is the name of this condition, and when it arises death rapidly results from suppression of the secretion of bile. It brings about a state of things called acholia; the patient is actually poisoned by the non-removal of those ingredients from the blood which it is the duty of the liver to remove. This corresponds in effect to the condition which alcohol can bring about by slow degrees."

The liver is the first important organ, next to the stomach and bowels, to receive the poisonous influence of alcohol.

"If alcohol is used habitually, though only in small quantities at a time, the liver may become the seat of serious changes. There may be a great increase of fat deposited in the cells, producing what is called 'fatty liver,' or it may lead to a great increase of connective tissue (membrane) between the cells, and surrounding the blood-vessels. This newly-developed connective tissue gradually contracts, and in so doing crushes the cells and obstructs the blood-vessels, making the organ much smaller than natural, and causing the surface to be covered with little projecting knobs, consisting of portions of liver-tissue that have been less compressed than the part that separates them. The pressure upon the liver-cells and the destruction of many of them, prevents the proper formation of bile and liver-sugar. The contraction of the newly-developed tissue, by obstructing the blood-vessels, interferes with the circulation. Malt liquors seem to produce fatty degeneration, while the stronger liquors cause the development of connective tissue."--Tracy's Physiology.

Speaking of diseases of the liver, Dr. Trotter said in his Essay on Drunkenness:--

"The chronic species is not a painful disease; it is slow in its progress, and frequently gives no alarm, till some incurable affection is the consequence. Hence, the fallacy and danger of judging merely by the feelings of the beneficial effects of the use of intoxicating drinks; for the liver and stomach may be seriously diseased, while a man imagines himself in moderate health."

Hardening of the liver, or "hob-nailed" liver, is said to be the result, largely, of taking liquor upon an empty stomach. Dr. E. Chenery, of Boston, in his excellent book, Facts for the Millions, tells of a patient of his who was well up to the evening before, when he went out and drank with some companions, taking the liquor on an empty stomach. That night, vomiting and pain in the right side came on, with high fever. Headache began and increased, followed by delirium and a general jaundiced condition. He died as a result. The disease was acute inflammation of the liver, brought on by the one broadside of alcohol poured "point blank" into the organ.

Dr. Chenery says further on in the same book:--

"There is another disorder of a very serious nature which science is now laying at the doors of the liver--diabetes mellitus, or sugar in the urine. Till quite recently, this formidable affection has been regarded as having its seat in the kidneys; and it is so classified in medical writings. Later researches, however, show that the sugar has been formed in the economy before it reaches the kidneys, and that these organs act only as strainers with respect to it, removing it from the blood as they remove salt and various other substances. In seeking for the fountain-head of diabetic sugar, it is found that the liver is the great glycogenic, or sugar-originating factory of the body. In an ordinary state of health this substance is produced in just the proper amount for the uses for which it is intended, so that it is all disposed of in the organism, and does not pass off by the kidneys. If any cause interrupts the processes by which the sugar is consumed, while its manufacture goes on normally, there will come to be an over-supply of sugar in the blood, which, when it reaches 3 parts to 1,000 of the blood, will begin to pass off by the kidneys and appear in the urine. On the other hand, if an undue amount of it is formed, the consumption remaining normal, it will also accumulate in the circulation, and be eliminated by the kidneys. In either case we have diabetes, the sugar irritating and diseasing the kidneys as it passes."

Dr. Harley, of the Royal Society of London, has made the subject of alcohol and diabetes matter for considerable study. He says a small quantity only of alcohol injected into the portal (liver) circulation of healthy animals will cause diabetic urine.

"If any one doubt the truth of the assertion that alcohol causes diabetes, let him select a case of that form of the disease arising from excessive formation, and after having carefully estimated the daily amount of sugar eliminated by the patient, allow him to drink a few glasses of wine, and watch the result. He will soon find the ingestion of the liquor is followed by an increase of sugar. If alcoholics increase the amount of saccharine matter in the urine of the diabetic, we can easily understand how their excessive use may induce the disease in individuals predisposed to it."--DR. HARLEY.

Some physicians claim that in jaundice and certain other bilious disorders even medicines prepared in alcohol are decidedly prejudicial and aggravating.

Dr. J. H. Kellogg, and other writers draw attention to the effects of alcohol in hindering the liver in its duty of destroying the toxic substances generated within the system of a sick person by the specific microbes to which the disease owes its origin, saying that the activity of the liver in destroying these poisons is one of the physiologic processes which stand between the patient and death.

The more this question is studied the more apparent is it that, other things being equal, the sick person who is cared for by a non-alcoholic physician has a much better chance of recovery than the one dosed by "a brandy doctor."

EFFECTS OF ALCOHOL UPON THE KIDNEYS.

"The kidneys, being the chief organs for the excretion of nitrogen waste, are among the most important organs of the body. Any defect in their healthy activity leads to serious interference with the working of many organs, due to the accumulation in the body of nitrogenous waste products. If both kidneys be cut out of an animal, it dies in a few hours from blood-poisoning, due to the accumulation of waste poisonous substances which the kidneys should have got rid of. Serious kidney-disease amounts to pretty much the same thing as cutting out the organs, since they are of little use if not healthy. It is always fatal if not checked, and often kills in a short time. The things which most frequently cause kidney disease are undue exposure to cold, and indulgence in alcoholic drinks."--Martin's Human Body.

"The kidneys are supplied with arterial blood, which, having given up water, urea, salt, and certain other substances, either secreted or simply strained from it, returns to the kidneys nearly as bright and fresh as when it entered them. While the lungs are concerned in removing carbonic acid--the ashes of the furnace--it is the peculiar province of the kidneys to remove the products of the wear and tear of the bodily machinery--the wasted nerve and muscle--in the form of urea, or other crystallizable substances, the presence of which in the economy for any considerable time is attended with disastrous results.

"Now, nature has put these organs, charged with so important work, as far away as possible from any source of irritation. Could alcohol get as direct access to them as to the liver, there is no doubt that their function would be destroyed almost at once, since the change in arterial blood by alcohol is much more extensive and damaging than that wrought in such venous blood as the liver receives from the portal veins. Thus while the liver takes the alcohol immediately from the alimentary canal, the kidneys receive it only after it has passed through the liver, the heart, the lungs, and the heart again; by which time much of it has escaped, while the remainder has been greatly diluted by the blood of the general circulation; yet coming to the kidneys even so considerably diluted, it has power to congest, irritate, and excite them to the excretion of an unusual amount of the watery elements of the urine, as if to wash the irritant away.

"But it is only the watery element that is increased, not the urea, which is the substance representing the waste of vital action, and is a poison to the system; this it is the special office of the kidneys to remove. Not only does alcohol not increase its elimination, but actually lessens the discharge. And should the irritation of the spirit continue, or be augmented in force, inflammation would follow, and the excretion of urea nearly or entirely cease and life be in the greatest jeopardy. Relief or death then must speedily follow."--Dr. E. Chenery, of Boston, in Alcohol Inside Out.

"Alcohol causes kidney-disease in several ways. In the first place it unduly excites the activity of the organs. Next, by impeding oxidation it interferes with the proper preparation of nitrogen wastes: they are brought to the kidneys in an unfit state for removal, and injure those organs. Third, when more than a small quantity of alcohol is taken, some of it is passed out of the body unchanged, through the kidneys, and injures their substance. The kidney-disease most commonly produced by alcohol is one kind of "Bright's disease," so called from the physician who first described it. The connective tissue of the organ grows in excess, and the true excreting kidney-substance dwindles away. At last the organ becomes quite unable to do its work, and death results.

"The three most common causes of Bright's disease are an acute illness, as scarlet fever, of which it is a frequent result; sudden exposure to cold when warm (this often drives blood in excessive quantity from the skin to internal organs, and leads to kidney-disease); and the habitual drinking of alcoholic liquids."--Dr. Newell Martin in The Human Body.

"Every physician knows or should know, that the quantity and quality of the effete, or waste, material separated from the blood by the kidneys and voided in the urine, is such as to render a knowledge of the action of any remedy or drink on the function of these organs, of the greatest importance in the treatment of all diseases, and especially those of an acute febrile character. As was long since demonstrated by clinical observation, and more recently by patient and accurate experiments by Bouchard and others, the amount of toxic, or poisonous, material naturally separated from the blood by the kidneys and passed out in the urine is so great that if wholly retained by failure of the kidneys to act for two or three days, speedy death ensues. Equally familiar to every observing physician is the fact that in all the acute febrile and inflammatory diseases, not only is the quantity of the urine secreted generally diminished, but its quality or constituency is also changed to a greater degree than even its quantity. Thus, some of the more important constituents are increased, others diminished, and often new or foreign elements are found present, all resulting from the disordered metabolic processes taking place throughout the system during the progress of these diseases.

"It is, therefore, hardly necessary to remind the physician that it is of the greatest importance to know as correctly as possible both the direct and the indirect influence of every medicine or drink on the action of the kidneys and all other eliminating organs and structures, lest he unwittingly allow the use of such as may not only retard the elimination of the specific causes of disease, but also favor auto-intoxication by retarding the elimination of the natural elements of excretion.

"That the presence of alcohol in the living system positively lessens the reception and internal distribution of oxygen, and consequently retards the oxidation processes of disassimilation by which the various products for excretion are perfected and their elimination facilitated, is so fully demonstrated, both by observation and experiment, as no longer to admit of doubt.

"As nearly all the toxic elements of urine are the results of these oxidation processes, the presence of alcohol in the system could hardly fail to interfere with them in a notable degree.

"The direct and somewhat extensive series of experiments instituted by Glazer, as published in the Deut. Med. Wochensch., Leipsic, Oct. 22, 1891, demonstrated this, as shown by the following conclusions:--'Alcohol, in even relatively moderate quantities, irritates the kidneys, so that the exudation of leucocytes and the formation of cylindrical casts may occur. It also produces an unusual amount of uric acid crystals and oxalates, due to the modified tissue changes produced by the alcohol. The effect of a single act of over-indulgence in alcohol does not last more than thirty-six hours, but it is cumulative under continued use.'

"Dr. Chittenden kept several dogs under the influence of alcohol eight or ten days, and found it to increase the amount of uric acid in their urine more than 100 per cent. above the normal proportion.

"Mohilansky, house-physician to Manassein's clinic, in the conclusions drawn from his interesting experiments on fifteen young men to determine the effects of alcohol on the metabolic processes generally, stated that 'it does not possess any diuretic action: but rather tends to inhibit the elimination of water by the kidneys.' It is further stated that this result is owing to the coincident effect of diminished systemic oxidation and of blood pressure.

"On the other hand, several observers have reported that the flow of urine was increased by the use of alcohol. From as full an examination of the subject as I have been able to make, it appears that the diverse results obtained have depended upon the previous habits of those experimented on, and the widely varying quantities of water drank with the alcohol. When the alcohol is taken with large quantities of water, as is usual with those who use beer and fermented drinks generally, the total amount of urine passed is usually increased, but not more than is found to result from taking the same quantity of water without any alcohol. When alcoholic drinks are taken by those already habituated to its use, it has less marked effect on the quantity and quality of the urine than when taken by those who had previously been total abstainers. This was illustrated by the experiments of Mohilansky on the fifteen men, some of whom were habitual drinkers, some occasional drinkers, and others total abstainers. When all were subjected to the same diet and drinks, with alcohol, in two the daily amount of urine voided remained unaltered, in five it was increased seven per cent., and in eight it decreased twelve per cent. But whatever may be the variations in the mere quantity of urine voided under the influence of alcohol, the alterations in quality pretty uniformly show an increase in the products of imperfect internal metamorphosis or oxidation, such as uric acid, oxalates, casts, leucocytes, albumen and potassium, with less of the normal products, as urea and salts of sodium.

"During the past year I have met with three cases in which the regular daily use of alcoholic drinks for several months, in quantities not sufficient to produce intoxication, had so altered the blood, and the renal function, that the urine contained both casts and albumen, and some degree of oedema was observable in the face and extremities. These changes were so marked as to justify a diagnosis of incipient nephritis, or Bright's disease. Yet after totally abstaining from the use of alcoholic drinks and remedies, and taking such vasomotor tonics as strychnine and digitalis, with a regulated diet and fresh air, they completely recovered.

"When it is remembered that in diphtheria, pneumonia and typhoid fever, the acute diseases in which a large part of the profession administer most freely alcoholic remedies, the function of the kidney is altered in almost the same direction as are found to take place under the influence of alcohol, it should certainly cause every practitioner to pause and critically review the pathological basis on which he has been prescribing. An an鋰thetic, like alcohol, may certainly render a patient with diphtheria, pneumonia or typhoid fever more quiet, and cause him to say he feels better, but if it at the same time diminishes the internal distribution of oxygen, retards the oxidation and elimination of waste and toxic products through the kidneys and lungs, and lessens vasomotor force, it cannot fail to protract the duration of disease, and increase the ratio of mortality."--Dr. N. S. Davis, A. M. T. A. Quarterly, April, 1894.

Dr. J. H. Kellogg, by a series of carefully executed experiments, conclusively demonstrated that alcohol hinders the elimination of poisonous matter by the kidneys. This property of alcohol is one of the objections which he sees to its use as a medicine. He says:--

"Water applied externally stimulates elimination by the pores of the skin, and employed freely internally by water drinking, and enemas to be retained for absorption, aids liver and kidney activity. If the patient dies it is because his liver and kidneys have failed to destroy and eliminate the poisons generated with sufficient rapidity to prevent their producing fatal mischief in the body."

CHAPTER VI.

ALCOHOL AS A MEDICINE.

Although nearly all of the foremost scientific investigators of the effects of alcohol upon the body have lost faith in the old views of the usefulness of alcoholic liquors as remedial agencies a considerable proportion of the medical profession do not seem yet to have learned how to treat disease without recourse to the alcohol therapy. This is largely due to the fact that the new thought has not yet crystallized to any large extent in the medical text-books, and also to the widely variant views held by professors of medicine.

The medical use of alcohol has been, and still is, the great bulwark of the liquor traffic. The user of alcoholics as beverages always excuses himself, if hard pressed by abstainers, upon the ground that they must be of service or doctors would not recommend them so frequently. In all prohibitory amendment, and no-license campaigns, the cry of "Useful as Medicine" has been the hardest for temperance workers to meet, for they have felt that they had to admit the statement as true, knowing nothing to the contrary. Indeed, thousands of those who advocate the prohibition of the sale of liquor as a beverage, use alcohol in some form quite freely as medicine, and are as determined and earnest in defence of their favorite "tipple" as any old toper could well be. Many use it in the guise of cordials, tonics, bitters, restoratives and the thousand and one nostrums guaranteed to cure all ills to which human flesh is heir.

The wide-spread belief in the necessity and efficacy of alcoholics as remedies is the greatest hindrance to the success of the temperance cause. It is impossible to convince the mass of the people that what is life-giving as medicine can be death-dealing as beverage. The two stand, or fall, together. Hence there is no more important question before the medical profession, and the people generally, than that of the action of alcohol in disease, and, as a goodly number of the most distinguished and successful physicians of Europe and America declare it to be harmful rather than helpful, it behooves thoughtful people to carefully study the reasons they assign for holding such an opinion. Certainly it is true that if physicians and people would all adopt the views of the advocates of non-alcoholic medication the temperance problem would be solved, and the greatest source of disease, crime, pauperism, insanity and misery would be driven from the face of the earth.

To understand the arguments advanced in favor of non-alcoholic medication it is needful to make some study of the effects of alcohol upon the body, and of the purposes for which alcoholics are prescribed medically.

Alcohol is used in sickness as a food, when solid foods cannot be assimilated, "to support" or sustain, the vitality; it is used as a stimulant, a tonic, a sedative or narcotic, an anti-spasmodic, an antiseptic and antipyretic; it is used in combination with other drugs, in tinctures and in pharmacy. It is not wonderful that the people esteem it above all other drugs, for none other is so variously and so generally employed. Those who discard it as a remedy teach that only in human delusions is it a food or a stimulant, and for the other uses to which it is put, outside of pharmacy, there are different agents which may be more satisfactorily employed.

IS ALCOHOL FOOD?

So well agreed are all the scientific investigators that alcohol has no appreciable food value that it would seem foolish to spend time upon a discussion of alcohol as food were it not that the idea of its "supporting the vitality" in disease, in some mysterious way is deeply rooted in the professional, as well as the popular mind.

Foods are substances which, when taken into the body, undergo change by the process of digestion; they give strength and heat and force; they build up the tissues of the body, and make blood; and they induce healthy, normal action of all the bodily functions.

Alcohol does none of these. It undergoes no change in the stomach, but is rapidly absorbed and mixed with the blood, and has been discovered hours after its ingestion in the brain, blood and tissues, unchanged alcohol. In many of the experiments made with it upon animals, considerable quantities of the amount swallowed were recovered from the excretions of the body, without any change having taken place in its composition. This, of itself, is sufficient evidence to show that it is a substance which the body does not recognize as a food.

Foods build up the tissues of the body. All physiologists are agreed that since alcohol contains no nitrogen it cannot be a tissue-forming food; there is no difference of opinion here. Dr. Lionel Beale, the eminent physiologist, says that alcohol is not a food and does not nourish the tissues.

"There is nothing in alcohol with which any part of the body can be nourished."--Cameron's Manual of Hygiene.

"Alcohol contains no nitrogen; it has none of the qualities of the structure-building foods; it is incapable of being transformed into any of them; it does not supply caseine, albumen, fibrine or any other of those substances which go to build up the muscles, nerves and other active organs."--SIR B. W. RICHARDSON.

"It is not demonstrable that alcohol undergoes conversion into tissue."--DR. W. A. HAMMOND.

If it is a food why do all writers and experimenters exclude it from the diet of children, and why is the caution always given people to not take it upon an empty stomach? Foods are supposed to be particularly suited to an empty stomach.

Foods induce healthy, normal action of all the bodily functions.

The chapter upon "Diseases Produced by Alcohol" is evidence that by this test alcohol shows up in its true nature as a poison, and not a food. Alcohol destroys healthy normal action of all the bodily functions, and builds up impure fat, fatty degeneration, instead of strong, firm muscle. Dr. Parkes, one of the most famous of English students of alcohol, says:--

"These alcoholic degenerations are certainly not confined to the notoriously intemperate. I have seen them in women accustomed to take wine in quantities not excessive, and who would have been shocked at the imputation that they were taking too much, although the result proved that for them it was excess."

Dr. Ezra M. Hunt, late secretary of New Jersey State Board of Health, remarks:--

"The question of excess occurs in sickness as well as in health, and all the more because its determination is so difficult and the evil effects so indisputable. The dividing line in medicine, even between use and abuse, is so zigzag and invisible that common mortals, in groping for it, generally stumble beyond it, and the delicate perception of medical art too often fails in the recognition."

All non-alcoholic writers assert that the continuous use of alcohol as a medicine is equally injurious to all the bodily functions as the employment of it as a beverage. Calling it medicine does not change its deadly nature, nor does the medical attendant possess any magical power by which a destructive poison may be converted into a restorative agent.

Dr. Noble, writing recently to the London Times, said:--

"The internal use of alcohol in disease is as injurious as in health."

Since foods induce healthy, normal action of all the bodily functions, and alcohol injures every organ of the body in direct proportion to the amount consumed, by this test it is proved to not be a food.

Foods give strength. Alcohol weakens the body. This has been determined again and again by experiments upon gangs of workmen and regiments of soldiers. These experiments always resulted in showing that upon the days when the men were supplied with liquor they could neither use their muscles so powerfully, nor for so long a time, as on the days when they received no alcoholic drink. Of the results of such tests Sir Andrew Clark, late Physician to Queen Victoria, said:--

"It is capable of proof beyond all possibility of question that alcohol not only does not help work but is a serious hinderer of work."

So satisfied are generals in the British army of the weakening effect of alcohol that its use is now forbidden to soldiers when any considerable call is to be made upon their strength. The latest example of this was in the recent Soudan campaign under Sir Herbert Kitchener. An order was issued by the War Department that not a drop of intoxicating liquor was to be allowed in camp save for hospital use. The army made phenomenal forced marches through the desert, under a burning sun and in a climate famous for its power to kill the unacclimated. It is said that never before was there a British campaign occasioning so little sickness and showing so much endurance. Some Greek merchants ran a large consignment of liquors through by the Berber-Suakim route, but Sir Herbert had them emptied upon the sand of the desert. A reporter telegraphed to England:--

"The men are in magnificent condition and in great spirits. They are as hard as nails, and in a recent desert march of fifteen miles, with manoeuvring instead of halts, the whole lasting for five continuous hours, not a single man fell out!"

This was in decided contrast to the march in the African war some years before when, as they passed through a malarial district, and a dram was served, men fell out by dozens. Dr. Parkes, one of the medical officers, prevailed upon the commander-in-chief to not allow any more alcoholic drams while the troops were marching to Kumassi.

Experiments in lifting weights have also been tried upon men by careful investigators. In every case it was found that even beer, and very dilute solutions of alcohol, would diminish the height to which the lifted weight could be raised. As an illustration of the deceptive power of alcohol upon people under its influence, it is said that persons experimented upon were under the impression, after the drink, that they could do more work, and do it more easily, although the testing-machine showed exactly the contrary to be true.

Athletes and their trainers have learned by experience that alcohol does not give strength, but is, in reality, a destroyer of muscular power. No careful trainer will allow a candidate for athletic honors to drink even beer, not to speak of stronger liquors. When Sullivan, the once famous pugilist, was defeated by Corbett, he said in lamenting his lost championship, "It was the booze did it"; meaning that he had violated training rules, and used liquor. University teams and crews have proved substantially that drinking men are absolutely no good in sports, or upon the water. Football and baseball teams, anxious to excel, are beginning to have a cast-iron temperance pledge for their members. So practical experience of those competing in tests of strength and endurance teach eloquently that alcohol does not give strength, but rather weakens the body, by rendering the muscles flabby.

Sandow, the modern Samson, wrote his methods of training in one of the magazines a few years ago, and stated that he used no alcoholic beverages. The ancient Samson was not allowed to taste even wine from birth.

A question worthy of serious consideration is: how are the sick to be strengthened and "supported" by drinks which athletes are warned to specially shun as weakening to the body? Either the sick are mistakenly advised, or the athletes are in error. Which seems the more likely?

Dr. Richardson says in Lectures on Alcohol:--

"I would earnestly impress that the systematic administration of alcohol for the purpose of giving and sustaining strength is an entire delusion."

In another place he says:--

"Never let this be forgotten in thinking of strong drink: that the drink is strong only to destroy; that it never by any possibility adds strength to those who drink it."

Sir William Gull, late physician to the Prince of Wales, said before a Select Committee of the House of Lords on Intemperance:--

"There is a great feeling in society that strong wine and other strong drinks give strength. A large number of people have fallen into that error, and fall into it every day."

Any unprejudiced person can readily see that experience and experiment unite in testifying that alcohol does not give strength, hence differs radically from most substances commonly classed as foods. Yet millions of dollars are spent annually by deluded people upon supposedly strength-giving drinks, and thousands of the sick are ignorantly, or carelessly, advised to take beer or wine to make them strong and to support them when solid food cannot be assimilated. Truly, "My people is destroyed for lack of knowledge."

Foods give force to the body.

Dr. Richardson says:--

"We learn in respect to alcohol that the temporary excitement is produced at the expense of the animal matter and animal force, and that the ideas of the necessity of resorting to it as a food, to build up the body or to lift up the forces of the body, are ideas as solemnly false as they are widely disseminated."

Dr. Benjamin Brodie says in Physiological Inquiries:--

"Stimulants do not create nerve power: they merely enable you, as it were, to use up that which is left."

Dr. E. Smith:--

"There is no evidence that it increases nervous influence, while there is much evidence that it lessens nervous power."

Dr. Wm. Hargreaves, of Philadelphia:--

"It is sometimes said by the advocates and defenders of alcohol, that by its use force is generated more abundantly. This it certainly cannot do, as it does not furnish anything to feed the blood or to store up nourishment to replenish the expenditure. For by their own theory, the increase of action must cause an increase of wear and tear; hence alcohol instead of sustaining life or vitality, must cause a direct waste or expenditure of vital force."

Dr. Auguste Forel, of Switzerland:--

"All alcoholic liquors are poisons, and especially brain-poisons, and their use shortens life. They cannot therefore be regarded as sources of nourishment or force. They should be resisted as much as opium, morphia, cocaine, hashish and the like."

Dr. W. F. Pechuman, of Detroit, in his valuable little treatise, Alcohol--Is it a Medicine? says clearly:--

"When alcohol or any other irritant poison is put into the system, the conservative vital force, recognizing it as an enemy, at once makes an effort through the living matter to rid the system of the offender;--the heart increases in action and new strength seems to appear. Now, right here is where the great mass of people and a large number of physicians are deluded. They mistake the extra effort of the vital force to preserve the body against harmful agencies for an actual increase in strength as the result of the agent given; we wonder that they can be so blind as not to see the reaction which invariably occurs soon after the administration of their so-called stimulant."

Dr. F. R. Lees, of England:--

"All poisons lessen vitality and deteriorate the ultimate tissue in which force is reposited. Alcohol is an agent, the sole, perpetual and inevitable effects of which are to avert blood development, to retain waste matter, to irritate mucous and other tissues, to thicken normal juices, to impede digestion, to deaden nervous sensibility, to lower animal heat, to kill molecular life, and to waste, through the excitement it creates in heart and head, the grand controlling forces of the nerves and brain."

If alcohol is a destroyer of bodily force, as any ordinary observer of drinking men can readily see, it is a problem beyond solving, how it is going to give force to, or sustain vitality in, the patient hovering between life and death. Too often has it been the means of hastening into eternity those who, but for its mistaken use, might have recovered from the illness affecting them.

Food gives heat to the body.

Alcohol does not, but really robs the body of its natural warmth. This finding of science was received with the utmost incredulity when first presented to the medical world, but the invention of the clinical thermometer settled it beyond controversy. It is now believed by all but a very few of those who have knowledge of the physiological effects of alcohol. While Dr. N. S. Davis, of Chicago, was the first to demonstrate this fact, it was Dr. B. W. Richardson, of England, who succeeded in putting it prominently before the attention of physicians.

The normal temperature of the human body is a little over 98 degrees by Fahrenheit's thermometer. If the temperature is found to be much above or below 98 degrees the person is considered out of health; indeed by this condition alone physicians are able to detect serious forms of disease. By the use of the clinical thermometer, placed under the tongue, it is easy to determine what agents acting upon the body will cause the temperature to vary from the natural standard. When alcohol is swallowed there is at first a decided feeling of warmth induced; if the temperature be taken now it will be found that in a person unaccustomed to alcohol the warmth may be raised half a degree; in one accustomed to alcohol the warmth may be raised a full degree, or even a degree and a half beyond the natural standard. But this warmth is only temporary, and is soon succeeded by chilliness.

Dr. Richardson says in his Temperance Lesson Book:--

"The sense of warmth occurs in the following way: When the alcohol enters the body, and by the blood-vessels is conveyed to all parts of the body, it reduces the nervous power of the small blood-vessels which are spread out through the whole of the surface of the skin. In their weakened state these vessels are unable duly to resist the course of blood which is coming into them from the heart under its stroke. The result is that an excess of warm blood fresh from the heart is thrown into these fine vessels, which causes the skin to become flushed and red as it is seen to be after wine or other strong drink has been swallowed and sent through the body. So, as there is now more warm blood in the skin than is natural to it, a sense of increased warmth is felt. The skin of the body is the most sensitive of substances and the sense of warmth through, or over the whole surface of the skin is conveyed from it to the brain and nervous centres of the body, by which we are enabled to feel.

"The warmth of surface which seems to be imparted by alcohol, only seems to be imparted. Positively the warmth is not imparted by the alcohol, but is set free by it.

"In a short time the sense of warmth is succeeded by a feeling of slight chilliness. Unless the person is in a very warm room, or has recently partaken of food, the thermometer will now show a decided decrease in temperature, reaching often to a degree. Should the person go out into a cold air, and especially should he go into a cold air while badly supplied with food, the fall of temperature may reach to two degrees below the natural standard of bodily heat. In this state he easily takes cold, and in frosty weather readily contracts congestion of the lungs, and that disease which is known as bronchitis. If the person drinks to drunkenness his temperature will be found to be from two and a half to three degrees below the natural standard. It takes from two to three days, under the most favorable circumstances, for the animal warmth to become steadily re-established after a drunken spree.

"The excitement of the mind in the early stages of drunkenness is not natural; it is exhaustive of the bodily powers, and exhaustive for no useful purpose whatever. * * * * *

"As nothing has been supplied by the alcohol to keep up the supply of heat the vital energy is rapidly exhausted, and if the person is exposed to cold, the exhaustion becomes extreme, sometimes fatal. All great consumers of alcohol are chillier during winter than are abstainers, and as they labor under the delusion that they must take wine or ale or spirits to keep them warm, they keep on making matters worse by constantly resorting to their enemy for relief."

Dr. Newell Martin makes this very clear in his physiology, The Human

Body.

"Our feeling of being warm depends on the nerves of the skin. We have no nerves which tell us whether heart or muscles or brain, are warmer or cooler. These inside parts are always hotter than the skin, and if blood which has been made hot in them flows in large quantity to the skin, we feel warmer because the skin is heated. As alcoholic drinks make more blood flow through the skin, they often make a man feel warmer. But their actual effect upon the temperature of the whole body is to lower it. The more blood that flows through the skin, the more heat is given off from the body to the air, and the more blood, so cooled, is sent back to the internal organs. The consequence is that alcohol, in proportion to the amount taken, cools the body as a whole, though it may for a time heat the skin."

If other evidence that alcohol is not heat-producing in the body were necessary it could be found in the fact that the products of combustion are decreased when it is present in the body. The quantity of carbonic acid exhaled by the breath is proportionately diminished with the decline of animal heat.

Arctic explorers learned by experience what science discovered by experiment. Dr. Hayes, the explorer, says:--

"While fresh animal food, and especially fat, is absolutely essential to the inhabitants and travelers in Arctic countries, alcohol, in almost any shape, is not only completely useless, but positively injurious."

Lieutenant Johnson, who accompanied Nansen upon his northern expedition, said, when interviewed by a reporter of the London Daily News:--

"The common opinion that alcohol becomes in some way a necessity in cold countries is entirely a mistaken one. This has been conclusively proved by the expedition. In making up his list of the Fram's equipments, Nansen did not include any spirits, with the exception of some spirits of wine for lamps and stoves."

In the list of stores taken upon the long sledging expedition after leaving the Fram no liquors are mentioned. See Farthest North, by Nansen. The omission of spirits was not because of any "temperance fanaticism," but because the experience of former Arctic expeditions had shown clearly that men freeze more readily after partaking of alcohol than when they totally abstain from it.

That wine is not a fuel-food was shown conclusively in the Franco-Prussian war during the siege of Paris. Food was scarce in the French Army, and wine was liberally supplied. The men complained bitterly of the extreme chilliness which affected them. Dr. Klein, a French staff surgeon, was reported in the Medical Temperance Journal of England, October 1873, as saying of this:--

"We found most decidedly that alcohol was no substitute for bread and meat. We also found that it was no substitute for coals. We of the army had to sleep outside Paris on the frozen ground. We had plenty of alcohol, but it did not make us warm. Let me tell you there is nothing that will make you feel the cold more, nothing which will make you feel the dreadful sense of hunger more, than alcohol."

There is no evidence against alcohol stronger than that which shows it to be not heat-producing, as commonly believed, but a reducer of heat in the body. Indeed, this question of bodily temperature is used in recent times to decide whether a man who has fallen upon the street is troubled by apoplexy, or influenced by alcoholism. If the clinical thermometer shows the temperature to be above normal, it is apoplexy; if below normal, it is alcoholism.

"Alcohol is clearly proved to be not a fuel-food, for if it were it would enable the body to resist cold, instead of making it colder; and in the extreme degrees of cold it would go on burning like other fuel-foods, and would maintain, instead of helping to destroy, life."--Richardson's Lesson Book.

Yet because it creates a glow of warmth in the skin immediately after drinking it, thousands of people will discredit all evidence that it is a reducer of bodily heat. Clinical thermometers, and after-sensations of chilliness, are unheeded, for "Wine is a mocker," and multitudes are willing to be deceived by it.

So, also, with the conclusions against it as a strengthening agent; because it dulls the sense of hunger and of fatigue, those who crave it will declare in the face of all scientific testimony that it strengthens them, and takes the place of food. They will cite, too, the cases of people who "lived upon whisky" during an illness of greater or less duration. Of the sustaining of life upon alcohol only, Dr. N. S. Davis has said:--

"The falsity of all such stories is made apparent by the fact that nineteen-twentieths of all the alcoholic drinks given to the sick are given in connection with sugar, milk, eggs or meat-broths, which furnish the nutriment, and would support the patients better if given with the same perseverance without the alcohol than with it. While we have quite a number of examples of men living on nothing but water forty or fifty days, I have never seen or learned of a well-authenticated case of a man's taking or receiving into his system nothing but alcohol for half of that length of time, without becoming sick with either gastro-duodenitis, nephritis, or delirium tremens."

Some of the defenders of the medicinal use of alcohol claim that since it has been shown to reduce tissue waste it should be classed as an indirect food, a conserver of tissue. Of this claim, Dr. N. S. Davis says in the Bulletin of the A. M. T. A., November, 1895:--

"A careful study of the conditions and processes necessary for both tissue building or nutrition, and tissue waste or disintegration, in all the higher order of animals, will show that neither process can be materially retarded without retarding or preventing the other. Both processes take place only in bioplasm or vitalized matter, supplied with oxygen, water and heat. Neither the assimilation of new material food, nor its use in tissue building can be effected without the presence of free oxygen and nuclein, or corpuscular elements of the blood. And without the presence of the same elements we can have no natural tissue disintegration and removal of the waste. The processes of tissue building and tissue disintegration, are therefore, so intimately related, and dependent upon the same materials and forces, that neither can be hastened or retarded from day to day without influencing the other. When alcohol or any other substance, introduced into the blood, retards the tissue waste, as shown by the diminished amount of excretory products, it must do so by either diminishing the amount of free oxygen in the blood, by impairing the vasomotor and trophic nerve functions or by direct impairment of the properties of the nuclein or protogen elements of the blood and tissues. The popular idea, both in and out of the profession is, that the alcohol, by further oxidation in the blood, lessens the amount of oxygen to act on the tissues, and generates heat or 'some kind of force.' Those who advocate this theory of saving the tissues by combining the oxygen with alcohol seem to forget that in doing so they are diverting and using up the only agent, oxygen, capable of combining with, and promoting the elimination of, all natural waste products as well as the various toxic elements causing disease.

"But the theory that alcohol directly combines with the oxygen of the blood by which it would be converted into carbonic acid and water with evolution of heat is completely refuted by the well-known fact that its presence in the blood diminishes both temperature and elimination of carbonic acid as already stated. Physiologists of the present day very generally agree that the capacity of the blood to receive oxygen from the lungs, and convey it to the systemic capillaries and various tissues, depends chiefly on its hemoglobin (red coloring matter), protein, or albuminous and saline elements.

"Both experimental and clinical facts in abundance show that alcohol at all ordinary temperatures displays a much stronger affinity for these elements of the blood and tissues, than it does for oxygen. And when present in the blood, it rapidly attracts both water and hemoglobin from the corpuscular and albuminoid elements of that fluid, and thereby diminishes its reception and distribution of oxygen. We are thus enabled to see clearly how the alcohol diminishes the oxygenation and decarbonization of the blood, and retards all tissue changes both of nutrition and waste without itself undergoing oxidation with evolution of heat. Consequently, instead of acting as a shield or conservator of the tissues by simply combining with the oxygen, the alcohol directly impairs the properties and functions of the most highly vitalized elements of the blood itself, and thereby not only retards tissue waste but also equally retards the highest grades of nutrition, and favors only sclerotic, fatty and molecular degenerations, as we see everywhere resulting from its continued use. Can an agent displaying such properties and effects be called a food, either direct or indirect, without a total disregard for the proper meaning of words?"

In another place he says:--

"This lessening of the elimination of tissue waste is simply an evidence of the accumulation of poisonous substances within the body, through the lessened activity of liver and kidneys and the impairment of the blood."

Dr. Ezra M. Hunt says in Alcohol as Food and as Medicine, page 37:--

"It sounds conservative of health to say of a substance that it delays the breaking down of tissue, but the physiologist does not allow a substance which occasions such delay, to possess, because of that, either dietetic or remedial value. To increase weight by prolonged constipation is not a physiological process."

Dalton says:--

"The importance of tissue change to the maintenance of life is readily shown by the injurious effects which follow upon its disturbance. If the discharge of the excrementitious substances be in any way impeded or suspended, these substances accumulate either in the blood or tissues, or both. In consequence of this retention and accumulation they become poisonous, and rapidly produce a derangement of the vital functions. Their influence is principally exerted upon the nervous system, through which they produce most frequent irritability, disturbance of the special senses, delirium, insensibility, coma, and finally, death."

The power to retard the passage of waste matter from the system is one of the gravest objections to the use of alcohol in sickness, as the germs of disease are thereby caused to remain longer in the body than they would, were no alcohol or drug of similar action, used. Thus recovery is delayed, if not effectually hindered.

The preponderance of scientific evidence is all against alcohol as possessing food qualities. It contains no elements capable of entering into the composition of any part of the body, hence cannot give strength; it is not a fuel-food as it does not supply heat to the body, but decreases temperature; and its classification as indirect food because it retards the passage of waste matter is shown to be utterly unscientific, as any agent which interferes with the natural processes of assimilation and disintegration is a dangerous agent, a poison rather than a food.

The question naturally arises:--

If these drinks are not liquid food, as we have been taught to believe, how is it, since they are made from food, as barley, corn, grapes, potatoes, etc?

These drinks are not food, although made from food, because in the process of manufacturing them the food principle is destroyed. The grain is malted to change starch into sugar--loss of food principle begins here--then the malted grain is soaked in water to extract the saccharine matter. When the sugar is all in the water the grain goes to feed cattle or hogs, and the sweetened water is fermented. The fermentation changes the sugar into alcohol.

Analyses of beer by eminent chemists show an average of 90 per cent. water, 4 per cent. alcohol, and 6 per cent. malt extract. The malt extract consists of gum, sugar, various acids, salts and hop extract. Starch and sugar are all of these capable of digestion, and the amount of them would be equal to 39 ounces to the barrel of beer. Liebig, the great German chemist, said:--

"If a man drinks daily 8 or 10 quarts of the best Bavarian beer, in a year he will have taken into his system the nutritive constituents contained in a 5 pound loaf of bread."

Eight quarts a day for a year would be 2,920 quarts, or a little more than 23 barrels. If sold to the consumer at the low rate of five cents a pint, it would cost him $292; a high price for as much nourishment as in a 5 pound loaf!

Analyses of wine by reliable chemists show that the consumer must pay $500 for the equivalent in nourishment of a 5 pound loaf of bread, wine being higher priced than beer. Wines average 80 per cent. water, about 15 per cent. alcohol, and 5 per cent. residue. This residue is composed of sugar, tartaric, acetic and carbonic acids, salts of potassium and sodium, tannic acid, and traces of an ethereal substance which gives the peculiar or distinguishing flavor. The only one of these ingredients possessing food value is sugar; this exists chiefly in what are called sweet wines. Yet how many thousands of people spend money they can ill afford for wines and beers to build up the failing strength of some loved one! A costly delusion, and too often a fatal one!

"Distilled liquors, if unadulterated, contain literally nothing but water and alcohol, except traces of juniper in gin, and the flavor of the fermented material from which they have been distilled."--Influence of Alcohol, by N. S. Davis, M. D.

It is the solemn duty of those to whom the people look for instruction in matters of health to undeceive the toiling masses as to the food-value of alcoholic liquids. Some of the medical profession are faithful in this regard, but too many others are themselves deceived, or care not for the destruction of the people.

IS ALCOHOL A STIMULANT?

A lady asked her family physician several years ago what he thought of the views of those medical writers who class alcohol as a narcotic, and not a stimulant. He answered with some heat, "Any one who says alcohol is not a stimulant is either a fool or a knave!" He could not have been aware that some of the most distinguished professors in American medical colleges teach that alcohol is not, properly speaking, a stimulant, but a narcotic.

The accepted definition of a stimulant in medical literature is some agent capable of exciting or increasing vital activity as a whole, or the natural activity of some one structure or organ.

Dr. N. S. Davis has said repeatedly that both clinical and experimental observations show that alcohol directly diminishes the functional activity of all nerve structures, pre-eminently those of respiration and circulation, thus decreasing the internal distribution of oxygen, which is nature's own special exciter of all vital action.

"Consequently it is antagonistic to all true stimulants or remedies capable of increasing vital activity. Instead, therefore, of meriting the name of stimulant, alcohol should be designated and used only as an an 鎧 thetic and sedative, or depressor of vital activity."

The following is taken from an editorial article in the American Medical Temperance Quarterly for January, 1894:--

"Drs. Sidney Ringer and H. Sainsbury in a carefully executed series of experiments on the isolated heart of the frog, found that all the alcohol when mixed with the blood circulating through the heart, uniformly diminished the action of that organ in direct proportion to the quantity of alcohol used, until complete paralysis was induced. In closing their report in regard to the action of different alcohols, they say that 'by their direct action on the cardiac tissue these drugs are clearly paralyzant, and that this appears to be the case from the outset, no stage of increased force of contraction preceding.'

"Professor Martin, while in connection with the Johns Hopkins University, performed an equally careful series of experiments in regard to the action of ethylic, or ordinary alcohol, directly on the cardiac structures of the dog, and with the same results. He makes the following explicit statement of the results obtained by him. 'Blood containing one-fourth per cent. by volume, that is two and a half parts per 1000 of absolute alcohol, almost invariably diminishes, within a minute, the work done by the heart; blood containing one-half per cent. always diminishes it, and may even bring the amount pumped out by the left ventricle to so small a quantity that it is not sufficient to supply the coronary arteries.'

"In 1883, R. Dubois, by direct experimenting upon animals, found that the presence of alcohol in the blood much intensified the action of chloroform and thereby rendered a much less dose fatal.

"Prof. H. C. Wood of the University of Pennsylvania, in an address upon An鉎 thesia to the Tenth International Medical Congress, of Berlin, in 1890, said: 'In my own experiments with alcohol, an eighty per cent. fluid was used largely diluted with water. The amount injected into the jugular vein varied in the different experiments from 5 to 20 c. c.; and in no case have I been able to detect any increase in the size of the pulse or in the arterial pressure produced by alcohol, when the heart was failing during advanced chloroform an鉎 thesia. On the other hand, on several occasions, the larger amounts of alcohol apparently greatly increased the rapidity of the fall of arterial pressure, and aided materially in extinguishing the pulse.

"Sir Henry Thompson says: 'That alcohol is an an鉎 thetic and paralyzant is a fact too well established to be questioned or contradicted.'

"Dr. J. J. Ridge, of London, has published elaborate tables, showing that even small doses of alcohol, averaging one tablespoonful of spirits--not quite half a wineglass of claret or champagne, and not quite a quarter of a pint of ale--impair vision, feeling, and sensibility to weight, without the subject's being conscious of any alteration. Dr. Scougal, of New York, has repeated and confirmed these experiments, and also demonstrated that the hearing was similarly affected.

"Drs. Nichol and Mossop, of Edinburgh, conducted a series of experiments on each other, examining the eye by means of the ophthalmoscope while the system was under the influence of various drugs. They found that the nerves controlling the delicate blood-vessels of the retina were paralyzed by a dose of about a tablespoonful of brandy.

"Dr. T. D. Crothers, of Hartford, Conn., has deduced some valuable facts from his experiments with the sphygmograph, upon the action of the heart. He has found by repeated experiments that while alcohol apparently increases the force and volume of the heart's action, the irregular tracings of the sphygmograph show that the real vital force is diminished, and hence its apparent stimulating power is deceptive."--Extract from the Annual Address before the Medical Temperance Association at San Francisco, Cal., June 8, 1894, by Dr. I. N. Quimby, of Jersey City, N. J.

Dr. J. H. Kellogg, of Battle Creek, Mich., has made extensive experiments as to the effects of alcohol. In summing up the results of these he says:--

"It would seem that no further evidence could be required that alcohol is a narcotic and an an 鋥 thetic, rather than a stimulant, and that its use as a supporting and tonic remedy is a practice without foundation in either scientific theory or natural clinical experience."

Sir B. W. Richardson at a medical breakfast in London in 1895, stated that though alcohol produced an increase in the motion of the heart it was ultimately weaker in its action, so he resolved to give up using such an agent.

Dr. A. B. Palmer of the University of Michigan prepared a "Report" upon alcohol in 1885 for the Michigan State Medical Society in which he cited experiments showing that the opinion that alcohol stimulates the heart by an increase of real force, is an error. It creates a flutter, but decreases power.

"Increased frequency of pulsation is often the strongest evidence of diminished power--as the fluttering pulse of extreme weakness."

He classes alcohol with chloroform.

"If chloroform is a narcotic, alcohol is a narcotic. If chloroform is an an 鋥 thetic, alcohol is an an 鋥 thetic. If one is essentially a depressing agent, so is the other. Their strong resemblance no one can question. The chief difference is that the alcoholic narcosis is longer continued, and its secondary effects are more severe."

In closing his summary of the changes in scientific knowledge of this drug he says:--

"We said it was a direct heart exciter. We now know it is a direct heart depressor. We said, and nearly all the text-books still say, it is a direct cardiac stimulant. We know from most conclusive experiments it is a direct cardiac paralyzant."

The following is taken from one of the many excellent papers upon alcohol written by that Nestor among physicians, Dr. N. S. Davis:--

"Alcoholics are very generally prescribed in that weakness of the heart sometimes met with in low forms of fever and in the advanced stage of other acute diseases. It is claimed that these agents are capable of strengthening and sustaining the action of the heart under the circumstances just named, and also under the first depressing influence of severe shock.

"There is nothing in the ascertained physiological action of alcohol on the human system, as developed by a wide range of experimental investigation, to sustain this claim. I have used the sphygmograph and every other available means for testing experimentally the effects of alcohol upon the action of the heart and blood-vessels generally, but have failed in every instance to get proof of any increased force of cardiac action.

"The first and very transient effect is generally increased frequency of beat, followed immediately by dilatation of the peripheral vessels from impaired vasomotor sensibility, and the same unsteady or wavy sphygmographic tracing as is given in typhoid fever, and which is usually regarded as evidence of cardiac debility. Turning from the field of experimentation to the sick-room, my search for evidences of the power of alcohol to sustain the force of the heart, or in any way to strengthen the patient has been equally unsuccessful. I was educated and entered upon the practice of medicine at a time when alcoholic drinks were universally regarded as stimulating and beat-producing, and commenced their use without prejudice or preconceived notions. But the first ten years of direct clinical or practical observation satisfied me fully of the incorrectness of those views, and very nearly banished the use of these agents from my list of remedies. While it is true that during the last thirty years I have not prescribed for internal use the aggregate amount of one quart of any kind of fermented or distilled drinks, either in private or hospital practice, yet I have continued to have abundant opportunity for observing the effects of these agents as given by others with whom I have been in council; and simple truth compels me to say that I have never yet seen a case in which the use of alcoholic drinks either increased the force of the heart's action or strengthened the patient beyond the first thirty minutes after it was swallowed. * * * * *

"Nothing is easier than self-deception in this matter. A patient is suddenly taken with syncope, or nervous weakness, from which abundant experience has shown that a speedy recovery would take place by simple rest and fresh air. But in the alarm of patient and friends something must be done. A little wine or brandy is given, and, as it is not sufficient to positively prevent, the patient in due time revives just as would have been the case if neither wine nor brandy had been used."

In the Medical Pioneer of November, 1895, Prof. E. MacDowel Cosgrave, Professor of Biology, Royal College of Surgeons in Ireland, says:--

"The result of all recent investigation is to show that the use of alcohol when a stimulant effect is desired, is an error; and that, from first to last alcohol acts as a narcotic."

Dr. Edmunds, of London, said in an address given in Manchester:--

"By giving alcohol as a stimulant in exhausting diseases, I believe we always do as we should in giving a dose of opium and brandy and water to comfort a half suffocated patient; i. e., increase his danger. If that be so, we reduce alcohol not only from the position of food medicine, but we reduce it from the position of a goad; and we say that the supposititious stimulating or goading influence of alcohol is a mere delusion; that in fact alcohol always lessens the power of the patients, and always damages their chance of recovery, when it is a question of their getting through exhausting diseases."

Many more such quotations might be adduced. Enough are given to show that the popular use of alcohol, when a stimulant is required, is considered a grave error by those who have most thoroughly studied the effects of this drug.

ALCOHOL AS A TONIC.

Dr. J. J. Ridge, of London, says:--

"The action of alcohol in relaxing unstriped muscular fibre, which entitles it to be called an anti-spasmodic, robs it of all claim to give tone. The sense of exhilaration which follows small doses of alcohol has been mistaken for real strength and increase of vitality. It is well known that relaxation of the blood-vessels throughout the body is one of the first effects of alcohol. The arteries of the retina have been observed to dilate after very small doses of alcohol. The diminution of tone is well seen in the tracings of the pulse under the influence of alcohol. If one needs a tonic, therefore, alcohol is one of the things to be shunned altogether.

"But alcoholic beverages contain other things beside alcohol. Beer contains infusion of hops, or other bitter stomachics. Some wines contain tannin. These ingredients, by creating or stimulating the appetite, increase the strength and vital power in certain cases. But we have a large number of drugs which will do the same without the disadvantages arising from the presence of alcohol, and, if the flavor be objected to, many of them can be taken in the form of coated pills.

"The external use of cold, either by a dripping sheet, cold sponging, or a shower-bath, according to the power of reaction, is a valuable means of giving real tone.

"Wine is frequently prescribed for those young persons who are growing rapidly, and whose strength does not seem to keep pace with their growth. It is important to know that alcohol is not desirable in such circumstances. There is often found in such cases a defective appetite, perhaps even sub-acute gastric catarrh, which may be due to imperfect mastication through bad teeth, or aggravated by it. There are other causes, such as late hours, bad habits, improper food or irregular meals. In such cases those means must be resorted to which are so effectual in improving the condition and strengthening the heart of athletes. Regular and regulated meals, exercise in the fresh air, a good amount of rest and sleep--these will do more than anything else to invigorate the bodily health."

Dr. N. S. Davis says:--

"Although I was taught, like all others, to use alcohol as a tonic when patients were sick, to hasten their recovery and promote their strength, yet it did not take me very long to find out that here and there was one already a teetotaler who would not take wine long, nor any kind of alcoholic drink unless prescribed, just as castor-oil, dose by dose, but who, when he got beyond the necessity of having it as a medicine, took no more. What was the comparison? My patients who refused, or did not take alcohol, got strong quicker and had less tendency to relapse than those who continued its use. Here was the first step in progress, and consequently I came soon to cease the recommending it merely to hasten recovery of strength. As a tonic, I found it of no value."

Dr. James Miller, of Edinburgh, says in Alcohol, Its Place and Power, written many years ago:--

"It may be well here to correct an important error, yet very current, in regard to the medicinal use of alcohol. People regard it as a simple and common tonic; and are ready to accept its supposed help as such in every form of weakness and general disorder of health. But it is ordinarily, no true tonic."

Dr. Ernest Hart, editor of the British Medical Journal, stated some years ago at a meeting of the British Medical Temperance Association that "the medical profession were nearly all agreed that alcohol is neither a food nor a tonic."

Many drunkards have been made, especially among women, by the delusion that alcohol has tonic effect. As a sample of these sad cases the following is given, taken from a recent number of The National Advocate:--

"There is in the jail at Elizabeth, N. J., a woman who was arrested while participating in wild drunken orgies with a gang of tramps in the woods near the town. She appears nothing but a besotted hag, but was only a short time ago a dutiful wife of a respectable man, and the mother of three beautiful children. Her father, who is said to be living in a village in New York State, is a highly respected minister of the Methodist Episcopal Church. Her children are in an asylum, and her husband is a wanderer in the West. The cause of her ruin was beer, prescribed for her by the family physician as a tonic. At first she refused to take it, having always been a teetotaler, but persuaded to obey the physician, she soon acquired a taste for the drink that speedily developed into the overmastering appetite, which has brought her and hers to this sad condition."

ALCOHOL AS A SEDATIVE.

Dr. J. J. Ridge says in the Medical Pioneer, April, 1893:--

"Alcohol, chiefly in the form of spirits, is often given to procure sleep and to relieve pain, such as that of neuralgia, dyspepsia, colic and diarrhoea. It is as a sedative that alcohol is so insidious and seductive in cases of chronic disease, as, if frequently resorted to, the drink craving is almost certainly developed. Hence the importance in many cases of rather bearing the ills we have than of flying to others that we know not of. It is clear that other narcotics, such as opium, morphia, chorodyne, chloral, are open to the same objection, and the victims of these drugs are terribly numerous. * * * * * In many instances some form of dyspepsia is the cause of the sleeplessness, palpitation or other uneasy feeling for which a sedative is desired, and when this is cured the symptoms vanish."

A prominent minister in a large American city was afflicted with insomnia a few years ago, and, after trying various remedies, was advised by a physician to try whisky "night-caps." He became a hopeless drunkard. A young medical student in New York appealed to one of his professors for aid in overcoming aggravated insomnia. The professor advised whisky and morphine! The advice led to the ruin of the young man.

ALCOHOL AS AN ANTIPYRETIC.

"By the power of alcohol to retard the evolution of heat in retarding molecular changes in the tissues, the liquids containing it may be used as antipyretics when the temperature is too high, and to retard the processes of waste when these are too rapid. But the antipyretic influence of alcohol is so feeble in comparison with the proper application of water to the surface, or with the internal administration of sulphate of quinia, salicylic acid, digitalis, etc. that no one thinks of using it for antipyretic purposes."--Dr. N. S. Davis in Principles and Practice of Medicine.

PROFESSOR ATWATER'S CONCLUSIONS UPON ALCOHOL AS A FUEL-FOOD.

In 1899 a decided sensation was caused by the announcement that Prof. Atwater, of Middletown, Conn., had proved that alcohol is a fuel-food equal in value to carbohydrates and fats. The study later of Prof. Atwater's report of his investigations led to prolonged discussions among medical men interested in the alcohol question, and his theory that alcohol is a food because it is oxidized in the body was vigorously opposed by many scientists of high standing. Professor Abel, of Johns Hopkins University, Baltimore, an investigator of alcohol who worked with the Committee of Fifty, said on this point:--

"Oxidizability cannot be made the measure of usefulness in regard to this substance."

Professor Gruber, president of the Royal Institute of Hygiene, Munich, said:--

"Does alcohol truly deserve to be called a food substance? Obviously, only such substances can be called food material, or be employed for food, as, like albumen, fat, and sugar, exert non-poisonous influence in the amounts in which they reach the blood and must circulate in it in order to nourish * * * * Although alcohol contributes energy it diminishes working ability. We are not able to find that its energy is turned to account for nerve and muscle work. Very small amounts, whose food value is insignificant, show an injurious effect upon the nervous system."

Sir Victor Horsley, the well-known London surgeon, said:--

"We know that alcohol lowers the temperature of the body. It can only do that by diminishing the activity of the vital processes. It also diminishes very greatly the power of the muscles, and it diminishes the intellectual power of the nervous system. To call an agent that causes such diminution of activity throughout the whole body a food is ridiculous."

An editorial in the Journal of the American Medical Association said:

"The fallacy of the reasoning which would place alcohol among the foods is very apparent when we put it in the form of a syllogism: All foods are oxidized in the body; alcohol is oxidized in the body; therefore alcohol is food. As logically we might say: 'All birds are bilaterally symmetrical; the earthworm is bilaterally symmetrical; therefore the earthworm is a bird.' Oxidation within the body is simply one of several important properties of food, as bilateral symmetry is one of several important characteristics of a bird."

Schafer's Physiology says:--

"It cannot be doubted that any small production of energy resulting from the oxidation of alcohol is more than counterbalanced by its deleterious influences as a drug upon the tissue elements, and especially upon those of the nervous system."

The Bulletin of the A. M. T. A. for July, 1899, contained an article upon Prof. Atwater by Dr. J. H. Kellogg, from which the following is taken:--

"Starch, sugar and fats become foods or fuels only through their assimilation. Abundant physiological evidence attests that no substance can act as a food, or as a true source of energy, unless it has first entered into the composition of the body. It must be assimilated. The forces manifested by the body, the muscular forces, or nervous energy, are the result of the breaking down of organized structure into simpler forms. For example, in the case of nervous energy, material from which nerve energy is derived is stored up in the nerve cell, and can be seen with the microscope in the form of minute granules, which disappear as the cell energy is expended, leaving the cell blank and shriveled when in a state of extreme fatigue from overwork. The same is essentially true of the muscle cell. The source of muscular energy is glycogen, an organized substance which becomes a part of the muscle tissue in a well-nourished muscle in a state of rest.

"Experiments have clearly shown that fat, sugar and starch must all alike be converted into the form of glycogen and enter into the muscle structure before they can become a source of energy.

"Professor Atwater tells us that alcohol can not form tissue, hence the query is pertinent, How can it be a source of vital energy? The body does not burn food as a stove does fuel. Food can be called fuel only in a highly figurative sense. The oxidation of food in the body does not take place directly. Food is assimilated, becoming a part of the tissue. Oxygen is also assimilated, entering into the composition of the tissue along with the food elements under the action of special organic ferments brought into play by nervous impulses received from the central ganglia.

"The molecules of these residual tissues which form the storehouse of energy in the body are rearranged in simpler forms, thereby giving up a portion of the energy which holds them together in the state in which they exist in the tissues, and this energy thus set free appears as muscle force, mental activity, glandular work and various other forms of functional activity."

CHAPTER VII.

ALCOHOL IN PHARMACY.

In the Journal of the American Medical Association for November 13, 1897, Dr. T. D. Crothers, editor of the Journal of Inebriety, says in a paper upon "Concealed Alcohol in Drugs":--

"A very important question has been repeatedly raised, and answered differently by persons who claim to have some expert knowledge. The question is, can strong tinctures of common drugs be given in all cases with safety; tinctures of the various bitters which contain from 10 to 40 per cent. of alcohol, and are used very freely by neurotic and debilitated persons? It is asserted with the most positive convictions that such tinctures are more sought for the narcotic effect of the alcohol than for the drugs themselves.

"In my experience a large number of inebriates who are restored, relapse from the use of these tinctures given for their medicinal effects. * * * * *

"The question is asked, how much alcohol can be used as a solvent in drugs without adding a new force more potent than that which is brought out by the alcohol? Opinions of experts differ. One writer thinks 10 per cent. of alcohol in any drug will, if given any length of time, develop the physiologic effect of alcohol in addition to that of the drug. An English writer says that in some cases a 5 per cent. tincture is dangerous from the alcohol which it contains.

"There is some doubt expressed by many authorities as to the potency of a drug which is covered up in a strong tincture. It is clear that the value of a drug is not enhanced, and it is certain that a new force-producing, or exploding agency, has been added to the body.

"In experience, any drug which contains alcohol can not be given to persons who have previously used it without rousing up the old desire for drink, or at least producing a degree of irritation and excitement that clearly comes from this source. It is also the experience of persons who are very susceptible to alcohol, that any strong tincture is followed by headache and other symptoms that refer to disturbed nerve centres.

"In many studies I have been surprised at the increased action of drugs when given in other forms than the tincture. Gum and powdered opium, have far more pronounced narcotic action than the tincture. Yet the tincture is followed by a more rapid narcotism, but of shorter duration, and attended with more nerve disturbance at the onset.

"I am convinced that a more exact knowledge of the physiologic action of alcohol on the organism will show that its use in drugs as tinctures is dangerous and will be abandoned.

"There are many reasons for believing that its use in proprietary drugs will be punished in the future under what is called the poison act."

Dr. J. J. Ridge published in May, 1893, in the Medical Pioneer, the following statement of the pharmacy of the London Temperance Hospital:--

"When the Temperance Hospital was first opened, it became a question of practical importance, what should be done with regard to the alcohol so largely employed as a vehicle and drug excipient. Not that the principle of the treatment of disease without the ordinary administration of alcoholic beverages precludes the employment of alcoholic tinctures, but it was felt that in such a test case as this it was important to obviate the objection that while withholding alcohol as a beverage, it was given in the medicine. As a matter of fact, it is surprising, when one looks into it, how much alcohol is often given merely as a vehicle for other drugs, and without the special action of alcohol being required or desired. In prescriptions which are to be seen in many text-books, it is not uncommon to find from one to two or three, or even four drachms of rectified spirit in the form of tinctures or spirits. This is very undesirable. If alcohol is needed it should be given in proper measured dose. But if it is not indicated, then it is not well to administer it in this indirect manner.

"Experiments were therefore made, partly at the hospital and specially by Messrs. Southall Bros. & Barclay, of Birmingham, with the result that new non-alcoholic tinctures were made replacing the following alcoholic tinctures and wines:--

Tinct. Aloes. " Arnic? " Aurantii. " Belladonn? " Buchu. " Calumb? " Camph. Co. " Capsici. " Cascarill? " Catechu. " Chirat? " Cinchon?Co. " " Flav. " Cinnamom? " Colchici Sem. " Conii. " Digitalis. " Ferri Acet. " Ferri Perchlor. " Gentiani Co. " Hyosciami. " Kino. " Krameri? " Limonis. " Lobeli? " Nucis Vomic? " Opii. " Quassi? " Rhei. " Scill? " Serpentari? " Stramonii. " Valerian? " " Ammon. Vin. Aloes. " Colchici Rad. " " Sim. " Ipecac. " Opii. " Rhei.

"These were made by extracting the principles of the drugs in the usual way except that instead of alcohol a mixture of glycerine and water was used in the proportion of one-fourth to one-third part of glycerine, and about five per cent. of acetic acid. These made very elegant preparations, and in the majority of cases appeared to have just the same, and just as great physiological action. Subsequently the ordinary tinctures were distilled, and the extracts thus obtained dissolved in the above menstruum, as far as was possible, in most cases the residuum being found to be inert.

"Gum resins and essential oils were found to be insoluble in this menstruum, and hence such drugs have been given in the form of pill, powder or mixture. Such tinctures are those of assafoetida, benzoin, cannabis indica, cantharides, castor, cubebs, lavender, myrrh, pyrethrum, sumbul, tolu and ginger. Out of 62 tinctures it was found that 46 made good preparations, and 16 did not.

"These were employed for several years. But for some time past, somewhat more reliable preparations have been made for us which contain all the constituents of the alcoholic tinctures without the alcohol. They are for the most part made by taking standardized tinctures, mixing with them sugar of milk, and distilling off the alcohol. The alcoholic extract remains behind in a finely divided condition mingled with sugar of milk. This is broken up, pulverized and compressed into tabloids of a definite dose, which can be taken either in that form or rubbed up and dissolved or suspended in gum water.

"The following have been made up in this form: aconite, belladonna, camph. co., cannabis indica, capsicum, cinchon. co., and cinchon. simpl., digitalis, gelseminum, hyosciamus, nux vomica, opium, strophanthus, ginger and Warburg. Other tinctures will be gradually added to this list.

"As external liniments those commonly used are the linimentum terebinthin?and the linimentum terebinthin?aceticum, which do not contain alcohol. A strong solution of iodine is made with iodide of potassium.

"The spiritus ammoni?aromaticus is made without the spirit, the aromatic oils being emulsionized by means of rubbing up with fine sand, but most of these subsequently rise to the surface. The spiritus etheris nitrosi is impossible without alcohol, but nitrite of amyl, and nitrites of potash or soda can be substituted. The spiritus chloroformi is replaced by aqua chloroformi, or as a sweetening agent by solution of saccharin. Thus a favorite expectorant mixture contains carbonate of ammonia five grains, acetum ipecac, ten minims, and solution of saccharin in each dose.

"As a special stimulant a subcutaneous injection of a drachm of pure ether has been given in a few cases; in others digitalis, or caffeine or ammonia in some form, such as the carbonate dissolved in a cup of hot coffee; or hot solution of Liebig's extract, or rectal injections of hot water."

It may be objected by some that glycerine belongs to the family of alcohols, hence hospitals using glycerine tinctures are not, strictly speaking, non-alcoholic. To this the answer is, that while glycerine certainly is classed in the family of alcohols, it is of a very different nature from ethyl alcohol, which is used for beverage purposes. Ethyl alcohol, the alcohol in all intoxicating beverages in common use, and the alcohol generally used in medicine, creates a fatal craving for itself, and is injurious to the body. Glycerine does not create any craving for itself, and has not been demonstrated to have injurious properties, and is not used for beverage purposes.

At the annual meeting of the New York State Medical Society, held in New York City, in October, 1898, a discussion was held upon the use of alcohol as medicine. Dr. E. R. Squibb, a leading pharmacist of Brooklyn, stated that during the last two or three years much had been accomplished in retiring alcohol as a menstruum for exhausting drugs. Of the other menstrua experimented with up to the present time, that which had given the best results was acetic acid, in various strengths. It had been discovered that a ten per cent. solution of acetic acid was almost universal in its exhausting powers. There were now in use in veterinary practice, and in some hospitals, extracts made with acetic acid. They were made according to the requirements of the pharmacopoeia, except that acetic acid was substituted for alcohol. Acetic acid, when used with alkaloids gives the physician some advantages in prescribing, owing to there being fewer incompatibles. In small doses, the percentage of acetic acid in the extract is so small as to be hardly appreciable, and when larger doses are required, the acetic acid can be neutralized by the addition of potash or soda.

Dr. Noble said, in article to London Times before referred to:--

"Modern science has shown that those drugs which are soluble in alcohol only, are, in all probability, more hurtful than useful."

The following from Dr. Jas. R. Nichols, editor Boston Journal of Chemistry, is too good to be omitted, although it should be familiar to temperance students:--

"The facetious Dr. Holmes has said, that if the contents of our drug-stores were taken out upon the ocean and thrown overboard, it would be better for the human race, but worse for the fishes. This statement may be a little sweeping; but it is true that all the showy bottles in drug-stores which contain alcoholic decoctions and tinctures might be submerged in the ocean, and invalids would suffer no detriment. Since the active alkaloidal and resinoidal principles of roots, barks and gums have been isolated and put in better and more convenient forms, there is no longer need of alcoholic tinctures and elixirs. Laudanum, which is a tincture of opium, might be banished from the shelves of every apothecary, as it is not needed. It is now known that the valuable narcotic and hypnotic principles of opium are contained in certain crystalline bodies, which can be isolated, and used in minute and convenient forms, and that they can be held in aqueous solutions. Alcohol is no longer needed to hold the active principles of opium, Peruvian bark or other indispensable drugs. As regards the vegetable tonics so called, the best among them is the columbo (Radix columbo) and this readily yields its bitter principle to water, as does quassia, gentian, senna, rhubarb and most other valuable substances. A careful survey of the contents of a well-appointed modern pharmacy leads to the conclusion that there is no one indispensable medicinal preparation which requires alcohol as a free constituent.

"The catalogue of modern remedies is almost endless, and many of them hold alcohol in some form; but every intelligent physician knows that 90 per cent. of these alleged remedies have little or no intrinsic value. The nostrums of the quack, the bitters, elixirs, cordials, extracts, etc. nearly all contain alcohol, and this is the ingredient which aids their sale. The whole unclean list might, with advantage to mankind, be thrown to the fishes.

"The chemist, more particularly the pharmaceutical chemist, may inquire how he is to conduct his processes without alcohol. It is from the pharmaceutical laboratory we derive some of the most important substances used in medicines and the arts. Among them may be named ether, chloroform and chloral hydrate, three of the most indispensable agents known to science, and the employment of alcohol is essential to their production. Alcohol is a laboratory product; it is a chemical agent which belongs to the laboratory; it is the handmaid of the chemist, and, so long as it exists, should be retained within the walls of the laboratory. In the manufacture of most of the important products in which alcohol is either directly or indirectly used, its production may be made simultaneous with the production of the agent desired. In the manufacture of ether and chloroform, the apparatus for alcohol may be made a part of the devices from which the ultimate agents, ether and chloroform, result. Fermentation and distillation may be conducted at one end, and the an鉎 thetics received at the other. It is true that in a chemical laboratory alcohol is an agent very convenient in a thousand ways. But, if it were banished utterly, what would result? There are other methods of fabricating the useful products named, and many others, without the use of alcohol, but the processes would be rather inconvenient and more costly. The banishment of alcohol would not deprive us of a single one of the indispensable agents which modern civilization demands, and neither would chemical science be retarded by its loss."

"It must be remembered that modern science has given us glycerine, naptha, bisulphide of carbon, pyroligneous products, carbolic acid and a hundred other agents which are capable of taking the place of alcohol in a very large number of appliances and processes."

The sale of liquor in drug-stores is beginning to be deplored by the more respectable pharmacists. At the annual meeting of the Massachusetts State Pharmacists' Association in 1895 the president said in his address:--

"One thing that every pharmacist, who has the best interests of his calling at heart, must bear in mind is that the liquor part of their business is being, and must be, slowly crowded out. Public sentiment has changed greatly in the last few years, and instead of all being classed alike, the line has been sharply drawn, and the stores that sell the least amount of liquor that they possibly can are gaining the confidence and esteem of the public, and consequently their business is growing from year to year, while the others are losing ground and dropping lower and lower."

The Evening Record of Boston contained the following in its issue of March 7, 1896:--

"The number of flagrant offences on the part of druggists in certain no-license towns--offences not only against the liquor laws, but also against the laws of decency and humanity--brought before the board of pharmacy, would appall the public if they were known. The Looker-On has seen the record of several of these druggists as transcribed from the police courts and they are very black records. One druggist after selling liquor over and over again to one customer, and several times getting him completely intoxicated, finally deposited him one night in a snowbank, in a state of frozen stupor, where he would have frozen to death had not the wife of the druggist's clerk threatened to complain to the police unless he was rescued.

"The story is told of one of the druggists of a neighboring no-license town. A man came in and asked for a pint of whisky. He was asked what he wanted it for. His reply was that he wanted it to soak some roots in. He got it, and as he went out he dryly remarked, 'I should have told you that it was the roots of me tongue that I want to soak.'"

CHAPTER VIII.

DISEASES, AND THEIR TREATMENT WITHOUT ALCOHOL.

The question, "What shall I take instead of wine, beer or brandy?" is frequently asked by those who have been trained to think some form of alcohol really necessary to the cure of disease, but, who, from principle would prefer other agents, if they knew of any equal in effect. This chapter deals somewhat with the answer to that question.

ALCOHOLIC CRAVING:--The craving for alcohol may be present for a time after a person has commenced to abstain from all beverages containing it. Or, it may occur periodically, as a sort of irresistible impulse. For the periodical craving Dr. Higginbotham, of England, recommends that a half drachm of ipecacuanha be taken so as to produce full vomiting. He says the desire for intoxicating drinks will be immediately removed. The craving is caused by vitiated secretions of the stomach; the vomiting removes these. Dr. Higginbotham says:--

"If a patient can be persuaded to follow the emetic plan for a few times when the periodical attacks come on, he will be effectually cured."

Some men in trying to abstain have found the use of fresh fruit, especially apples, very helpful. Nourishing and digestible food should be taken somewhat frequently. A cup of hot milk or hot coffee taken at the right moment has saved some.

AN 芃 IA:--In this complaint there is a deficiency of the red corpuscles of the blood. It may be the result of some fever or exhausting illness; it may accompany dyspepsia, and is then due to imperfect digestion and assimilation of the food. The poverty of the blood produces shortness of breath, and often palpitation of the heart also, especially on a little exertion. There is generally more or less weariness, languor and debility, sometimes also giddiness, sickness, fainting and neuralgia.

"In the treatment of an 鎚 ia, port wine and other alcoholic liquors are worse than useless."--DR. J. J. RIDGE, London.

"The common prescription of wine or some form of spirits for states of general exhaustion and an 鎚 ia, is a serious mistake. It assumes that the temporary increase in the action of the heart is renewed vigor, and that some power is added to the failing energies. This theory rests solely on the statement of the patient that he feels better. In reality the exhaustion is intensified, though covered up."--Medical Pioneer.

"Deficiency of nutrition, of light and of pure air may be mentioned as common causes of an 鎚 ia. * * * * * It is evident that the first step in the treatment of this disease is to remove the cause. If the cause is dyspepsia, this must receive attention; if intestinal parasites, they must be dislodged; if prolonged nursing, nursing must be interdicted; if too little food, a larger quantity of nourishing, wholesome food must be employed. Such simple and easily digested foods as eggs, poached or boiled, boiled milk, kumyzoon, good buttermilk, pur 閑 of peas, beans or lentils, boiled rice, well-cooked gruels and other preparations of grains are suitable. Beef tea and extracts are worthless. * * * * *

"A careful course of physical training is essential to securing perfect recovery in cases of chronic an 鎚 ia due to indigestion, or any other serious disturbance of the nutritive processes."--DR. J. H. KELLOGG.

APPETITE, LOSS OF:--"There is often disinclination for food because it is not required. Many cannot eat much breakfast, because they have had a hearty supper. Or having had both a hearty breakfast and luncheon, they feel but little desire for a dinner of four or five courses. Generally the stomach is right and the habits wrong. What is to be done then, for such lack of appetite? Simply go without food until appetite comes.

"When ale or beer is taken regularly with meals the stomach learns to expect them, and the food is not relished without them. The appetizing power of beer and bitter ales is chiefly due to the hop or other bitter ingredients which they contain. When it seems necessary to assist the appetite temporarily, a small quantity of simple infusion of hops may be taken.

"Sometimes appetite fails because of exhaustion of body and mind. This may be nature's warning against overwork, and cannot be neglected with impunity. Life will inevitably be shortened if it is found necessary to rely upon the aid of alcohol in any form in order to do a day's work.

"Bouillon, or beef soup, at the beginning of a meal are incentives to appetite. Change of scene, and life in the open air are the very best aids to appetite, when aids are really required."

APOPLEXY:--"There is a popular idea that whenever a person is taken ill with giddiness, fainting or insensibility, brandy should be at once procured and poured down his throat. Nothing can be more dangerous in apoplexy. This disease is due to the bursting of some blood-vessel in the head, and the poured-out blood presses on the brain and leads to more or less insensibility. If fainting occurs, it may possibly save the patient's life, because then the blood-vessels contract, and the flow of blood ceases immediately; time is thus given for the ruptured blood-vessel to became sealed up by a clot, which will prevent further loss of blood. If brandy is given, there is, first, great risk of choking the patient; if that danger is escaped and the brandy is swallowed and absorbed, the vessels become relaxed and the heart recovers its force; hence the ruptured vessel, if not sufficiently sealed by clot, may be started again, and fatal hemorrhage result.

"The only treatment which unskilled hands can adopt is to lay the patient on his back on the floor or sofa with the head and shoulders somewhat raised; to loosen all the dress round the neck and body; to apply cold to the head and hot flannels or a hot bottle to the feet and hands, or to soak them in hot mustard and water, and to gently rub the arms and legs."--DR. J. J. RIDGE.

Dr. Alfred Smee, surgeon to the Bank of England, says:--

"Give nothing by the mouth. Apply a stream of cold water to the head. If the feet are cold apply warm cloths. If relief is not soon obtained, apply hot fomentations to the abdomen, keeping the head erect."

BED-SORES:--Some object to using alcohol even as an outward application. Dr. Ridge recommends that when a patient is confined to bed the parts pressed on be well washed every day with strong salt and water or alum water, and carefully dried. Glycerine of Tannin may then be applied. If any redness appears, especially if any dusky patch is formed, collodion may be applied with a brush, and all pressure should be taken off the part by a circular air-pillow or by a cushion; or small bran or sand-bags may be made and carefully arranged. If the skin is broken, zinc or resin ointment may be applied.

Some recommend finely powdered iodoform sprinkled over the surface of the sore.

BOILS AND CARBUNCLE:--"In many cases these troubles result from an overloaded condition of the system, which is the result of taking too much food, or some error in diet. The boils are an effort of nature to be rid of offending matter. In some cases they are due to the use of impure water, or the presence of sewer gas in the house. In others, overwork, or other debilitating causes, may have produced the state of the digestive organs which usually causes the boils. Carbuncle is, essentially, an extensive boil.

"Apply iodine early or a piece of belladonna plaster. The diet should be plain and unstimulating, condiments being avoided and plenty of fresh vegetables taken, if possible. Fresh-air, exercise and proper rest should be obtained, and late hours avoided.

"Medical advice is requisite in carbuncle. The popular notion that port wine is absolutely necessary is both erroneous and mischievous."--RIDGE.

CATARRH:--Among the causes are repeated colds; errors in diet, especially excess in the use of fats and sugar, and an inactive state of the liver.

Cut off from your bill of fare all salted foods, avoid fats and condiments; drink freely of pure water; live in the open-air and sunshine as much as possible, taking much out-door exercise. Take a cold sponge or towel bath every morning, beginning at the face and finishing by plunging the feet into a foot-tub. Follow with vigorous rubbing with a crash or Turkish towel. Those subject to sore throat should hold the head over a basin of cold water and lave the neck with the water for about two minutes. The writer was formerly subject to frequent sore throats, but has had none for over two years, as she believes, because of the adoption of this measure, together with the towel bath every morning, summer and winter.

Care should be taken to avoid exposure to draughts, or any other means which will produce liability to cold. Care in diet, good ventilation and the morning cold bath are essential if a radical cure is desired. Local measures, while giving relief, will not remove the predisposing causes. Dr. Kellogg recommends saline solutions in the form of the nasal douche, a teaspoonful of salt to a pint of soft water, adding twenty to thirty drops of carbolic acid, if there is offensive odor, as a relief measure.

Sleeping in a poorly ventilated room is said to be one cause of catarrh.

Hay Fever is a form of catarrh. The vapor bath is recommended as very helpful in this trouble. Nature Cure says that two vapor baths and a two or three days' fast will cure any case of hay fever. The use of pork and other clogging foods should be avoided by those afflicted with this trouble. The bowels should be kept in good condition. If constipated, the use of prunes, figs, grapes, apples and other such fruits will be very beneficial; walking, and massage of the bowels, being added if the fruits are not sufficient. No one able to walk should depend upon drugs to relieve a constipated condition.

COLDS:--"If the bowels are constipated, the skin over-burdened and clogged with bilious matter, and the lungs weak, it is as easy to take cold as to roll off a log. If, on the contrary, the lungs are well developed, and the respiratory power large, providing abundant oxygen to keep bright the internal fires, the colon clean, the skin daily washed, and the system hardened by the cold bath, taking cold is next to impossible.

"The first remedial agent for a cold should be a copious enema. Then open the pores of the skin by a hot bath; take a glass of hot lemonade and go to bed."--The New Hygiene.

CHILLS:--For chill, take a hot foot and hand bath, with mustard in the water, 1/4 pound to a gallon; then go to bed in a well ventilated room. Drink freely of hot lemonade or hot water. Catarrh, colds and hay fever may all be effectually relieved by hot baths. Relief may be gained also from inhaling the vapor from pine needles or hemlock leaves. Put them in a bowl, pour boiling water over them, hold the face down over the bowl, the head being covered, and inhale the vapor well up into the nostrils and head. A few drops of hemlock oil in the hot water will do as well.

COUGHS AND HOARSENESS:--Boil flaxseed in 1 pint water, strain, add two teaspoons honey, 1 ounce rock candy, and juice 3 lemons. Drink hot. Also; roast a lemon till hot, cut, and squeeze on 3 ounces powdered sugar.

COLIC:--This may arise from cold, or from error in diet. If the latter it is desirable to induce vomiting. For the pain, apply hot flannels or fomentations; drink hot water. In severe cases, sprinkle a little turpentine on flannel, wrung from hot water, and apply to abdomen. Colic resulting from the accumulation of fecal matter should be treated with hot enemas until relieved. A hot hip-bath is sometimes necessary to relief.

The colic of children and infants should never be treated with alcoholics. In infants it generally arises from excessive or improper feeding; care should be taken that the milk provided them is not sour.

In severe cases the babe should be immersed in warm water, keeping the head above water, of course. This is also the best remedy in convulsions. The hot bath, with a copious enema of warm water, has saved the lives of many babes.

For adults, hot water, with a pinch of red pepper added, will do all that brandy can do, and more.

CHOLERA:--Brandy has been considered by many a really necessary medicine in cholera. The following is a discussion upon Alcohol in Cholera which was held at the annual meeting of the British Medical Temperance Association, in May, 1893, and is taken from the Medical Pioneer of June, 1893:--

"Dr. Richardson opened a discussion on Cholera in relation to Alcohol. He said he would bring forward five points on the subject.

1. The negligence among the people at large produced by alcohol in the presence of a cholera epidemic. There was no doubt on the part of any who had seen an epidemic of cholera as to the mischief done by alcohol, apart from its action as a remedy. People rush to the public houses and take it to ward off the danger, or to relieve them when they begin to feel ill, and the result is very bad morally. He had seen this in different epidemics. Or people got in spirits to face the danger, and many became intoxicated and less able to resist.

2. Its misuse by those affected. It was often given to cheer them up and remove their fear and nervousness. In his opinion it invariably produced mischief.

3. He was unable to find any physiological reason for giving it. There was a constant drain of fluid, causing spasms and cramp, both of the muscles and blood-vessels, and difficult circulation through the lungs. Spasm may be relaxed by alcohol, but, on the other hand, alcohol is exceedingly greedy of water, and so increases the flux. But it also reduces animal temperature, which is a strong feature of cholera, so much so that he could almost diagnose cholera blindfold in the stage of collapse, by the icy coldness.

4. Its uselessness as a remedy during the acute stage. He had seen a great deal of cholera and never saw alcohol do any good whatever. There was a temporary glow which passed away in a few minutes, and then the evil it does in other ways was brought out. Water was far better, even if cold. The College of Physicians had given some instructions and ordered great care in

the administration of alcohol; this was not far enough, but good as far as it went. The recoveries were best where the treatment was simplest, such as external warmth with plenty of diluents. He had given creasote largely.

5. Its injuriousness during the stage of reaction. The reactive fever following collapse caused a great number of deaths. In this stage alcohol was absolutely poisonous. He could recall many such cases in which he had given alcohol through ignorance, and always with disaster.

"Brigade-Surgeon Pringle said that when he went out to India he thought alcohol was something to stand by, but he had soon found out his mistake; he had himself suffered from it. He could confirm what Dr. Richardson had said as to the demoralization produced by alcohol to which men resort to keep up their spirits, and men seized under these circumstances were in the greatest danger. Nature effects a cure in many cases without assistance, and often with wonderful rapidity. People apparently dead and about to be buried, he had known to get up and recover. When alcohol is given during collapse there is often no absorption until reaction occurs, and then the quantity accumulated speedily produces intoxication. It was the same with opium: he had found pills unchanged in the stomach for hours. He recommended hot drinks; he had tried every kind of medicine and had little faith in it. The nursing was very important, and it was important that the nurses should abstain.

"Dr. Morton said it was easy to see that on physiological grounds alone, alcohol, with its strong affinity for water and its tendency to lower temperature, could not be a useful drug in the treatment of cholera collapse, and with its powers of paralyzing vascular inhibition and checking elimination of effete matter, could not be otherwise than harmful in the stage of reaction. As these conclusions were corroborated by practical experience he did not think members would hesitate to banish it from their equipment against cholera.

"Dr. Ridge said it should be remembered that Doyen had made experiments on guinea-pigs and had found they were proof against cholera, unless they had previously had a dose of alcohol. This explained why drunkards and hard drinkers were so much more liable to have cholera, and have it badly as all observers declared to be the case. Another reason might be that small quantities of alcohol, such as would be found circulating in the blood, favored the growth and multiplication of bacteria, certainly those of decomposition, and probably those of cholera. Hence, other things being equal, the abstainer had a great advantage.

"Dr. Norman Kerr said that he had observed both in America and Glasgow that not only notorious drunkards but free drinkers suffered; abstainers were less liable unless they took contaminated water, and the less liquid taken the less chance of taking cholera; beer-drinkers often took more than abstainers. The alcohol-drinker uses up more water from his blood and so has less to flush out the system. Alcohol, given to a patient, disguised his condition so that he might seem better though really worse. Hence it is better and safer not to give any. The doctors and nurses ought to be abstainers. A doctor after dinner was more likely to take a roseate view of a case, looking at it through an alcoholic pair of spectacles. Alcohol was not really a stimulant, but a depressant, and this is a very depressing disease; it was important to have our vital resisting power as vigorous as possible. Hot water both relaxes and stimulates, and the whole cry of the sufferer is for water. Many persons who died in cholera did not die of the disease, but of the drugs such as alcohol and opium. Acid drinks should be given, as the bacilli could not live in acid mixtures. Cholera might come, but he believed we were better prepared to meet it and to treat it.

"Surgeon-General Francis sent a communication which was read by the Honorable Secretary. He said: 'Having had many opportunities of treating cholera in various parts of India and amongst all classes, I have no hesitation in affirming that alcohol in any shape is one of the very worst remedies. Life is, so to speak, paralyzed, and we give a remedy which, apparently stimulating, is in reality, a paralyzer and therefore mischievous; the death-rate might be considerably reduced provided alcohol were rigidly excluded.'"

Dr. Norman Kerr in a valuable paper upon Cholera says:--

"The first thing is to get rid of the poison. How? By assisting it out; but alcohol keeps it in by blocking the doors, just as the doors were blocked in the terrible calamity at Sunderland not long ago. The alcohol makes the heart and circulation labor more. Alcohol not only retains the cholera poison, but retards the action of the heart. Brandy and opium used to be employed, but the records show that if the object had been to make cholera as fatal as possible, that object was achieved by the indiscriminate administration of brandy and opium. Better leave the victim alone, and his chances of recovery will be greater than if he have a thousand doctors, and as many nurses, administering to him brandy and opium. Alcohol is especially dangerous in the third stage, that of reactive fever, because it adds to the fever. Then, alcohol is not only unsafe in the three stages of genuine cholera, but especially unsafe in the premonitory diarrhoea stage, which gives nearly every one warning before they are attacked by genuine cholera. Brandy is taken simply because it puts away the pain. If there are only the pain and slight diarrhoea, speaking medically, it is all right, but if there is anything behind the pain, it is all wrong. After the alcohol, the mischief is going on, only the patient does not know it, and valuable time is lost. All the alcohol does is to deaden sensation. * * * * * Here I can thoroughly recommend ice and iced water. I have always treated cholera patients with these. Let them drink iced water to their hearts' content; they can never drink too much; and this opinion is fortified by that of Professor Maclean, of Netley. There is no need of a substitute for brandy in cholera, because in ordinary circumstances in that disease the action of a stimulant is bad. Flushing of the blood is required, and water will do it. Milk will not do it, because it is too thick-- nothing but pure, cold water, all the better if iced."

In 1893 Dr. Ernest Hart, editor of the British Medical Journal, read an able paper upon Cholera before the American Medical Association. His argument was that the introduction of such a substance as alcohol, itself being a product of germ action, into a system already suffering from the toxic influence of a ptomaine, could not be otherwise than pernicious.

CHOLERA MORBUS:--Dr. Kellogg says: "The stomach should be washed by means of the stomach-tube when possible. A large hot enema should be given after each evacuation of the bowels. The addition of tannin, one drachm to a quart of water, is serviceable. When the vomited matter no longer shows signs of food, efforts should be made to stop the vomiting. Give the patient bits of ice the size of a bean to swallow every few minutes. At the same time apply hot fomentations over the stomach and bowels. If the patient suffer much from cramp, put him into a warm bath. The first food taken should be farinaceous. Oatmeal gruel, well boiled and strained, is useful."

CHOLERA INFANTUM:--"Iced water may be given in very small quantities every few minutes. Give the stomach entire rest for at least twenty-four hours. There will be no suffering for want of food as long as the stomach is in such a condition. Withhold milk until nature has had time to rid the alimentary canal of the poison-producing germs. White of egg dissolved in water is an excellent preparation in these cases. Egg enemata may also be advantageously used.

"Warm baths, the hot blanket pack when the surface is cold, and the hot enema are all useful. Keep the child wrapped warmly.

"Great care should be taken in returning to the milk diet. The milk should be thoroughly sterilized by boiling for half an hour, and should be mixed with some barley water so as to avoid the formation of large curds in the stomach. Cream, diluted with water, may be used instead of milk."

CONSUMPTION.

Dr. Koch, the celebrated German microscopist, pronounces consumption contagious, because during its progress a very minute bacterium is developed which may be transmitted from one person to another.

It is said that a person with healthy lungs might daily breathe millions of tubercle bacilli without any danger, and that the best preventive of this disease is to live much in the open air, or if this is impossible to spend ten or fifteen minutes a day in deep breathing exercises in the open air. "Fresh-air and disease-germs are antagonistic."

Alcohol, chiefly in the form of whisky, was for many years considered of great value in the treatment of consumption of the lungs. Indeed, it was looked upon not only as a curative, but also as a prophylactic, or preventive, of great service to those predisposed to this disease by reason of narrow chest and weak lungs.

Sir Benjamin Ward Richardson was the first medical scientist who showed plainly that alcohol, instead of being a preventive of consumption, is really the sole cause of one type of this disease, the type now classed under the head of "alcoholic phthisis." For this kind of phthisis there is no hope of cure.

French physicians some years ago came to the conclusion that alcohol was a prolific cause of tuberculosis and that the administration of alcoholic liquors in tubercular troubles was a great error, and in the International Anti-Tuberculosis Congress held in Paris in 1905, about 2000 medical scientists being present, they presented the following resolution, which was adopted: "In view of the close connection between alcoholism and tuberculosis, this Congress strongly emphasizes the importance of combining the fight against tuberculosis with the struggle against alcoholism."

Since that time a great crusade against tuberculosis has been carried on by means of exhibits and lectures, and in connection with these, almost invariably the people are warned against intemperance. For example, a pamphlet sent out by the Boston Association for the Relief and Control of Tuberculosis says: "Do not spend money for beer or other liquors, or for quack medicines or 'cures.' Self-indulgence and intemperance are very bad. Vice which weakens the strong kills the weak." The New York State

Charities Aid Association, working with the State Board of Health, says in a pamphlet: "Patent medicines do not cure consumption. They are usually alcoholic drinks in disguise, and the use of alcoholic drinks is dangerous to the consumptive." At the great exhibit in Washington in September, 1908, in connection with the International Anti-Tuberculosis Congress different warnings against alcohol were upon the walls. Among these was a large poster of white cloth on which was printed the opinions on alcohol, in brief, of some of the best-known authorities on consumption. The opinions as given on that poster are given here, with others, in order to show the great change of sentiment regarding alcohol and consumption which has come about within a few years:--

"Alcohol has never cured and never will cure tuberculosis. It will either prevent or retard recovery. It is like a two-edged weapon; on one side it poisons the system, and on the other it ruins the stomach and thus prevents this organ from properly digesting the necessary food."--S. A. KNOPF, M. D., New York, Honorary Vice-President of the British Congress on Tuberculosis.

Dr. Knopf in his prize essay on "Tuberculosis and How to Combat It," says in several places: "Avoid all alcoholic beverages." He says also, "Alcohol should never be given to children even in the smallest quantities."

"It is a recognized fact in the medical profession that the habitual use of alcoholic drinks predisposes to tubercular infection. It is also recognized, I think, by most physicians that alcohol as a medicine is harmful to the tubercular invalid."--FRANK BILLINGS, M. D., Chicago, Ill., Former President American Medical Association.

"Alcoholic liquors are of damage to consumptives because they tend to impair nutrition, disturb the action of the stomach, and give a false strength to the invalid on which he is sure to presume. Besides, we know that in countries where drinking prevails most, the ravages of tuberculosis are most marked."--EDWARD L. TRUDEAU, M. D., Adirondacks Sanitarium for

Consumptives, Saranac Lake, N. Y.

"In my judgment whisky should not be used by people who have consumption, and in my practice I prohibit its use absolutely. At the White Haven Sanitarium and Henry Phipps Institute we do not use alcohol in any form in the treatment of our patients."--LAWRENCE F. FLICK, M. D., Vice-President of the National Association for the Study and Prevention of Tuberculosis, Philadelphia, Pa.

"I do not feel that I can emphasize strongly enough the harm that can be done by the use of alcohol in tuberculosis, and the indiscriminate use of it certainly borders on the criminal. I do not believe that any legitimate reason can be given for the routine employment of alcohol in the treatment of tuberculosis. I furthermore know of no emergency in which it is indispensable. My experience with patients who have been accustomed to the use of alcohol, especially moderately, is very unsatisfactory. They seem to show an abnormally low resisting power to the tubercle bacillus. The fact has been established that alcoholism is a very potent factor in the causation of tuberculosis. I find it not only unnecessary in treatment but believe it to be contraindicated."--F. M. POTTENGER, M. D., Superintendent the Pottenger Sanitarium for Diseases of the Lungs and Throat, Monrovia, California.

"I have met with a small class of consumptive patients who could take alcoholic liquors freely for a length of time, without deranging either the stomach or the brain, and with a decided amelioration of the pulmonary symptoms, and an arrest of the emaciation. Some of these have actually increased in embonpoint, and for three to six months were highly elated with the hope that they were recovering. But truth compels me to say that I have never seen a case in which this apparent improvement under the influence of alcoholic drink was permanent. On the contrary, even in those cases in which the emaciation seems at first arrested, and the general symptoms ameliorated, the physical signs do not undergo a corresponding improvement; and after a few months the digestive function becomes impaired; the emaciation begins to increase rapidly; and in a short time the patient is fatally prostrated."--DR. NATHAN S. DAVIS, SR., of Chicago.

"The use of whisky in this disease positively interferes with digestion which must under all circumstances be kept as perfect as possible in order that the patient may assimilate the food which is so necessary to the upbuilding of the system and to gain strength to fight the onslaught of the disease.

"Its constant use would not only interfere with digestion but would have a tendency to create disease in other organs of the body so that we therefore consider the use of whisky in tuberculosis positively contraindicated.

"Wishing you success in your laudable campaign."--DR. M. COLLINS, Superintendent National Jewish Hospital for Consumptives, Denver, Colorado.

"It is difficult for many people to adapt themselves to a methodical plan of life long enough to establish a permanent cure in consumption. I have known many a young fellow with only a slight trouble in his lungs to die in the Adirondacks more from the effects of whisky than from the disease itself."-- DR. HENRY P. LOOMIS, of New York City, in a Lecture on Consumption. (See page 232, of Handbook, on the Prevention of Tuberculosis.)

"The majority of our patients receive no medication whatsoever. The stomach is rarely in condition to bear excessive medication, and the promiscuous use of creosote and similar preparations is to be condemned. Milk and raw eggs are the best articles of diet in addition to a regular diet of simple food."--JAMES ALEXANDER MILLER, M. D., of the Vanderbilt Clinic, New York. (From Medical Record.)

"In my specialty, the treatment of pulmonary diseases, I rarely prescribe alcohol in any form, and in the sanitaria with which I have been connected it is the exception where alcohol in any form is prescribed. I have advised against its use where such has been the custom, believing that as a rule alcoholic liquors do more harm than good in the treatment of this disease."--PROF. VINCENT Y. BOWDITCH, M. D., Harvard Medical School, Boston.

"From personal experience in handling pulmonary tuberculosis, not only at the Nordrach Ranch Sanitorium, for the past five years, but in an active practice of thirteen years, I am more than convinced that whisky and liquor, in any form, are absolutely poisonous to the consumptive.

"Whenever we admit a patient to the Nordrach Ranch Sanitorium, we ascertain whether the individual is an alcoholic or not; and we invariably find that such an individual is lacking in vitality enough to combat the disease. They may look fat and strong, pulmonary tuberculosis usually makes quick work of them.

"It is also a noticeable fact, proven by various statistics, that a very large percentage of alcoholics become tubercular; and if we ever stamp out tuberculosis, we will also have to stamp out intemperance.

"Trying to cure consumption with whisky is like trying to put out a fire with kerosene. This is very easy to understand when we stop to consider the nature of this disease. In the first place, we have a very rapid heart's action, dating from the very earliest manifestations of the disease. The pulse is often in excess of 100, even in incipient cases, and if the stimulation of alcohol is added, we have what might be called a 'runaway heart'; and if there is one thing needed in the long combat against tuberculosis, it is a good heart."--JOHN E. WHITE, M. D., Medical Director Nordrach Ranch Sanitorium, Colorado Springs, Colorado.

"You ask me my opinion as to the use of whisky in the treatment of consumption. In reply permit me to say that I regard its use in this disease as most universally pernicious."--PROF. CHARLES G. STOCKTON, M. D., Buffalo Medical College, Buffalo, N. Y.

"It was formerly thought that alcohol was in some way antagonistic to tuberculous disease, but the observations of late years indicate clearly that the reverse is the case, and that chronic drinkers are more liable to both acute and pulmonary tuberculosis. It is probably altogether a question of altered tissue soil, the alcohol lowering the vitality and enabling the bacilli more readily to develop and grow."--DR. OSLER, formerly Professor of Medicine in Johns Hopkins University, Baltimore, Md., now of Oxford University, England.

"Upon investigation I found 38 per cent. of our male tubercular patients were excessive users of alcohol, 56 per cent. moderate users. From my study of the cases I am led to believe that in a vast majority of these cases drink has been a large factor in producing the disease, by exposure, lowering of vitality, etc. I believe that alcohol has no place in the treatment of tuberculosis. Many patients are deceived by the false strength it gives them."--O. C. WILLHITE, M. D., Superintendent of Cook County Hospital for Consumptives, Dunning, Ill.

"In tuberculosis there is a state of over-stimulation of the circulatory system due to the toxins. The use of alcoholics simply makes the condition worse. It reduces resistance and makes the person more susceptible to the disease."--H. J. BLANKMEYER, M. D., Sanatorium Gabriels, in the Adirondacks, N. Y.

"The practice of taking alcoholics of any sort, and in any quantity, over a considerable length of time, is certain to produce more or less injury to a tubercular patient, and their use by tubercular people cannot be too strongly condemned."--H. S. GOODALL, M. D., Lake Kushaqua, N. Y.

Most of these opinions were written for the author of this book in response to letters of inquiry. Are they not indicative of a day when the medical profession will lay aside alcoholic liquors in the treatment of all diseases? It is acknowledged that the past usage of giving whisky and cod-liver oil to consumptives was an error; some day, it may be not far distant, a larger acknowledgment may be made, and the medical use of alcoholic liquors will be entirely a thing of the past.

Rev. J. M. Buckley, D.D., editor of The Christian Advocate, was in early manhood considered an incurable consumptive. Being a man of great will power and indomitable perseverance, he resolved to try the open-air cure, together with the use of an inspirator. The result was perfect restoration to health, so that, as is well known, he can be easily heard by audiences of thousands at Chautauqua and other places where he is greatly in request for lectures. He has written a pamphlet giving a full history of his case. It can be obtained from Eaton & Mains, 150 Fifth Avenue, New York, for fifty cents, and should be read by all consumptives who have any "grit" in their composition.

Dr. Forrest, a hygienic physician, says:--

"What is to be done if the germs have already obtained lodgement in the lungs? Increase the general nutrition of the body in every way, and then the lungs can resist the inroads of the disease. The first thing necessary to improve the nutrition of the body is to stimulate the digestive and absorbent functions of the stomach and intestines. Naturally then, you must throw the so-called cough medicines out of the window. The drugs used to stop a cough are sedatives. Now, no sedative or nauseant is known that does not lock up the natural secretions and thus lessen the digestive powers. The cough is nature's method of expelling offending matter from the lungs and bronchial tubes. It is infinitely better to have this stuff thrown out of the lungs than retained there."

Keep the bowels clean is this physician's next recommendation.

Sweet cream is preferable to cod-liver oil as it is not so likely to derange the stomach. Easily digested food is necessary, as the organs of digestion are in weakened condition.

Again Dr. Forrest says:--

"The consumptive should live as much as possible in the open air.

"Dr. Trudeau inoculated twelve rabbits with tubercle or consumptive germs. Six of these he turned loose on an island where they ran wild. The other six were kept confined in hutches such as rabbits are usually kept in. Results-- All the six rabbits in the open air recovered from the inoculation and remained well. Five of the confined rabbits died of tubercles in the lungs and different parts of the body. The sixth was still lingering, badly diseased, when the experiment was brought to a close. Fresh air and exercise enabled the first six to overcome the disease germs. Confinement gave full play to the disease in the others.

"Now, you house lovers, sleepers in close bedrooms, people afraid of cold air, you are the rabbits in the hutches. Beware, lest the verdict be in your case, 'Died of tubercles in the lungs.' If you are not able to leave your home, live with open windows, day and night, summer and winter.

"Exercise systematically, especially those exercises, accompanied by deep breathing, that open and strengthen the lungs--exercises without fatigue.

"If you are hoping that some wonderful, mysterious drug has been or will be discovered, a drug that will cure consumption without your help, you are hoping against hope. Improved nutrition is your salvation, and that must come through exercise, diet and fresh air."

Dr. J. H. Kellogg, in his Home Hand-Book of Hygiene and Medicine, recommends a salt sponge bath upon retiring, to arrest night sweats, or sponging with hot water. He adds:--

"It is important that patients should know that the sweats are greatly aggravated by opium in any form, and hence are increased by cough mixtures of any sort which contain this drug. Very simple remedies are often effective to relieve the most distressing cough, such as gargling of water in the throat, holding bits of ice in the mouth, taking occasional sips of strong lemonade, and similar remedies. As a general rule, patients run down and the disease progresses much more rapidly, after beginning the use of opium in any form. Sometimes it is best that the cough should be encouraged instead of being repressed. When the patient expectorates very freely, the cough is a necessary means of relieving the chest of matters which would seriously interfere with the functions of the lungs if retained, by filling up the bronchial tubes and air-cells. The kind of cough needing relief is an irritable, ineffective cough, unaccompanied by any considerable degree of expectoration. Loaf sugar, honey or a mixture of honey and lemon juice, and other simple, familiar remedies are often effective in relieving such a cough.

* * * * *

"It is perhaps needless to add that the numerous quack remedies for consumption advertised in the newspapers are wholly without merit. There is no known drug which will cure this disease, or in any certain degree influence its progress. Numerous remedies have been recommended as curative, but not one has thus far stood the test of experience."

DISPLACEMENTS OF THE UTERUS:--These conditions are not among those for which alcoholic liquors are likely to be advised by a physician, but women frequently resort to Lydia Pinkham's Compound and other alcoholic preparations in the vain hope of finding the relief so positively promised in the nostrum advertisements. Women are sometimes seriously injured by using the nostrums specially advised for uterine weaknesses, for this reason: a drug which may be of service in an an 鎚 ic condition of the womb may do much damage in an inflamed or engorged condition, yet the nostrum vendors advise their preparations for all alike, without a word of warning as to possible dangers.

Ordinary displacements may be recovered from by cleanliness of the parts and by exercises which strengthen the muscles in the pelvic region. The writer has known a considerable number of women who have been restored to health by exercises after months, in some cases, and several years in others, of weakness and misery. One of these women was a close relative of a celebrated specialist in women's diseases. He said he could not do any more for her, and gave permission for her to try the exercises, which were given her by a well-equipped teacher of physical training.

There are three kinds of displacements: anteversion, retroversion, and prolapsus. The causes of these troubles are various; lack of proper care in child-bearing, miscarriages, heavy lifting, a hard fall, jumping out of a carriage, straining, too violent exercise in gymnasium work, and tight-lacing, also gradual weakening of the ligaments which sustain the uterus in position.

An abdominal supporter should be worn constantly during the day for a year or so, then left off gradually an hour or two at a time. It should be worn during the second year whenever any extra work is to be done.

There is a supporter sold by the Battle Creek Sanitarium which is highly recommended, but any physician can get one for a patient.

Perfect cleanliness is necessary. For this purpose a hot vaginal douche should be taken two or three times a day. This douche should be made astringent by adding to a pint of water a quarter ounce of alum or tannin. The hot astringent injections tone up the lower supports of the uterus, and cleanse the passage. The patient should remain in a recumbent position for some hours after the douche if possible. Considerable rest hastens a cure. Take the rest in the fresh air when weather permits. Persistent use of sitz baths will be found helpful.

For prolapsus the simplest form of internal supporter is a small roll of cotton. After the organ is carefully put into position this supporter should be pressed up against the mouth of the womb, the patient meanwhile lying upon her back. The ball of absorbent cotton should be large enough to be retained in position, and should be saturated with a weak solution of glycerine and alum or glycerine and tannin before being applied. A piece of white cord should be tied firmly around the centre of this tampon by which it may be removed. Remove before taking the douche.

Persons who feel unable to purchase an elastic or other abdominal supporter can make a substitute (not so good, but of considerable service) from unbleached muslin made in the shape of the letter T, and having the cloth double. It should go up to the waist and be made to fit over the hips, then should be fastened firmly in front with safety-pins, and the cross-piece be drawn up from the back and fastened securely in front.

The daily exercises are the most important part of the treatment. They must be begun gradually, and taken at greater length as strength is gained. Those for prolapsus will be given first:--

The patient should lie upon a rug, or on a firm long sofa or couch. The feet should be drawn up as close to the body as possible. Now lift the lower part of the body so that the hips and lower portion of the trunk will have no support but what comes from the feet and shoulders. Hold this position for a minute or two (longer when able without much fatigue). After a few minutes' rest repeat. This exercise may be continued from twenty to thirty minutes, according to patient's strength. The elevation of the hips in this exercise aids in the restoration of the organ to its natural position. This exercise should be continued daily, the number of times being increased as strength increases.

A second exercise which is very helpful in prolapsus is to support the body on the toes and elbows with the face downward, and the hips raised as high as possible. Another exercise may be taken with an assistant; the patient should lie face downward, supporting the body by the chest, and keeping the limbs rigid while the assistant lifts the feet as high as possible without hurting. These movements strengthen the abdominal muscles and draw fresh blood to the weakened parts, and cause quickened circulation in addition to restoring the displaced organ to natural position. They should be taken at night just before retiring after a hot douche. The bowels should be kept open by the free use of fruit. The patient should sleep with the hips elevated as much as can be endured without real discomfort and sit with the feet on a stool. When strength sufficient is acquired the exercises for anteversion will be found useful, and any other exercises which strengthen the abdominal muscles, such as bending backward and forward, and sideways. Kneading and percussing the abdomen by an osteopath or masseur strengthens, and also relieves constipation. Rest during the day should be taken with the feet higher than the head.

Prolapsus due to laceration in child-birth may require a surgical operation.

In case of antiflexions the first exercise given for prolapsus should be taken daily. (The advice for the prolapsus treatment and the exercises are taken from the writings of Dr. J. H. Kellogg, superintendent of the Battle Creek Sanitarium.).

ANTEVERSION:--Persons suffering from anteversion or retroversion should sleep without pillows under the head, and lie flat upon the back; they should sit with the feet as high as convenient and avoid high seats which hinder the feet from touching the floor. They should discard corsets and tight stocking supporters which push or hold down the organs which need to be replaced. Stocking supporters should be fastened over the hips and comfort waists can be bought in place of corsets.

It is well to have an attendant to prepare weak patients for first exercises in all uterine troubles by the use of towels wrung from hot water applied to the back and abdomen for a few minutes to relax the muscles, or a hot water bottle, or hot salt bag may be used. Then, with the patient lying with head low, the attendant should give the abdomen and small of the back a thorough rubbing or kneading for ten minutes or less according to strength of patient. Olive oil can be used on the hand in the rubbing.

FIRST EXERCISE FOR ANTEVERSION:--Lie on bed or rug; fold arms on chest; hold trunk of body still; stretch legs, and hold the position about half a minute, then relax at the knee and ankle. Then point the toes down and stretch upper leg muscles; relax; then stretch under leg muscles by stretching heel out. The patient will feel the exercise as far as the shoulders, and should be careful not to lift the body from the floor at first. When patient can hold stretching exercise for a minute then lift first the right, then the left leg, and take same exercise until the person can give a quick little kick for, say, twelve times, as the leg is straightened.

SECOND EXERCISE:--Lying on the back, stretch to full length; move the left leg out at the side, then up and back to position, forming a semi-circle, keeping muscles tense throughout. Then move right leg out at the side--left-- stretch toes long--relax--stretch heel--, lift a little higher and bring back to place in a circle and rest. Same with left leg and then both together. Few people can do this easily at first, the weight of the legs is too much for the weak muscles at the back; but some one can hold the foot at first. When the patient can do this easily without bringing on any pain or ache, she may sit in a low chair and take arm lifting exercises.

Raise both arms out at the sides, then slowly raise them up close to the head and consciously lift all the organs of the body up, relax, and lower arms down front and repeat slowly, six or ten times at first, until for five minutes the patient can do this sitting. Then take it standing for ten minutes or more. Stand with feet wide apart. Dr. Anderson says, "A woman who will do this twenty times each day can never have anteversion, if she dresses properly, for it lifts the organs in place each time." It lifts the chest and abdomen up, and brings a feeling of exhilaration if done in the open air.

After the patient has taken exercises for five or six weeks she may lie flat on the back, fold arms and raise body up to sitting position without unfolding arms. Then turn on right side and do the same, then on left side and do the same. This is fine for back and abdomen muscles.

Anteversion needs the Rest Cure, and resting with the body in a position in which nature can right things is an important thing to remember. Rest always after exercise, either with a pillow under the knees or with the legs hanging over a low foot-board, or lying on a couch with the feet higher than the head. Exercise will relax the muscles and call for blood which will revitalize and stimulate the weakened conditions. A woman with this trouble should be careful about bending quickly over, or climbing stairs, until she gains strength.

RETROVERSION:--Place the patient with face downward on bed or mat and with a small pillow under the lower part of the abdomen. Relax the muscles by applying a hot towel, hot salt bag or hot water-bottle just below the small of the back, and lower part of the abdomen for ten or fifteen minutes. (Hot salt bags are most effective and are easy to handle.) Then rub the back briskly with a circular movement; if tender in front, do not rub the abdomen. The circulation will gradually carry away any inflammation as soon as the muscles reach a normal condition, though kneading of back and abdomen, using sweet oil on the hand, is helpful if the patient can bear it.

The patient must remember that these conditions have been months in coming and only painstaking work and time can restore the weakened organs. The manner of dress is very important; loose, comfortable clothing must be worn. Sleep with the face down as much as possible; nature will correct itself, if allowed, many times.

FIRST EXERCISE:--Fold arms under forehead and draw right knee up close to body and hold two minutes (unless painful) and slowly straighten, and stretch very slowly. Do the same with the left leg until the patient can repeat the exercise twelve times with each leg and hold five minutes instead of two, with the knee close to the body. It will probably take two weeks to gain strength for this. After that time raise the body up on hands, and move legs just as a baby does when creeping, except that the patient only follows the movement and does not move along.

SECOND EXERCISE:--Patient take sitting position on floor and clasp hands under knees, and bring knees up, so that chin and knees meet and hold. Then straighten legs, slide hands toward the heels as far as hands can reach, (stretch hands toward heels); make a continuous movement of this.

THIRD EXERCISE:--Sit on floor. Place the hands on floor at sides, legs straight out in front, lift the body from the floor with the arms, up and down. This is a fine exercise for raising up the misplaced organs.

FOURTH EXERCISE:--Place the patient flat on back and push the body up to sitting position with hands quite far back and palms down, recline again, up and down until arms and back are very tired. Then sit up, legs straight in front, raise the body from the floor, (an inch) and move backward, resting weight on hands, then move over on knees as at first exercise and creep, then sit up and move backward again. These will take a month to perfect. Begin by exercising five minutes and gradually work up to half an hour, rest between, always. The patient must have the right mental attitude, must think that she is trying to replace the uterus by lifting it to its natural position. The exercises must not be lazily done.

Sitting in a tub of hot water is most helpful where there is much tenderness, or inflammation. Witch-hazel in hot water douches or a weak solution of hot salt water is a wonderful tonic in some cases.

EXERCISE FOR REPLACING UTERUS TO BE TAKEN JUST BEFORE RETIRING:--Kneel on the bed; bend forward until the chest is touching the bed and the hips are elevated as high as possible. The inlet of the vagina should then be opened so as to admit air. As soon as the air enters the womb falls into position. Lie down at once and give nature a chance to regain strength while you sleep.

The tampon soaked in glycerine and alum, and the douches of hot water, in which a little alum is dissolved, are both of great service in controlling the flooding which so frequently accompanies change of life and miscarriages. (Exercises for anteversion and retroversion supplied by a successful teacher of such work.)

The writer of this book asked a well-known medical writer why physicians do not advise exercises for the cure of displacements instead of operations. He said it is because women are not willing to do anything to help themselves. They expect the physician to cure them, and the only way a physician can "cure" is to operate. Sensible women, however, will be glad to practice helpful exercises.

DEBILITY:--"The debility of convalescence requires fresh air, easily digested food, the avoidance of over-exertion, with a gradually increasing amount of exercise. Such debility is only aggravated by alcohol, though it may for a time be partially masked thereby. Milk, eggs, fresh fruit and farinaceous articles are the best foods. General debility without obvious cause, may be treated by cold or tepid bathing. Salt added to the bath is helpful. Change of air is a good tonic. Port wine and other alcoholics while giving a false sensation of increased vigor, really reduce the tone of the pulse, and therefore tend to enfeeble the system. Alcohol is a relaxant, not a tonic."

DEPRESSION OF SPIRITS:--"Learn the Delsarte exercise for the 'blues,' and practice them daily. Hot air baths. Avoid rich food. Take out-door exercise."

DIARRHOEA:--"This is a symptom of the presence of an irritant of which the stomach is trying to be rid. Do not arrest it prematurely, but assist it. If it persists, arrowroot, or corn starch, or flour, mixed with cold water to the consistency of cream may be taken, a tablespoonful at a time. 2. Bread charcoal with cold milk. 3. A tablespoonful of cinnamon water with a teaspoonful of lime water, mixed, every one, two or three hours. Smaller dose for a child. Diet should be confined to toast, milk toast, milk, cold or boiled. Tea, broth, meat, etc., are sure to renew the trouble. Diarrhoea in infants is generally due to errors in feeding, either over-feeding or the use of improper kinds of food. Boiled milk thickened with flour is a simple remedy in light cases. Alcoholics are utterly unnecessary in diarrhoea, and to order them for young children is quite wrong. A full enema of water, as hot as can be borne, will remove offending substances from the bowels.

"Beware of diarrhoea medicines containing opium in any form. They are unnecessary and dangerous, particularly for young children."

DYSENTERY:--"At the beginning of the disease the stomach should be relieved by the use of a large warm-water emetic. The quantity of food should be restricted to the smallest amount compatible with comfort. Ripe fruits, especially grapes, and most stewed fruits, may be used in abundance to keep the bowels regular. Salads, spices and other condiments, fats and fried foods should be strictly avoided, together with tea, coffee, alcoholics and all other narcotics.

"The diet should consist chiefly of simple soups, well boiled oatmeal gruel, egg beaten with water or milk, and similar foods. In many cases regulation of the diet is sufficient. Either the hot or the cold enema may be employed.

"The use of opium, which is exceedingly common in this disease, is not advisable, as it produces a feverish condition of the system, decidedly prejudicial to recovery. Herroner, an eminent German physician, very strongly discourages the use of opium in this disease."--DR. J. H. KELLOGG.

DYSPEPSIA:--"It is commonly supposed that a little good whisky or brandy aids digestion, while on the contrary it has been proved conclusively by observing the processes of digestion upon persons who have fistula of the stomach, or by evacuating the contents of the stomach by means of a stomach-pump about an hour after taking a meal--in one instance after taking an ounce of alcohol, and in another where no alcohol was taken--that alcohol coagulates the albuminoids, throws down the pepsin, decreases the acidity (the combined chlorin and free hydrochloric acid), and increases the fixed chlorids. Any one can make the observation upon himself, that a meal taken without alcohol is more quickly followed by hunger than one with it.

"Blumenau says: 'On the whole, alcohol manifests a decidedly unfavorable influence on the course of normal digestion even when ingested in relatively small quantities, and impairs the normal digestive functions.'

"Dr. Chittenden, professor of physiologic chemistry in Yale College, as a result of some investigations made by himself and Dr. Mendel, states in the American Journal of Medical Sciences, that he finds that as small a quantity as three per cent. of sherry, porter, or beer lessens the activity of the digestive powers."--Bulletin of A. M. T. A.

"It should be observed that doses of alcohol which have no appreciable effect in delaying digestion, are so small as to be practically useless for any beneficial action."--Medical Pioneer.

One doctor writes:--

"What makes dyspepsia so hard to cure? This very alcohol taking. The best cure is to refuse all alcoholic drinks, at meals and all other times, and drink nothing but water."

The causes of dyspepsia are various; errors of diet being the most common. Others are mental worry, care and anxiety, and the use of drugs. An eminent writer upon this disease says:

"My main object in the treatment is to prevent the sufferers from resorting to drugs, which in such cases, not only produce their own morbid conditions, but also confirm those already existing.

"The extensive and often habitual use of alkalies for acidity, of purgatives for constipation, nervines and opiates for sleeplessness, and after-dinner pills to goad into action the lagging stomach, has been a potent factor in the production of a large class of most inveterate dyspepsias."

Underdone bread, cake, and pie, are unfit for any stomach, yet are seen upon many tables. "Breakfast foods," cooked for ten or twenty minutes, are also dyspepsia producers. All breads, cakes, pies and cereals, require thorough cooking to fit them for digestion. Most cereals are better for supper than for breakfast, as they should be cooked in a double boiler for several hours. A young man, troubled with dyspepsia, learned to his amazement that the oatmeal, which he supposed was his best food, had much to do with the giddiness which often overcame him. He was advised to use dry foods, such as toast, zwieback and shredded wheat. This diet, together with the abandonment of nostrums, led to a cure. Zwieback is bread sliced, and dried in a moderate oven until light brown. Whole wheat bread is best. It is very delicious and is quite easily digested. In the case of the young man, it is probable that the difficulty with the oatmeal was the lack of sufficient cooking. Oatmeal made into gruel, well cooked, and diluted with a large quantity of scalded milk is easy of digestion.

Eating between meals, and excess in eating, lead to stomach derangement.

"The best remedy for acidity of the stomach is hot-water drinking. Two or three glasses should be taken as hot as can be sipped, one hour before each meal, and half an hour before going to bed. The effect of the hot water is to wash out the stomach, and so remove any fermenting remains of the previous meal. Heartburn may be treated the same as acidity."

Persons troubled with slow digestion are better to eat only two meals a day. The writer has personal knowledge of a goodly number of women who have been benefited wonderfully by adopting the two meal a day plan.

Some persons, much troubled with dyspepsia, have adopted the plan of prolonged fasting advocated by Dr. Dewey, and testify to a cure by this method. While heroic, it is certainly more rational than drug treatment. For acute dyspepsia a fast is requisite.

All that alcoholics can do for dyspepsia is to allay the uneasy sensations for a time, while adding to the trouble. It has been abundantly proved that alcohol must pass from the stomach before digestion can begin.

Dr. Ridge says:--

"Many cases which seem to be relieved by the use of beer are really benefited by the hop, or other bitter, which the ale or beer contains. Hop tea is a useful stomachic, and a quarter of a pint, or half that quantity, may be taken cold. It is made in the same way as tea, using a handful of hops to a pint of boiling water. Make fresh every day."

Dr. Kellogg says:--

"In cases of chronic dyspepsia the use of alcohol seems to be particularly deleterious, although not infrequently prescribed, if not in the form of alcohol or ordinary alcoholic liquors, in the form of some so-called 'bitters,' 'elixir' or 'cordial.' Nothing could be further removed from the truth than the popular notion that alcohol, at least in the form of certain wines, is helpful to digestion. Roberts showed, years ago, that alcohol even in small doses, diminishes the activity of the stomach in the digestion of proteids. Gluzinski showed, ten years ago, that alcohol causes an arrest in the secretion of pepsin, and also of its action upon food. Wolff showed that the habitual use of alcohol produces disorder of the stomach to such a degree as to render it incapable of responding to the normal excitation of the food. Hugounencq found that all wines, without exception, prevent the action of pepsin upon proteids. The most harmful are those which contain large quantities of alcohol, cream of tartar or coloring matter. Wines often contain coloring matters which at once completely arrest digestion, such as methylin blue and fuchsin.

"A few years ago I made a series of experiments in which I administered alcohol in various forms with a test meal, noting the effect upon the stomach fluid as determined by the accurate chemic examination of the method of Hayem and Winter. The result of these experiments I reported at the 1893 meeting of the American Medical Temperance Association. The subject of experiment was a healthy young man whose stomach was doing a slight excess of work, the amount of combined chlorin being nearly fifty per cent. above normal, although the amount of free hydrochloric acid was normal in quantity. Four ounces of claret with the ordinary test meal reduced the free hydrochloric acid from 28 milligrams per 100 c. c. of stomach fluid to zero, and the combined chlorin from .270 to .125. In the same case the administration of two ounces of brandy with the ordinary test meal reduced the combined chlorin to .035, scarcely more than one eighth of the original amount, the free hydrochloric acid remaining at zero. Thus it appears that four ounces of claret produced marked hypopepsia in a case of moderate hyperpepsia, whereas two ounces of brandy produced practically apepsia."

FAINTING OR SYNCOPE:--The following letter from the late Sir B. W. Richardson was addressed to a lady who had sought the great physician's advice on the subject:--

"25 Manchester Square, W., July 18, 1896.

"DEAR MADAM: There is no substance which acts as a substitute for alcohol, nor is anything like it wanted. The human body is a water engine, as I have often described it, and alcohol plays no part in its natural motion. The idea that when it begins to fail, a stimulant has to be called for, springs merely from habit, and if, whenever any of the symptoms of fainting you speak of occur, the person merely lies down on the side or back and drinks a glass of hot water, or hot milk and water, all that can be done is done. In the London Temperance Hospital I have been treating the sick for diseases of all kinds and during all stages, and have never administered a minim of alcohol, or any substitute for it, and we have got on better than when I--feeling it at all times at command--made use of it in the ordinary way.

"I am, dear Madam, faithfully yours, "B. W. RICHARDSON."

TREATMENT:--"Lay the patient down in a current of air with the feet raised higher than the head, preferably on one side in case of sickness occurring, or bend the head down to the knees, to restore the flow of blood to the brain. Loosen all clothing. Rub the limbs, chest and over the heart with the hand or a rough towel. Sprinkle cold water on the head and face. Smell ammonia, strong vinegar, smelling salts or any pungent odor. Put hot bottles to the feet, and in severe cases a mustard plaster over the heart. Sip hot milk, hot water, hot tea, hot black coffee, beef tea or a meat essence. Crowding round the patient and all excitement should be avoided. In 999 cases out of 1,000, no medicine is necessary.

"Faintness often proceeds from indigestion, flatulence inducing pressure on the heart."

FAINTNESS, WEAKNESS, EXHAUSTION, FATIGUE:--"The truth is that for simple weakness, faintness, exhaustion, fatigue, cold or wet, the best remedies are simple fresh air, pure water, digestible food and rest. These are nature's restoratives, and the sooner both physicians and people learn to rely upon them instead of upon drugs the better it will be for all parties. And as the effect of alcoholic liquors are directly depressing to the strength and activity of all the natural functions and processes of life, as shown by the most varied and scientific investigations, it is important that this fact be taught to both doctors and people everywhere."--DR. N. S. DAVIS.

FITS:--"Whether the fit be apoplexy or epilepsy all alcoholics are extremely bad, both at the time and afterwards. Alcohol, the 'genius of degeneration,' is the chief cause of apoplexy, and also a cause of epilepsy, especially when taken in the form of beer. It diminishes the tone of the arteries and blood-vessels, and thus tends to cause, aggravate and maintain a congested state of the capillaries throughout the whole body. In the treatment of epilepsy, therefore, neither alcohol nor any so-called substitute should be given. * * * * *

"In the convulsions of children alcohol is equally injurious."--DR. RIDGE.

FLATULENCE:--"Many uneasy sensations or pains, even in distant parts of the body, are due to wind in the bowels, resulting from indigestion. Asthma, cramps, depression of spirits, faintness, giddiness, hiccough, prostration, sinking sensations and sleeplessness, are all frequently due to the same cause. The diet needs careful attention where there is much flatulence; tea is often a cause. Charcoal biscuits are useful in some cases; lemon juice in others. Fluid Magnesia may be taken. Watch for the cause and remove it."

HEADACHE:--The New Hygiene says: "This is the manifestation of a deeper-seated trouble, usually in the stomach. The use of stimulants is a sure promoter of headache. All users of alcoholic liquors are, I believe, subject to headache, and it is also a sure result of overindulgence in tea and coffee.

"To prevent the attacks, live regularly, avoid late hours and excessive brain work; avoid tea, coffee and alcoholic beverages, also sweets of all kinds, including sauces and pastries, and anything fried in fat. Eat plenty of good, plain food, including fruit, especially oranges. Eat none late at night. Exercise regularly in such a way as to bring all the muscles into play, at least once a day.

"To relieve an attack flush the colon.

"Headaches, which so largely result from the retention of impure matter in the body, will be cured if a good quantity, say two or three glasses, of hot water be drank in the morning or at night, and then the next regular meal omitted, so that an interval of house-cleaning can be had before other material is moved in."--Life and Health.

"Avoid pills and powders. Persons suffering from headache need to be warned against taking remedies that contain opium and alcohol, and also against the use of a recent popular remedy, usually called a 'white powder' or 'white tablet.' They take the latter readily because the druggist or physician says it contains no opium. This is true, but it is one of the lately discovered coal tar preparations (anti-febrine, acetanilid, etc.) and is very depressing to the human system. Headache is usually a symptom of trouble somewhere else, often in the alimentary canal, an overloaded stomach, constipation, or tight clothing. Learn the cause and remove that, and the headache will disappear."--DR. H. J. HALL, Franklin, Ind.

"Gentle massage is helpful and the use of cold compresses. Lack of sufficient sleep will cause headache. Women often bring on nervous headache by overwork and worry."

HEMORRHAGE:--"Never give alcohol in a case of profuse hemorrhage. The faint feeling, or irresistible inclination to lie down is nature's own method of circumventing the danger, by quieting the circulation and lessening the expulsive force of the heart, thus favoring the formation of clot at the site of the injury."--Clinique.

"For uterine hemorrhage an emetic to induce vomiting is the best cure."-- Dr. Higginbotham in British Medical Journal.

"If the faint is dispelled too quickly, and the blood-vessels are relaxed by alcohol, or the heart aroused to energetic action by any remedy, the hemorrhage may recommence, and may prove fatal. Quiet, the application of cold, pressure, the elevation of the wound where possible, and the absence of stimulants, are the cardinal points of treatment in most cases."--DR. RIDGE.

"If then, it seems absolutely necessary to rouse a person out of a dead faint, what can be done? Swallowing is out of the question, lest the patient choke. The head must be laid low, and the face and chest flapped with a cold wet cloth, or alternately with hot wet cloths; smelling salts (not too strong) may be applied to the nose.

"When the faint has been recovered from, but the hemorrhage continues so much that it is feared another faint may occur, and, perhaps, be fatal, it may be warded off by drinking any hot liquid; if Liebig's extract of meat, or strong beef tea, is at hand and can be given hot, there is nothing better."

HEART DISEASE:--Dr. Ridge says: "I trench here on a delicate subject, because, when there is real disease of the heart, medical advice will of course have been obtained, and very probably a doctor may have said that some alcoholic liquor is essential. There are, also, several different forms of heart disease which require altogether different treatment, and only a physician can tell the difference, or appreciate the necessity for the particular treatment required. But it may be pointed out that alcohol is utterly unable to 'strengthen' the heart, or give tone to the blood-vessels, or to the system at large.

"The alteration in the pulse due to alcohol is chiefly owing to its paralyzing action on the blood-vessels, and when they are too contracted, and thereby cause the weakened heart to labor too much, the alcohol will give relief for the time. But we have in nitrite of amyl, a fluid which will act more quickly and more powerfully; but this must not be employed without medical direction. It is very useful in cases of angina pectoris, or breast pang, but is rarely required in the majority of cases in which the valves of the heart are diseased. The paralyzing action of alcohol is not generally produced by less than half a wine-glassful of brandy or whisky, or twice that quantity of wine, and often much more is required. The relief to uneasy sensations which much smaller quantities sometimes produce is due to their an鑵 thetic or benumbing action, by which the nerves of the patient are rendered less sensible, although the danger is by no means diminished. * * * *

"The only sensible way to avert the evil consequences of heart disease is to strengthen the heart, and that is to be done by strengthening the body generally. The amount of exercise, the kind of baths, etc., which should be taken, have to be modified in accordance with the nature of the case. If these natural health-giving measures cannot be employed nothing is an effectual substitute.

"Weak or feeble heart is a common complaint, and is as ordinary an excuse for resorting to alcoholic liquors as 'Timothy's stomach.' If there is no organic disease; if the valves of the heart are healthy and act properly, all anxiety on this point may be entirely banished. The slow pulse, the feeble pulse, the cold feet, the want of energy, these are not to be got rid of by such a mere temporary agent as alcohol, even if relief can be thus obtained from day to day. The constant application of alcohol to the tissues of the body alters them gradually by its chemical action. In addition to this, the balance of the nervous system is altered, an unnatural condition is produced, and the unhappy patient becomes more liable to disease and more easily succumbs when attacked.

"Many of these 'feeble hearts' mean too little exercise, very often also, too much or improper food and drink.

"The best remedies are cold sponging (according to the season); avoidance of coddling; plain, wholesome food; abstinence from tea, hot drinks and condiments; regular out-of-doors exercise and all similar true tonic measures."

Dr. Kellogg says:--

"Persons subject to attacks of angina pectoris should carry with them a small bottle containing a sponge saturated with nitrite of amyl, and place it to the nose when necessary.

"Sympathetic palpitation may be relieved by bending the head downward, allowing the arms to hang down. The effect of this measure is increased by holding the breath a few seconds while bending over. Another ready means of relief is to press strongly upon the large arteries on either side of the neck.

"Palpitation of the heart is often mistaken for real organic disease of the organ. * * * * * A careful regulation of the diet is in most cases all that is necessary to effect a cure."

Dr. Edmunds, of London, was asked during a medical discussion what he thought of the use of alcohol in heart disease. His answer is embodied in the following:--

"With regard to the use of brandy in cases of heart disease, he was convinced it was a mistake to use it in such cases. There were many forms of heart disease, but the most common kind arose from the heart being too fat. Excess of fat debilitated the heart and injured its working, just as a piece of wax attached to a tuning fork would impair its usefulness. In such cases he dieted his patients in order to reduce their weight. Every dose of brandy taken for heart disease increased the evil. The moment brandy was taken for heart disease, or any other chronic complaint of a similar kind, the disease was increased. If doctors recommended alcohol to their patients, he had been asked what abstainers should do. In such cases, as had been suggested, he thought the patients might ask what the alcohol was to do for them, and if the reply was not satisfactory, they should get another doctor."

Dr. T. D. Crothers, of Hartford, Conn., has deduced some valuable facts from his experiments with the sphygmograph, upon the action of the heart. He has found by repeated experiments that while alcohol apparently increases the force and volume of the heart's action, the irregular tracings of the sphygmograph show that the real vital force is diminished, and hence its apparent stimulating power is deceptive.

Dr. C. W. Chapman, of the National Hospital for Diseases of the Heart, wrote in the Lancet:--

"The very thing (alcohol) which they supposed had kept their heart going was responsible for many of its difficulties."

Of cases of palpitation and irregularity caused by business anxieties or indigestion, he said:--

"To give alcohol is only to add fuel to the fire."

HEART FAILURE:--"In cases of cardiac weakness, the thing needed is not simply an increased rate of movement of the heart, or an increased volume of the pulse, but an increased movement of the blood current throughout the entire system. In the application of any agent for the purpose of affording relief in a condition of this kind, the peripheral heart as well as the central organ must be taken into consideration. In fact, the whole circulatory system must be regarded as one. The heart and the arteries are composed of essentially the same kind of tissue, and have practically the same functions. The arteries as well as the heart are capable of contracting.

"Both the heart and the arteries are controlled by excitory and inhibitory nerves. These two classes of nerves are kindred in structure and in origin, the vagus and the vasodilators being medullated, while the accelerators of the heart and the vasoconstrictors of the arteries are non-medullated and pass through the sympathetic ganglia on the way to their distribution.

"Winternitz and other therapeutists have frequently called attention to the value of cold as a cardiac stimulant or tonic. The tonic effect of this agent is greater than that of any medicinal agent which can be administered. The cold compress applied over the cardiac area of the chest may well replace alcohol as a heart tonic. The thing necessary to encourage the heart's action is not merely relaxation of the peripheral vessels, but, as Winternitz has shown, increased activity of the peripheral circulation in the skin, muscles and elsewhere. Alcohol paralyzes the vasoconstrictors, and so dilates the small vessels and lessens the resistance of the heart action; but at the same time it lessens the activity of the nerve centres which control the heart, diminishes the power of the heart muscle, and lessens that rhythmical activity of the small vessels whereby the circulation is so efficiently aided at that portion of the blood circuit most remote from the heart. A continuous cold application applied to that portion of the chest overlying the heart stimulates the nerves controlling the walls of the vessels, and at the same time energizes the corresponding cardiac nerves. It is wise to remember that the vasoconstrictor nerves are one in kind with the excitor nerves of the heart, while the vasodilators are in like manner associated with the vagus. With this in mind, it is clear that while alcohol paralyzes the vasoconstrictors, it at the same time weakens the nerves which initiate and maintain the activity of the heart; while, on the other hand, cold excites to activity those nerves which produce the opposite effect.

"The apparent increase of strength which follows the administration of alcohol in cases of cardiac weakness is delusive. There is increased volume of the pulse for the reason that the small arteries and capillaries are dilated, but this apparent improvement in cardiac action is very evanescent. This is a natural result of the fact that while the heart is relieved momentarily by sudden dilation of the peripheral vessels, the accumulation of the blood in the venous system, through the loss of the normal activity of the peripheral heart, gradually raises the resistance by increasing the amount of blood which has to be pushed along in the venous system. This loss of the action of the peripheral heart more than counterbalances the temporary relief secured by the paralysis of the vasoconstrictors.

"Thermic applications, general and local, may safely be affirmed to be the true physiological heart tonic. In the employment of the cold pericardial compress as a heart tonic, the application should generally be continued not more than half an hour at a time, and its use may be alternated with general cold applications to the surface. A cold towel rub, or the cold trunk pack is the best form for application if the patient is very feeble.

"The cold towel rub is applied thus: wring a towel as dry as possible out of very cold water, and spread it quickly and evenly over the surface; rub vigorously outside until the skin begins to feel warm; then remove, dry the moistened surface, rub until it glows, and make the same application to another part; and so on until the whole surface of the body has been gone over. The procedure should be rapid and vigorous.

"If the cold trunk pack is employed, a sheet of not more than one thickness should be wrung as dry as possible out of very cold water, and wrapped quickly about the body, after first dipping the hands in water, and rubbing the trunk vigorously. In cases of extreme cardiac weakness, very cold and very hot applications may be alternately applied over the region of the heart. The duration of the hot and cold applications should be about fifteen seconds each.

"Any one who has ever witnessed the marvelous effects of applications of this sort in reviving a flagging heart will never doubt their efficacy, and will have no occasion to resort to alcohol, or any other intoxicant, to stimulate a flagging heart. The writer has employed these measures for stimulating the heart for more than twenty years, and might cite hundreds of instances in which their efficiency has been demonstrated. They are applicable not only to the cardiac depression encountered in the adynamic stage of typhoid and other fevers, but in cases of heart failure from hemorrhage, of surgical shock, collapse under chloroform or ether, opium poisoning, coal gas asphyxia, drowning, etc."--Dr. J. H. Kellogg, in Bulletin of the A. M. T. A., Jan., 1899.

Dr. N. S. Davis tells of a case of threatened collapse where he was called in consultation. Patient was in a small, unventilated room.

"It was easy to see that what she needed was fresh air in her lungs. Instead of giving alcohol in any form she was moved into a large, well-ventilated room. All symptoms of 'heart failure' disappeared. Had she begun to take whisky or brandy, physician and friends would have attributed her recovery to that, when in fact it would have retarded recovery by hindering oxygenation of the blood."

"It would also be a very great mistake to suppose that when reaction follows collapse, in cases in which alcohol has been given, this result is always due to the alcohol. I have seen so many cases of severe collapse recover without alcohol that I cannot but be skeptical as to its necessity, and even as to its value. I was much struck many years ago by a case of post partum hemorrhage which was so severe that convulsions set in. I should then have given brandy if there had been any to give, but there was none in the house and none to be got. I administered teaspoonfuls of hot water and the patient revived and recovered; next day, except for an 鎚 ia, she was as well as ever, with no reactionary fever or other disturbance, as would almost certainly have been the case if brandy had been given.

"In collapse from hemorrhage, we have learned the value of injections of warm saline water, either into the veins, the skin or the rectum, and the same treatment is available in other cases of collapse with contracted vessels.

"Another measure which has proved most efficacious is the inhalation of oxygen gas. This is especially useful in cases in which alcohol is decidedly injurious, namely, those in which there is increasing congestion of the lungs, which the heart, though doing its utmost, is unable to overcome. Alcohol only increases the congestion, and the heart is already over-exerted and nearly exhausted. The effect of the oxygen is apparent in a few seconds, and cases have been rescued in which death appeared to be inevitable and imminent."--DR. RIDGE.

HEART STIMULANTS:--"The advantage of beef extract over alcohol as a stimulant was demonstrated on a large scale in the Ashantee war."--DR. RIDGE, London.

For those who must have a drug: aqua ammonia, 8 drops to 1/2 cup of hot water, or 20 grains carbonate ammonia to 1/2 cup water. Hot water alone is a useful stimulant; also water, hot or cold, with a few grains of Cayenne pepper added. The latter is good, not only to start the heart's action in collapse, but also to relieve violent pain. Hot milk is a most valuable stimulant. Many persons to whom hot milk has been given during the extreme weakness of acute disease have testified afterward to its good effects in comparison with the wine formerly administered. The wine caused an after-feeling of chilliness and weakness, while the milk gave warmth and added strength.

INSOMNIA OR SLEEPLESSNESS:--"A person who suffers from sleeplessness should avoid the use of tea and coffee, tobacco, alcoholic liquors and all other disturbers of the nervous system. Eating immediately before retiring has been recommended, but the ultimate result may be an aggravation of the difficulty instead of relief. If a person suffers from 'all gone feelings' so that he cannot sleep, he should take a few sips of cold water or a glass of lemonade. As complete relief will generally be obtained as from eating, and the stomach will be saved work when it should be resting. A warm bath just before retiring, a wet-hand rub, a cool sponge bath, gentle rubbing of the body with the dry hand, a moist bandage worn about the abdomen during the night, are all useful measures. When the feet are cold, they should be thoroughly warmed by a hot foot or leg bath, and thorough rubbing. When the head is congested, these measures should be supplemented by the application of cold to the head, as the cold compress or the ice-cap."

A walk in the evening, or gentle calisthenics, may help those of sedentary habits. Bicycle riding and horse-back riding in the evening have helped many.

The practice of long deep breathing will often put persons to sleep when all other devices fail. The lungs should be filled to their utmost capacity, and then emptied with equal slowness, repeating the respiration about ten times a minute, instead of eighteen or twenty, the natural rate. Those who fall asleep upon first going to bed, and after a few hours awake, and are unable to sleep again, may find relief by getting out of bed, and rubbing the surface of the body with the dry hand. Or walk about the room a few minutes, exposing the skin to the air, go back to bed and try the deep breathing.

"The use of drugs for the purpose of inducing sleep should be avoided as much as possible. Opium is especially harmful. Sleep obtained by the use of opiates is not a substitute for natural sleep. The condition is one of insensibility, but not of natural refreshing recuperation. Three or four hours of natural sleep will be more than equivalent to double that amount of sleep obtained by the use of narcotics. When a person once becomes dependent upon drugs of any kind for producing sleep, it is almost impossible for him to dispense with them. It is often dangerous to resort to their temporary use, on account of the great tendency to the formation of the habit of continuous use. The use of opiates for securing sleep is one of the most prolific means by which the great army of opium-eaters is annually recruited. Chloral, bromide of potash, whisky and other drugs are to be condemned almost as strongly as opium."--DR. KELLOGG.

Dr. Furer, of Heidelberg, Germany, in a paper before the International Congress against alcohol, held in Basle, Switzerland, in Sept., 1895, said:--

"The sleep from alcohol does not act as a mental tonic, but leaves the mind weaker next day."

Some noble specimens of manhood have become wrecks through accepting the advice to try "whisky night-caps." Edison recommends manual labor, instead of going to rest, for aggravated insomnia. He says sleep will soon come naturally.

LA GRIPPE:--"Alcohol has no place in the treatment of la grippe; on the contrary it is because of the too frequent use of this, and other narcotics, that epidemics make such fearful headway in our land, and such must be the rule until the people study the laws of health and obey them. Profuse sweating, followed by a careful bathing of the body in tepid water, gradually cooling it to a normal temperature, and avoiding unnecessary exposure, will relieve. The patient should sleep in pure air and eat as little as possible, and that only when hungry. * * * * * Quinine is essentially a nerve poison, and capable of producing a profound disturbance of the nervous centres. A drug of such potency for evil should be employed with the greatest care, and never when a milder agency will secure the result. Exceedingly pernicious is the habit of dosing children with this drug."--DR. CHARLES H. SHEPARD, Brooklyn, N. Y.

"A late surgeon of the gold coast of Africa wrote the following to the London Lancet of Jan. 2, 1890: 'Some of the worst cases of this disease, the grippe, remind me of an epidemic I saw among the natives of the swamps of the Niger. * * * * * Irrespective of disinfectants and inhalations there is a simple, effective and ready remedy, the juice of oranges in large quantities, not of two or three, but of dozens. The first unpleasant symptoms disappear, and the acid citrate of potash of the juice, by a simple chemic action decreases the amount of fibrine in the blood to an extent which prevents the development of pneumonia.'"

The Syracuse (N. Y.) Post-Standard contained the following during the epidemic of 1899:--

"Dr. George D. Whedon declared to a Post-Standard reporter yesterday that there is practically no subsiding of the grippe in this city. Dr. Whedon said that the weather conditions have little, if anything, to do with the disease, and that it is impossible to define the conditions which produce it. It is some morbific agency, the influence of which, Dr. Whedon said, is exerted upon the pneumogastric nerve.

"Dr. Whedon was emphatic in denouncing treatment by means of alcoholic stimulants, and coal tar derivatives. In discussing the subject at some length he said:--

'I find that infants and young children are practically exempt from the disease, and the liability increases with age. In my own experience, which has since 1889 amounted to an aggregate of 3,000 cases, alcoholic stimulants have appeared to be usually of little or no value; their usual stimulating effect does not seem to be realized in this condition. Unless malarial complications exist quinine appears of no benefit, and then should not be used in larger than two grain doses. Large doses depress the weakened heart, and in all cases increase the terrible confusion and headache constantly present in severe cases.

'From the views I entertain of its pathology, and from the terrible fatality which has attended the extensive use of the coal tar derivatives in treatment of la grippe, I argue that the manner in which they have been prescribed in the beginning of the disease, to reduce fever, and relieve the often intense suffering, lowers the heart's action, which is already sufficiently incapacitated by the toxic agent producing the disease.

'The intention is usually to stimulate later, but later is in many cases unfortunately too late. The heart being overwhelmed by the poison, and by the added depression of all coal tar preparations, cannot keep up the pulmonary circulation. The swelling of the lungs increases, and the result is fatal.

'I am aware of the weight of authority for their administration and of the relief they afford, but am just as well assured that were their use discontinued, the greatly increased death-rate from la grippe would cease to appear.

'These coal tar remedies are being used everywhere, and the medical journals recommend them despite the fatal results. They are being used every hour in the day in Syracuse, and, as a result, are knocking out good people. Among the most popular coal tar derivatives I might mention anti-kamnia, salol-phenacetine, anti-pyrine and salicylate of soda.

'Prognosis is favorable at all ages. Patients should be kept warm, and perfectly quiet in bed, and supplied with such nutritious and easily digested food, at frequent intervals, as the partially paralyzed stomach can take care of. All nourishment must be fluid and warm rather than cold.'"

The Journal of Inebriety for April, 1889, says:--

"The present epidemic of influenza has proved to be very fatal in cases of moderate and excessive alcoholic drinkers.

"Pneumonia is the most common sequel, breaking out suddenly, and terminating fatally in a few days. Heart failure and profound exhaustion, is another fatal termination. One case was reported to me of an inebriate, who, after a full outbreak of all the usual symptoms, drank freely of whisky and became stupid and died. It was uncertain whether cerebral hemorrhage had taken place, or the narcotism of the alcohol had combined with the disease and caused death.

"A physician appeared to have unusual fatality in the cases of this class under his care.

"It was found that he gave some form of alcohol freely, on the old theory of stimulation. Another physician gave all drinking cases with this disease alcohol, on the same theory, and had equally fatal results. It has been asserted that alcohol, as an antiseptic, was useful in these bacterial epidemics, but its use has been followed by greater depression, and many new and complex symptoms. The frequent half domestic and professional remedy, hot rum and whisky, has been followed by more serious symptoms, and a protracted convalescence. Many facts have been reported showing the danger of alcohol as a remedy, also the fatality in cases of inebriates who were affected with this disease.

"The first most common symptom seems to be heart exhaustion and feebleness, then from the catarrhal and bronchial irritation, pneumonia often follows."

The vapor or Turkish bath is the best means of "breaking up" this disease, together with hot lemonade and rest in bed for a day or two. The inhalation of hot steam should be tried when there is much bronchial irritation.

LIFE-SAVING STATIONS, THE USE OF ALCOHOL IN:--"There is no possible useful place for alcoholic liquors in connection with a life-saving station. Applied externally the rapid evaporation of alcohol reduces the temperature; taken internally it diminishes the efficiency of both respiration and circulation, and by increasing congestion of the kidneys it directly increases the danger of secondary bad effects from exposures of any kind.

To restore warmth and circulation to the surface, light, rapid friction and the wrapping with dry flannel is the safest, cheapest and most efficient, while free breathing of fresh air, and frequent small doses of milk, beef-tea, ordinary tea or coffee, or even simple water, will afford the greatest amount of strength and endurance, and leave the least secondary bad consequences. It is just as easy to keep at hand a jug or flask of any one of the articles named as it is to keep a flask of whisky or brandy. There is no need of keeping them hot, as they act well at any temperature at which they can be drunk."--DR. N. S. DAVIS, Chicago.

MEASLES:--"In mild cases, very little treatment is required, except such as is necessary to make the patient comfortable. Good nursing is much more important than medical attendance. If the eruption is slow in making its appearance, or is repelled after having appeared, the patient should be given a warm blanket pack.

"The old-fashioned plan of keeping the patient smothered beneath heavy blankets, and constantly in a state of perspiration is wholly unnecessary. The irritation of the skin, as well as the sensitiveness to cold, may be relieved by rubbing the skin gently two or three times a day with vaseline or sweet oil. There is no danger from the application of cold water to the surface except in the last stages of the disease, after the eruption has disappeared.

"The patient should be allowed cooling drinks as much as desired. During the disease a simple but nutritious diet should be allowed, but stimulants of all kinds should be prohibited."

"It is wholly unnecessary, and dangerous as well, to give whisky to bring out the eruption."--DR. I. N. QUIMBY, Jersey City.

"Any hot drink, such as ginger tea or hot lemonade, may be used to hasten the eruption, if delayed."

MALARIA:--Observers of this disease in such regions as the gold coast of

Africa have noted the fact that malarial attacks are generally preceded by impaired digestion. The disease is said to be due to animal parasites. These parasites are supposed to generate in the soil of certain regions, and thence, through the drinking water, or otherwise, find entrance to the human body.

"A healthy stomach is able to destroy germs of all sorts, hence the best protection from malaria is the boiling of all drinking water, and the maintenance of sound digestion and purity of blood by an aseptic dietary."

Dr. J. H. Kellogg says in The Voice:--

"It must be understood, however, that fruit in malarial regions, especially watermelons, may be thickly covered with malarial parasites and the parasites may sometimes find entrance to the fruit when it becomes over-ripe, so that the skin is broken. It is evident, then, that care must be taken to disinfect such fruit by thorough washing, or by dipping in hot water, which is the safer plan. The same remark applies to cucumbers, lettuce, celery, cabbage and other green vegetables which are commonly served without cooking. Not only malarial parasites but small insects of various kinds are often found clinging to such food substances, their development being encouraged by the free use of top dressing on the soil, a process common with market gardeners.

"The treatment of malarial disease is too large and intricate a subject for proper treatment in these columns. We will say briefly, however, at the risk of being considered very unorthodox, that the majority of cases of malarial poisoning can be cured without the use of drugs of any sort. In fact, in the most obstinate cases of chronic malarial poisoning, drugs are of almost no use whatever. Quinine, however, is certainly of value as a curative agent in these cases, either in destroying the parasites, or in preventing their development; but as it does not remove the cause, its curative effect is likely to be very transient. The practice of habitually taking quinine as a preventive of malarial disease is a most injurious one, as quinine is itself a non-usable substance in the system, and therefore must be looked upon as a mild poison, to be dealt with by the liver and kidneys the same as other poisons. By habitual use it may itself become a cause of disease. One or two periodical doses of quinine often prove of great service in interrupting the paroxysms of an intermittent fever, but other treatment must also be employed to develop the bodily resistance, and fortify the system against disease. The morning cold bath, followed by vigorous rubbing, is a most excellent measure for this purpose, but the old-fashioned German wet-sheet pack is one of the best remedies known. The paroxysm itself can generally be avoided by means of the dry pack, begun before the chill makes its appearance; but this requires the services of an expert nurse. In not a few cases it is wise for a person who suffers frequently from malarial disease to seek a change of climate to some non-malarial region.

"Col. T. W. Higginson of the First South Carolina Volunteers, in 1862, said of Dr. Seth Rogers, an eminent Southern physician, who was surgeon of the regiment: 'Fortunately for us, he was one of that minority of army surgeons who did not believe in whisky, so that we never had it issued in the regiment while he was with us, and got on better, in a highly malarial district, than those regiments which used it.'"

MATERNITY:--Dr. Ridge says:--"It is one of the greatest mistakes to make use of alcoholic beverages to 'keep up the strength' during labor. It is, of course, impossible to predict at the commencement how long the labor will last; if then brandy, or other similar drink, is resorted to early, it acts most injuriously. The desire for food is often entirely removed; the demand of the system being therefore unperceived, and so not supplied, a state of weakness and prostration is in time produced, if the labor should be protracted, which may be really serious. The nervous system becomes exhausted by the repeated action of the alcohol. If a fatal result is not occasioned, yet the prostration of body and mind after delivery is aggravated, and convalescence thereby retarded. Alcoholic drinks produce paralysis and congestion of the blood-vessels, and in this way largely increase the liability to flooding after the labor is over. Alcohol also increases the liability to a feverish condition.

"It is necessary to take small quantities of plain, nourishing food at regular intervals, and nothing is of greater value than well-cooked oatmeal: other farinaceous food may be substituted, if preferred. If there is much prostration, meat extracts or beef tea are of great value. Tea tends to produce flatulence and to prevent sleep.

"After the labor is over, the best restorative is a cup of hot beef tea or an egg beaten up in warm milk or a cup of warm gruel. Rest, and absence of excitement and worry are essential and alcohol is specially injurious."

MENSTRUATION, PAINFUL:--Young girls often resort to the use of brandy during the monthly period, and parents ask anxiously, "What can they use instead of the brandy?"

The very best thing that can be done is to go to bed, wrapped in flannels, with a hot-water bottle or other hot application to the abdomen, and to the feet. Take hot ginger tea, or pepper tea.

A warm hip-bath taken at the beginning may give relief, or a large hot enema retained for half an hour or so. Rest is necessary.

For those who must go to work, Dr. Ridge recommends five drops of oil of juniper, to be taken on sugar.

NEURALGIA:--"The principal cause of neuralgia is defective nutrition of the nerves. Disorders of digestion are very often accompanied by neuralgia in various parts of the body. It may also result from taking cold, from loss of sleep, from dissipation, and also from the use of tobacco, alcohol, tea and coffee.

"The patient's general health must be improved by a wholesome, simple diet, and the employment of tonic baths, as a daily sponge bath, and massage in feeble cases. Sun-baths and exercise in the open air are of first importance.

Ordinary neuralgia may almost always be relieved by either moist or dry heat. In some cases, cold applications give more relief than hot. As a rule, abnormal heat requires cold, and unnatural cold requires hot applications. In many cases it is necessary to give the patient a warm bath of some kind. Electricity often succeeds when all other remedies fail.

"For facial neuralgia apply hot fomentations, together with the use of sitz baths, or hot foot baths. The head may be steamed by holding it over hot water, adding pieces of hot brick occasionally to keep water steaming, head being covered.

"There is no complaint, perhaps, in the treatment of which the use of port wine will be more strongly urged by kind friends, with the assurance that it is impossible to get well without it. This is quite untrue, as thousands can testify."--DR. RIDGE.

"Avoid opiates of all sorts. 'It is better to bear the ills we have than fly to others that we know not of.' The pangs of neuralgia are as nothing to endure compared with the sufferings of an opium wreck. Build up the general health, and the neuralgia will disappear."

NAUSEA.--"A feeling of sickness is not uncommonly due to indigestion. If it is caused by rich food take a pinch of bicarbonate of soda in a little water, or a teaspoonful of fluid magnesia. The acidity of the food will thus be neutralized, and this course is far preferable to benumbing the stomach with brandy. If indigestion is the cause, it is often salutary to miss one or two meals, so as to allow the stomach to recover.

"When due to pregnancy, a little a 雛 ated water, or soda water is useful; sometimes a small wafer or a crust, eaten before rising in the morning, will check it. An early morning walk, if the weather is pleasant, is helpful.

"The moist abdominal bandage is a very excellent means of relieving nausea during pregnancy. It should be worn constantly for a week or two, and then omitted during the night. Daily sitz baths are also of great advantage. In many cases electricity relieves this symptom very promptly. In very urgent cases in which the vomiting cannot be repressed, and the life of the patient is threatened, the stomach should be given entire rest, the patient being nourished by nutritive injections. Fomentations over the stomach, and swallowing small bits of ice, are sometimes effective when other measures fail."--DR. J. H. KELLOGG.

OUTGROWING THE STRENGTH:--"There is sometimes debility or weakness in rapidly growing boys and girls which is attributed to this cause. It is popularly supposed that port wine or beer, is the great remedy; but nothing can be worse. It is true that gin given continuously to puppies will keep them small, but no one would advocate the amount of spirit required in proportion by a lad or girl to produce the same effect. If the growth could be checked by chemicals it would be most injurious to do so.

"In the treatment of such cases fresh air by day and night is essential; cold sponging, followed by friction with a rough towel, and exercise are desirable."

PNEUMONIA.

Dr. Julius Poheman says in Medical News:--

"The effect of alcohol upon nearly all the organs of the body has been carefully investigated. But, strange to say, literature contains only a few straggling hints upon the action of alcohol on the pulmonary tissue. It has long been known that the abuse of alcohol is a predisposing cause of death when the drinker is attacked with pneumonia. No experimental evidence has been published of the action of alcohol in producing pathological conditions in the lungs. In order to determine this action, a series of experiments was made upon dogs in the winters of 1890-1891 and 1892-1893. The dogs were a mixed lot of mongrels gathered in by the city dog catchers. They varied in weight from fifteen to twenty-five pounds, and were apparently in good health. In all, thirty animals were experimented on.

"The experiments were performed as follows:--A carefully etherized animal had injected into his trachea just below the larynx a quantity of commercial alcohol varying from one dram to one ounce in amount. The effects of equal amounts of alcohol upon animals of the same weight varies greatly. Two dogs, weighing twenty-five pounds each, were injected with two drams of alcohol. One died in one hour, and the other in six hours after the injection. Four other dogs, two weighing twenty-four pounds each, another eighteen pounds, and the fourth fifteen pounds, were all injected with the same amount, two drams. All four survived, and were as well as usual in four weeks. Another dog of eighteen pounds died five minutes after an injection of two drams, while another of fifteen pounds took one ounce and recovered.

"The symptoms in the dogs were all alike, dyspnea, increasing as the inflammation increased, until the accessory muscles of respiration were called into play. The stethoscope showed that air had great difficulty in entering the bronchi and air vesicles, and showed also the tumultuous beating of the heart in pumping blood through the lung. It was impossible to take the temperatures. Post-mortem examinations showed the lungs dark, congested and solid in some places. The air passages were filled with frothy, bloody mucus, even in the dog that died in five minutes. On section, the lungs were dark, congested, and full of bloody mucus. This shows how acutely sensitive the respiratory passages are to the action of alcohol. On microscopic examination of the lungs, the air tubes and vesicles were found filled with immense numbers of red and white corpuscles and much mucus. The same picture was presented as in a slide from the lungs of a broncho-pneumonic child.

"The striking similarity between the two is enough to prove that the pathological condition is the same, and that alcohol has produced a lesion very closely resembling, if not absolutely like, that of broncho-pneumonia in the human subject. This to some extent explains why drunkards attacked by pneumonia succumb more readily than the temperate. The sensitive lung tissue is enveloped in alcohol--flowing through the capillaries of the lung on one side, and exhaled, filling the air vesicles and tubes on the other. The condition must create a state of semi-engorgement or of mild inflammation, similar to the drunkard's red nose, or his engorged gastric mucous membrane. Such a state will reduce the vitality of the pulmonary tissue, and its power of resistance to external influences. Add to this an inflammation such as a pneumonia, and the lungs find themselves unable to stand the pressure."

As previous chapters contain much showing the reasons why alcohol is dangerous in pneumonia, space need not be taken here to do more than indicate briefly some points of non-alcoholic treatment.

Pneumonia is generally supposed to result from a cold; it is ushered in by the symptoms of a chill, followed by fever, headache, shortness of breath, pain in chest, etc. It sometimes occurs as a complication of typhoid fever and other acute diseases.

"It is not a very fatal disease in young and healthy subjects, but in weak children, old persons and habitual drinkers, it is a very fatal malady."

Nature Cure recommends a vapor bath immediately upon the appearance of the first symptoms, together with copious drinking of hot lemonade, and a good supply of pure fresh air in the room, together with the application of alternating hot and cold compresses, and no drugs.

Dr. Kellogg says:--

"Cool compresses or ice-bags, alternated every three hours by hot fomentations for ten minutes, should be applied to the chest, particularly to the affected side, the seat of pain. The hot fomentations relieve the pain, and the cold compresses check the diseased process. The compresses should be wrung out of cold water, and changed every five to eight minutes, or as often as they become warm. Although the cool compresses are not usually liked by the patient, they will soon give relief if their use is continued, and they do much towards shortening the course of the disease. Care should be taken to keep the patient's body from being wet except where the treatment is applied. The cold compress is much used in the large hospitals of Germany. When the pulse becomes as rapid as 95 to 110 or more, cool sponging, the wet-sheet pack, the cool full bath or the cool enema should be employed. When much chilliness is produced by the contact of water with the skin, the cold enema is a most admirably useful measure. The amount of water required is from half a pint to a pint. The temperature may be 40 to 60 degrees. The apartment should be kept as cool as possible without discomfort, and an abundance of fresh air should be continually supplied.

"The diet of the patient should consist of milk, oatmeal gruel, ripe fruit, and similar easily digested food. No meat, eggs or other stimulating food should be allowed.

"Discontinue the cold treatment after the first twenty-four to forty-eight hours. If the surface is cold, apply hot sponging or a hot pack. Avoid causing chilliness."

PRE-NATAL INFLUENCE OF ALCOHOL:--"The use of beer as a medicine during pregnancy is without doubt perilous to the health and vigor of the offspring. Children born under such conditions are sickly and feeble, and suffer from disease more severely than others, or die early. Alcoholic prescriptions to pregnant women are, from all present knowledge of the facts, both dangerous and reprehensible in the highest degree."--DR. T. D. CROTHERS, Hartford, Conn.

"M. Fere, an eminent French physician, recently reported to the Biological Society of Paris the results of experiments which he had been conducting for the purpose of throwing light upon this question. These experiments demonstrate that the exposure of hen's eggs to the influence of the vapor of alcohol, previous to incubation, retards the development of the embryo, and favors the production of malformations. It is evident from these experiments that alcohol may act directly upon the embryo when there is no marked influence of alcoholism in the parent."

PAIN AFTER FOOD:--"This may occur in acute or chronic gastric catarrh, or in a neuralgic or oversensitive condition of the stomach, or in ulcer or cancer of that organ. In all these it comes on soon after food has been swallowed; but, if occurring a long time after a meal, it is probably due to atonic dyspepsia. Alcohol will undoubtedly sometimes relieve this kind of pain by deadening the nerves of the stomach so that the pain is not felt so much; but this effect soon passes off, and if the cause of the malady is not removed by other means, increasing quantities of alcohol will be required to give relief. Many cases of drink-craving have originated in this way. Medical aid will generally be required. A small mustard poultice over the pit of the stomach is often useful, especially in inflammatory cases, or any other outward application of heat. Food should be fluid, or semi-fluid, and digestible. Ginger tea, or peppermint water, may serve to disperse gas."

POISON, ANIMAL.

The following by Dr. Chas. H. Shepard, of Brooklyn, who introduced the Turkish bath into America, is taken from the Journal of the A. M. A., for Nov. 13, 1897:--

"Animal poison is by no means uncommon, and so quick and mysterious is its action that a prompt remedy is a vital necessity. There is good reason to believe that the numerous remedies that have been recommended from earliest times as antidotes for animal poison are worthless, as they have not the properties commonly ascribed to them. The paucity of remedies is so great that alcohol is the one which comes most quickly to the mind of those who have been taught in the traditions of the past, and who are not fully aware of its action on the human system. We shall endeavor to show that the action of alcohol is not helpful, but on the contrary is really detrimental; and also that there is a better way out of the difficulty.

"If we get a splinter in the body, vital energy is aroused to get rid of the offending substance, inflammation is set up, and sloughing goes on until the splinter is voided. If the splinter is covered with acrid material, the same process is intensified, and nature endeavors to eliminate the offending substance through the natural excretions. Upon the peculiarity of the material depends the direction of this elimination.

"It is well known that some poisons are thrown off by the kidneys, some by the lungs, while others again are attacked by all the emunctories. The difference in the power of the system to absorb different substances, appropriate whatever can be utilized, and throw off whatever can not be used, is sometimes called idiosyncrasy, but more properly it may be called vital resistance, and upon the integrity of this power rests the ability to combat disease in all its forms, whether it be the absorption of any animal virus or the poison resulting from undigested food. This ability is in proportion to the integrity and soundness of every tissue and organ of the body. This may be illustrated by the fact that with a person suffering from kidney disease, which necessarily impedes elimination, the ordinary effects of a poison are intensified; therefore whatever aids in the promotion of good health, or in other words, the normal action of all the functions, will contribute to the safety of the individual in any and every emergency.

"When a person dies from the effect of poisoning, it is simply because the system was unable to eliminate the offending substance and was exhausted in the effort. There is a tolerance of some substances which frequently results in chronic disease, and again it is shown in what is called the cumulative effect or acute disease.

"Those who would hold that a substance is at one time a medicament, and at another time a poison, have much trouble in drawing the line between the beneficial and the poisonous effect. The idea that poisonous substances act on the system is responsible for many grave mistakes, whereas always, and under all circumstances, it is the system that does all the action.

"There might be some excuse for the idea that disease is an entity, from the facts that have been brought to light by the germ theory, but this theory is of recent date, while the entity theory is as old as superstition.

"Snake poison, which may be cited as a type of other animal poisons, takes effect through the circulation, and acts by paralyzing the nerve centres, and by altering the condition of the blood. In ordinary cases death seems to take place by arrest of respiration, from paralysis of the nerves of motion. The poison also acts septically, producing at a later period sloughing and hemorrhage.

"Dr. Calmette, a noted French scientist, claims that what is poisonous in the snake's bite, is not the venom absorbed into the blood, but a principle which the blood itself has developed out of the poison. This would necessitate very quick action when the poison is inserted in one of the large veins, as that is followed by instant death.

"The following cases fairly represent some of the tragedies that are occurring in our everyday life.

"A man 60 years old falls and dislocates his finger, he goes to the hospital, where in a short time he dies from blood poisoning. * * * * * Another man 48 years old, many years a wine merchant, whose great toe was severely crushed by a heavy man stepping on it, was taken with blood-poisoning and in spite of all treatment, even to the amputation of the leg, he soon succumbed to the disease. * * * * * A young woman 24 years old, picks a pimple on her chin and at once her face begins to swell. In vain was all medical treatment, for in a few days she died in terrible agony. * * * * * About a year ago there died in Brooklyn, N. Y., a physician in his 38th year, who six days previously received a slight scratch in his hand while performing a post-mortem examination. All that medical science could suggest was done to no avail. * * * * * In the summer of 1896 a young woman 22 years of age was bitten on the leg by an insect. Several physicians were called in but their treatment gave no relief; blood-poisoning set in; it was decided to amputate the leg, but before it could be done she died. * * * * * In July, 1896, a veterinary surgeon 34 years of age, while removing a cancer from a horse pricked his finger with his knife. The wound was so slight that he forgot all about it. A few days later blood-poisoning set in and in a short time his end came. * * * * * Some forty years ago a man named Whitney was teasing a rattlesnake in a Broadway barroom, was bitten by it, and, though whisky was poured down his throat by the quart, he soon died.

"Such results seem entirely unnecessary were the proper course pursued, and at the same time they are a fearful commentary on the medical resources of the day.

"The latest researches in regard to alcohol reveal it as a poison to the human system in whatever way it may be diluted or disguised. Its effect is always the same in proportion to the amount taken. It is impossible to habitually use it in any form, even in small quantities, without disease and degeneration resulting therefrom. When taken into the stomach the action is the same as with any other narcotic; the meaning of this word is to become torpid. It benumbs the nerves of sensation, and thus the vital resistance to any offending material is reduced, and while the patient feels less of any disturbance the real harm goes on with accumulated force because of the lack of vitality and non-resistance of the nervous system.

"When the body is in the throes of a vital struggle with a virulent poison it would seem, to any unprejudiced mind, the height of folly to further weaken the vital resistance by the administration of any narcotic, and especially alcohol.

"The eminent German, Professor Bunge, says: 'All the results which on superficial observation appear to show that alcohol possesses stimulant properties, can be explained on the ground that they were due to paralysis.' * * * * * Professors S. Weir Mitchell and E. T. Reichert, in Researches on Serpent Poison, make this notable statement: 'Despite the popular creed, it is now pretty sure that many men have been killed by the alcohol given to relieve them from the effects of snake bite, and it is a matter of record that men dead drunk with whiskey and then bitten, have died of the bite.'

"As a great contrast to the weakness of the mass of our people who are drug-takers and alcohol-consumers, and who are liable to almost any epidemic that comes along, and quickly succumb to a serious injury, may be mentioned the Turkish soldiers of to-day, who know nothing of drugs as we use them and never use alcohol in any form. During the late controversy with the Greeks, one of them who was reported as having been shot in the stomach, remained in the ranks, and afterward walked ten miles. Another one who was wounded twice in the legs and once in the shoulder, continued attending to his duties for twenty-four hours, until an officer noticed his condition and ordered him to the hospital. The heat was tremendous, but the troops endured it without complaint, and the doctors were astonished at the wonderful vitality of the wounded Turks, who recovered with remarkable rapidity. This, with good reason, is attributed to their abstemious lives.

"It has been stated that the Moqui Indians handle the rattlesnake with impunity, and are not inconvenienced by its occasional bite.

"The rational treatment of animal poison is to endeavor to prevent the entry of the virus into the circulation and to neutralize it in the wound before it is absorbed; but when it has entered the system everything should be done for its elimination.

"The most powerful aid to the human system, and the most perfect eliminator known to man is heat. It is used with much advantage, and great success by means of water, both internally and externally, but above all is its use by hot air, as in the Turkish bath, which works in harmony with every natural function, promoting the action of all the secretions, and more particularly the excretions. By this means will the system unload itself of an accumulation of impurities in an incredibly short space of time, while the heat aids in destroying whatever there may be of virus therein.

"Calmette, whom we have previously quoted, has shown that whatever be the source of snake venom, its active principle is destroyed by being submitted to a temperature of about 212 degrees for a variable length of time.

"In the not remote future thousands of human beings will owe to the Turkish bath not only an immunity from disease in general, but also an escape from the horrors of a premature death from hydrophobia, the poison of snake bite, or the slower action of infectious disease.

"The mass of testimony that has been accumulating for over thirty years past is more than sufficient to convince any reasonable mind that is willing to examine the facts.

"The medical profession has searched the world over and under for the means of controlling disease, while within the human body itself lies the vital power which needs only to be cultivated and exalted to its true function to banish the mass of disease from the land."

Dr. Shepard states in another article that Turkish baths are now used in London and Paris for the cure of hydrophobia.

Dr. J. H. Kellogg says:--

"A great number of remedies have acquired the reputation of being cures for snake bites. The partisans of each one of these have been able to produce a large number of cases, which apparently supported their claims; the uniform testimony of all scientific authorities upon this subject, however, is that all these so-called antidotes are worthless. Prof. W. Watson Cheyne, M. B., F. R. C. S., surgeon of Kings College Hospital, London, England, states, in the International Encyclopedia of Surgery, that 'there is no known antidote by which the venom can be neutralized, nor any prophylactic.' This eminent authority also remarks further: 'Hence medication with this view is to be avoided altogether, and the aim of treatment should be to prevent the poison from gaining access to the general circulation, and to avoid its prostrating effects if its entrance has already taken place.' The same writer asserts that the only aim of the constitutional treatment should be 'to sustain the strength until the poison shall have been eliminated.' The idea that the saturation of the body with whisky to the point of intoxication, if possible, is beneficial in these cases, is in the highest degree erroneous. Whisky intoxication, according to Dr. Cheyne, actually 'favors the injurious effect of the poison. What is required is to keep the patient alive until the poison has been eliminated.' Whisky will not do this, but actually aids the poison in its fatal work by lessening the resistance of the patient, and hence lessening his chances for recovery.

"The reputation of whisky as a remedy in these cases is due to the fact that on an average only one person in eight who is bitten by a rattlesnake is really poisoned; the reasons for this were fully explained in an interesting paper on 'Rattlesnakes,' by the eminent Dr. S. Weir Mitchell, and published in the Smithsonian Contributions to Knowledge for 1860. If the snake strikes several times before inflicting a wound, the sacs containing the venom may be emptied, so that the succeeding bite will introduce only the most minute quantity of poison--not enough to produce serious, or fatal results. If the part bitten is covered by clothing, the poison may be absorbed by the clothing, so that but very little enters the circulation. In various other ways the snake is prevented from inflicting a fatal wound. The popular idea, that every bite of a rattlesnake is necessarily poisonous, is thus shown to be erroneous. It is not at all probable that the administration of whisky has ever in any case contributed to the long life of a person bitten by a rattlesnake.

"Whisky is often recommended by physicians with the idea that it will sustain the energies of the patient, or will stimulate the heart, etc.; but it has been clearly shown that alcohol in all forms is not only useless for these purposes, but does actual damage, since it lessens the resistance of the patient, weakens the heart, and helps along the prostration which is the characteristic effect of the rattlesnake venom. Alcohol has, for many years, been used as an antidote for collapse under an an 鋥 thetic administered for surgical purposes, but no intelligent physician nowadays thinks of using alcohol for such a purpose; instead, alcohol is given before the an 鎔 thetic for the purpose of facilitating its effect. Errors of this sort which have once become established are very hard to uproot. Probably some physicians will continue to use alcohol for shock, exhaustion, general debility and similar conditions as well as for rattlesnake poisoning for another quarter of a century, but such use of alcohol does not belong to the domain of rational medicine and is not supported by scientific facts."

"Under the Pasteur method, a man who did not take alcohol was much more likely to recover from the bite of a mad dog than one bitten under the same conditions, who used that drug; while in lock-jaw there was absolute failure to secure immunity if the patient had taken alcohol. In India it used to be given in large quantities for snake bite, but it was found that it had a direct effect in interfering with the processes of repair, and so is being abandoned."--DR. SIMS WOODHEAD, of the Royal College of Physicians and Surgeons, London, Eng.

"Nothing could be more irrational and dangerous than the popular notion concerning the antagonism of whisky and snake-bites, and Willson reports that several of the fatalities in his series were directly due to alcohol rather than to the bite."--Editorial, Journal of the American Medical Ass'n.

RHEUMATISM:--"Unquestionably, the most active cause of rheumatism, as well as of migraine, sick-headache, Bright's disease, neurasthenia and a number of other kindred diseases, is the general use of flesh food, tea and coffee, and alcoholic liquors. As regards remedies, there are no medicinal agents which are of any permanent value in the treatment of chronic rheumatism. The disease can be remedied only by regimen,--that is, by diet and training. A simple dietary, consisting of fruits, grains, and nuts, and particularly the free use of fruits, must be placed in the first rank among the radical curative measures. Water, if taken in abundance, is also a means of washing out the accumulated poisons.

"An individual afflicted with rheumatism in any form should live, so far as possible, an out-of-door life, taking daily a sufficient amount of exercise to induce vigorous perspiration. A cool morning sponge bath, followed by vigorous rubbing, and a moist pack to the joints most seriously affected, at night, are measures which are worthy of a faithful trial. Every person who is suffering from this disease should give the matter immediate attention, as it is a malady which is progressive, and is one of the most potent causes of premature old age, and general physical deterioration. American nervousness is probably more often due to uric acid, or to the poisons which it represents, than to any other one cause."--Good Health.

"Alcohol favors the development of rheumatism. It does this by preventing waste matter from leaving the system. Beer and wine, because they contain lime and salts, are said to cause rheumatism, or at least to aid in its development. These salts are absorbed into the system, unite with the uric acid, and form an insoluble urate of lime, which is deposited around the joints, thus causing them to become enlarged and stiff. * * * * *

"The success of the Turkish bath treatment has been phenomenal. Of over 3,000 cases treated here at least 95 per cent. have been entirely relieved, or greatly helped. Some who were treated over twenty years ago have stated that they have not had a twinge of rheumatism since. Very few have persevered in the use of the bath without experiencing permanent relief."--DR. CHARLES H. SHEPARD, Brooklyn.

"Those having a bath cabinet can have a good substitute at home for the Turkish bath. Remember that if tobacco and alcohol are indulged in, there can be no permanent relief."

The New Hygiene says:--

"Under no circumstances take any of the thousand and one nostrums advertised as sure cures for this disease. Pure unadulterated blood is the only remedy. This can only be produced by cleansing the system of impurities, and giving it the right kind of material out of which to make it. Keep out the poisonous physic, clean out the colon, strengthen the lungs, and feed the system with proper food, and this disease will vanish like a fog before the rising sun."

The same book in advocating the use of the Turkish bath for rheumatism, says:--

"The fact, which is well attested, that when a person enters the bath the urine may be strongly acid, but, on leaving the bath, after half an hour, it is markedly alkaline, shows that the bath has a strong effect upon the system."

Dr. Ridge says of rheumatic fever:--

"I would urge most strongly the desirability of avoiding every form of alcoholic liquor, from the very commencement of the disease, as affording the best chance for a speedy and safe recovery. The highest authorities are agreed on this point, but there is a lingering practice which makes reference necessary in order to confirm the wavering."

In Mt. Sinai Hospital, New York, the hot blanket pack is used in acute rheumatism, almost to the exclusion of other methods. The pack should be continued two to four hours at least, and may be repeated two or three times within the twenty-four hours with advantage.

Nature Cure says that thorough massage, and half a dozen cups of hot lemonade will cure a severe case of sciatica:--

"The massage should be commenced moderately, and increased as the patient can bear it. Rubbing and slapping of the muscles with bare hands will hasten a cure, and be agreeable to the patient. One to two hours treatment, if vigorous, will effect a cure."

SEA-SICKNESS:--Brandy is a common resort in this trouble, many taking it under such circumstances who would under no other. Yet it frequently adds to the sickness, instead of relieving it.

"Be sparing in diet for two or three days before the expected voyage. If very sensitive, take to your berth as soon as you go on board, or lie down on deck; get near the centre of the vessel, and lie with your feet to the stern. Go to sleep if possible. Iced water may be sipped, but nothing solid should be taken at first; after a while a cracker or wafer may be taken."

It is said upon good authority that if two or three apples are eaten shortly before going on board, or before rough water is encountered, sea-sickness is entirely averted. It will be well to partake of no other food for some hours previous to the voyage when trying this.

Good Health says:--

"If any of our readers have occasion to cross the ocean in the stormy season, we recommend three things; keep horizontal, with the head low; put an ice-bag to the back of the neck, keep the stomach clean, free from greasy foods and meats, and eat nothing till there is an appetite for food. A habitually clean dietary before going on board is doubtless a good preparation for such a voyage, as well as for any other nerve strain, or test of endurance. It pays to be good--to your stomach, as well as in other ways."

The following is guaranteed by a Russian physician to be an effective cure and a means of avoiding sea-sickness when the symptoms first make their appearance. Take long and deep inspirations. About twenty breaths should be taken every minute, and they should be as deep as possible. After thirty or forty inspirations the symptoms will be found to abate. This is recommended for dyspepsia also.

SORE NIPPLES:--"Alum water, or tannin, used for several months in advance will harden as effectually as brandy. If there is soreness on commencing to nurse, put a pinch of alum into milk, and apply the curd to the nipple."

SPASMS:--"These are caused by flatulence, as a result of indigestion. A little hot ginger tea, or capsicum tea, may do all that is required. If these are not at hand, loosen every tight band, rub well the region of the heart and stomach, slap the face with the corner of a wet towel, and give sips of cold water."

SHOCK:--"In shock, or collapse, the state is similar in some respects to that which is present in fainting. Every function is almost at a standstill; absorption from the stomach and elsewhere is at its lowest point, because the circulation of the blood is so much interfered with. Hence much of the brandy which is so often given, and to such a wonderful amount, with very little apparent effect of intoxication, is really not absorbed at all, and is very often rejected from the stomach by vomiting, when reaction does occur, if not before.

"The patient should be wrapped up warmly, and put to bed as soon as possible. The limbs may be rubbed with hot flannels, and hot water bottles put to hands and feet. In some cases, also, towels wrung out of hot water may be wrapped around the head. Hot milk and water, hot water slightly sweetened, or with a little peppermint water in it, should be given as soon as the patient can swallow. Hot beverages will warm the skin more rapidly and powerfully than any alcoholic liquor.

"If the patient cannot swallow, an enema of hot water, or hot, thin gruel, should be administered, and may be of use in addition to hot drinks. Beef extract may be added to the hot water with advantage.

"In the vast majority of cases there need be no anxiety so far as the shock is concerned; reaction will occur in due time if ordinary care be taken, and will be more natural and steady if the system is not embarrassed by the presence of the narcotic alcohol. In the state of collapse the voluntary nervous system is depressed; alcohol diminishes the power and activity of the nervous centres of the brain, hence its action is undesirable in shock or collapse."--

DR. J. J. RIDGE, London.

"No procedure could be more senseless than the administering alcohol in shock. A stimulant of some kind is necessary in such cases, and alcohol, instead of being a stimulant is a narcotic. * * * * * Alcohol causes a decrease of temperature, the very thing to be avoided in cases of shock."--DR. J. H. KELLOGG.

"I am perfectly sure that a large dose of alcohol in shock puts a nail in the coffin of the patient."--DR. H. C. WOOD of the University of Pennsylvania.

SINKING SENSATIONS:--Many women have a feeling of weakness or "goneness" at about eleven o'clock in the morning, and are led by it to the injurious practice of eating between meals. It is often due to indigestion, or to the use of beer or wine. A few sips of hot milk, of fruit juice, or even of cold water will often relieve it, especially if total abstinence is persevered in.

SUDDEN ILLNESS:--"Those taken suddenly ill are likely to fare best if placed in a recumbent position, with head slightly elevated, all tightness of garments about the neck or waist relieved, and a little cold water given in case of ability to swallow. A mustard plaster on the back of the neck, or over the stomach, and hot water or hot bottles to the feet, are never out of place, while vinegar, or smelling salts, or dilute ammonia to the nostrils is reviving."--EZRA M. HUNT, M. D., late secretary of New Jersey State Board of Health.

"Both the popular and professional beliefs in the efficacy of alcoholic liquids for relieving exhaustion, faintness, shock, etc. are equally fallacious. All these conditions are temporary, and rapidly recovered from by simply the recumbent position, and free access to fresh air. Ninety-nine out of every hundred of such cases pass the crisis before the attendants have time to apply any remedies, and when they do, the sprinkling of cold water on the face, and the vapor of camphor or carbonate of ammonia to the nostrils, are the most efficacious remedies, and leave none of the secondary evil effects of brandy, whisky or wine."--DR. N. S. DAVIS.

SUNSTROKE:--"There has lately been a correspondence in the Morning Post on the subject of 'Sunstroke and Alcohol.' We quite agree with the statement that 'nothing predisposes people to sunstroke so much as this pernicious habit of taking stimulants (so-called) during the hot weather.' As far as this country is concerned, nearly every case of sunstroke might be more appropriately designated 'beerstroke.' One effect of alcohol is to paralyze the heat-regulating mechanism; the blood becomes overloaded with waste material, and the narcotism, and vasomotor paralysis, produced by the alcohol, is added to that produced by the heat. Abstainers, other things being equal, can always endure extremes of temperature better than consumers of alcohol."--Medical Pioneer, England.

"During the month of January, 1896, there occurred over three hundred deaths from sunstroke in Australia. When called upon to offer suggestions relative to its prevention, the medical board promptly informed the Colonial government that, of all the predisposing causes, none were so potent as indulgence in intoxicating liquors, and in its treatment nothing seemed to have a more disastrous effect than the administration of alcoholic stimulants."--Medical News.

The Bulletin of the A. M. T. A. for August, 1896, contained the following:--

"Recently a leading medical man, a teacher in a college, warned his student audience against the anti-alcoholic theories urged by extremists and persons whose zeal was greater than their intelligence. He affirmed positively that the value of alcohol was well known in medicine, and established by long years of experience.

"Not long afterward a man was brought into his office in a state of collapse from sunstroke, and this physician and teacher ordered large quantities of brandy to be administered; the patient died soon after."

Dr. T. D. Crothers tells of a case where alcohol was administered to a child for partial sunstroke, and says, "there were many reasons for believing that the profound poisoning from alcohol gave a permanent bias and tendency that developed into inebriety later."

"When a person falls with sunstroke (or heatstroke) he should at once be carried to a cool, shady place. His clothing should be removed, and cold applications made to the head, and over the whole body. Pieces of ice may be packed around the head, or cold water may be poured upon the body. Cold enema may also be employed. In case the face is pale, hot applications should be made to the head and over the heart and the body should be rubbed vigorously."--DR. J. H. KELLOGG.

TYPHOID FEVER.

As many lives are lost by this disease, its treatment must ever be one of intense interest, not only to physicians, but also to all humanity. Since non-alcoholic treatment has reduced the death-rate in typhoid to five per cent., the views regarding such treatment expressed by leading practitioners will doubtless be read with eagerness.

The following is a paper by Dr. N. S. Davis taken from the Medical Temperance Quarterly.

"ALLEGED INDICATIONS FOR THE USE OF ALCOHOL IN THE TREATMENT OF TYPHOID FEVER:--On the first page of the first number of a new medical journal bearing date July, 1895, may be found the following statement: 'The question of administering alcohol comes up in every case of typhoid fever. In mild cases, especially when the patient is young, healthy and temperate, stimulants are not needed so long as the disease follows the typical course. Here, as elsewhere, alcohol should be avoided when not absolutely demanded. There is, however, generally such a dangerous tendency toward nervous exhaustion, that in a majority of cases more or less alcohol is required. The indication which calls for its use is an inability to administer enough food. * * * * * Again, the existence of high temperature nearly always makes it necessary to stimulate the patient, as does threatened nervous exhaustion and heart failure, for immediate effect; likewise a weak, small, compressible, rapid pulse, with impaired cardiac impulse and systolic sound, is a frequent indication; other remedies may be required, but alcohol cannot be dispensed with.' The next paragraph continues: 'It is necessary to give alcohol in serious complications of typhoid fever, such as pneumonia, pleurisy, hemorrhage and severe bronchitis or diarrhoea. It is best to begin giving it early and in small quantities: two to six ounces is a moderate amount, eight to twelve ounces daily is not too much for adynamic or complicated cases.'

"The foregoing quotations purport to have been condensed from one of our recent authoritative works on practical medicine, and doubtless fairly represent the prevailing opinions concerning the use of alcohol in the treatment of typhoid and other fevers, both in and out of the profession. A careful reading will show that the whole is founded on the following four assumptions:

"1. That alcohol when taken into the living body acts as a general stimulant, and especially so to the cardiac and vasomotor functions. 2. That in mild, uncomplicated cases of typhoid fever in young and previously healthy subjects, stimulants are not required and no alcohol should be given. 3. That in a 'majority of cases' the tendency toward dangerous 'nervous exhaustion' and 'heart failure' is so great that the giving of 'more or less alcohol is required.' 4. The amount required may vary from two to twelve or more ounces per day.

"In the two preceding numbers of this journal, I have endeavored to show that the chief causes of nervous exhaustion and heart failure, in typhoid and other fevers were impairment of the hemoglobin and corpuscular elements of the blood, deficient reception and internal distribution of oxygen, and molecular degeneration of the muscular structures of the heart itself. These important pathological conditions are doubtless caused by the specific toxic agent or agents giving rise to the fever. Consequently the rational objects of treatment are to stop the further action of the specific cause, either by neutralization, or elimination, or both; to stop the further impairment of the hemoglobin and other elements of the blood; and to increase the reception and internal distribution of oxygen, by which we will most effectually prevent further fatty or granular degeneration of cardiac and other structures. The language of the paragraphs I have quoted, fairly assumes that alcohol is a stimulant capable of relieving nervous exhaustion and cardiac failures, regardless of the causes producing those pathological conditions, and consequently its use is necessary in the 'majority of cases' of typhoid fever.

"Can such an assumption be sustained by either established facts, or correct reasoning? Can nervous and cardiac exhaustion, induced by the presence of toxic agents in the blood, with deficiency of both hemoglobin and oxygen, be relieved by a simple stimulant, that neither neutralizes nor eliminates the toxic agents, nor increases either the hemoglobin or oxygen? That alcohol does not neutralize or destroy toxic ptomaines, or tox-albumins, is proved by abundant clinical experience, and also by the fact that chemists use it freely in the processes for separating these substances from other organic matters for experimental purposes. That its presence in the living body retards metabolic changes generally, and thereby aids in retaining instead of eliminating toxic agents of all kinds, has been so fully shown in the pages of preceding numbers of the Medical Temperance Quarterly, that the leading facts need not be repeated here. That its presence does not increase the hemoglobin, or favor oxy-hemoglobin or increased internal distribution of oxygen, but decidedly the reverse, has been equally well demonstrated by numerous and reliable experimental researches in this and other countries.

"Then it must be conceded that alcohol is not capable of fulfilling either of the important indications presented in the treatment of typhoid fever as stated above. Nevertheless, the advocates of its use apparently recognize but two ideas or factors in these cases, namely, the popularly inherited assumption that alcohol is a stimulant, and as the patient is in danger from nervous and cardiac weakness, therefore the alcohol must be given, pro re nata without the slightest regard to the existing causes of the weakness, or the modus operandi of the so-called stimulant.

"This is proved by the fact that they group together as stimulants, and give to the same patient in alternate doses, remedies of directly antagonistic action, as alcohol and strychnine, or digitalis, etc.

"The accepted definition of a stimulant in medical literature, is some agent capable of exciting or increasing vital activity as a whole, or the natural activity of some one structure or organ.

"For instance, both clinical and experimental observations show that strychnine directly increases the functional activity of the respiratory, cardiac and vasomotor nervous systems, and thereby increases the internal distribution of oxygen, which is nature's own special exciter of all vital action. Therefore it is properly a direct respiratory, cardiac and vasomotor stimulant and indirectly a stimulator of all vital processes. But the same kind of clinical and experimental observations show that alcohol directly diminishes the functional activity of all nerve structures, pre-eminently those of respiration and circulation, and also of all metabolic processes, whether respirative, disintegrative or secretory. Consequently it not only acts as directly antagonistic to strychnine, but equally so to all true stimulants or remedies capable of increasing vital activity. Instead, therefore, of meriting the name of stimulant, alcohol should be designated and used only as an an 鋞 thetic and sedative, or depressor of vital activity.

"And a thorough and impartial investigation will show that its use in the treatment of typhoid and other fevers, while deceiving both physician and patient, by its an 鋞 thetic effect in diminishing restlessness, both prolongs the duration and increases the ratio of mortality of the disease, by its impairment of vital activity in the organizable elements of both blood and tissues."

Equally interesting is the following outline of treatment pursued by Dr. W. H. Riley, of the Battle Creek Sanitarium.

"The purpose of the present paper is to give briefly an outline of the method of treatment of typhoid fever as used by the writer in a considerable number of cases.

"A consideration of the pathology of this disease does not properly come under this head, but we wish simply to call attention to the well-known fact that typhoid fever is a germ disease. The germ which causes this fever has generally been supposed to be the bacillus of Eberth. More recent bacteriological studies rather indicate that the bacillus coli may also cause the disease. These germs are usually carried into the body in food or drink, and, lodging in the small intestines, begin to grow and multiply, and by their life produce poisonous ptomaines which are absorbed and carried by the circulation to all the organs and tissues of the body.

"It is these ptomaines, thus carried to all parts of the body, that are largely the immediate cause of the pyrexia and attending symptoms. The organisms which produce these poisons for the most part remain in the intestines, although they have been found in the spleen.

"The indications for treatment are:--

"1. To remove or destroy the cause (to eliminate the germs and ptomaines from the body).

"2. To sustain the vital and resisting powers of the patient.

"If the patient is seen early in the disease, it has been my practice to immediately put him to bed and give a free dose of magnesium sulphate. This is preferably given in the morning or forenoon, and may be repeated once or twice on successive days. Besides this the patient should have a large enema of water at a temperature of from 75?to 80?F.; and this may be repeated daily or even oftener, for some time, if necessary, to keep the bowels empty of the poisonous substances.

"The salines and enemas thus used carry out bodily a large number of germs and ptomaines that are present in the intestines; and further, the salines, by producing an increased secretion of the mucous membrane of the intestines, tend to disentangle and set free many of the germs that have found a lodging place in the walls of the intestines.

"For the elimination of the ptomaines which have been absorbed into the circulation and carried to the tissues, nothing is better than the internal use of water. From three to five pints should be drunk during every twenty-four hours. It should be taken in small quantities--six to eight ounces every hour or two during waking hours, except when food is taken. I will refer to this point more in detail later.

"A consideration of the general care of the patient properly comes under the second head of the indications for treatment as given above. The patient should be put to bed in a large, light, well-ventilated room. At least two sides of the room should communicate directly by windows with out-of-doors, in order that the room may be properly ventilated.

"All unnecessary articles of furniture, such as carpets, couches, upholstered chairs, pictures, etc. should be removed.

"The room should be thoroughly cleaned before the patient is put into it.

"There should be two beds in the room for the use of the patient. These should be, preferably, narrow and so placed in the room that there is a free approach to both sides of the bed, for the convenience of the nurse in giving treatment. Iron bedsteads are preferable to wooden. The bedding should be firm, yet soft and smoothly drawn. There should be just sufficient covering to protect the body. The patient should be changed from one bed to the other daily. This may be done by placing the two beds side by side and carefully moving the patient from one to the other. The sheets on the bed from which the patient has been taken should be washed and disinfected at each change of the beds, and all other bedding should be thoroughly aired and exposed to the sunlight daily.

"The patient should have the care of a thoroughly educated, careful and competent nurse, one who understands perfectly the various methods of using water in the treatment of fevers.

"There is no other single remedy that I consider so valuable in the treatment of fever as the internal use of water. As above stated, the patient should drink six or eight ounces every hour during the waking hours, except for about two hours after food is taken. The water should be thoroughly sterilized, and as a rule may be taken either cool or hot. Ice water is objectionable. Hot water is often preferable. This is a simple remedy, but nevertheless is efficacious. It should be given to the patient whether he calls for it or not, and it should be considered an important part of his treatment. When water is taken into the stomach and absorbed into the circulation, it throws into solution the ptomaines which have been absorbed from the intestines and are present in the circulation and tissues, and thereby puts them in a favorable condition for elimination. It increases the activity of the kidneys, and thus hastens and increases the elimination of the poisons in the system.

"In the early stage of the fever, when the pulse is full, and the action of the heart increased, it is best to give the patient cool water. Later in the disease, when the action of the heart is weak, and the patient feeble, it is best to give the water hot.

"Winternitz, many years ago, demonstrated that hot water taken into the stomach acts as a cardiac stimulant, and the increased heart's action is immediate, or at least before the water has time to absorb, which indicates that the water in the stomach acts reflexly as a cardiac stimulant. The water after absorption also increases the circulation by filling the blood-vessels, and increasing arterial pressure. The writer has frequently noticed a decided increase in the fullness, and rapidity of the pulse, after a patient has drunk a glassful of hot water.

"The external use of water also forms an important part of the treatment. The patient should be sponged off with tepid water every hour or two when the temperature is 103? or above. When the temperature is less than this, it is not necessary to sponge the body so frequently. Sometimes a hot sponge bath is more efficacious in reducing the temperature than the tepid or cool bath. The sponge bath reduces the temperature, relieves many of the distressing nervous symptoms, is refreshing to the patient, and promotes sleep. The temperature of the body may also be reduced by the use of cool compresses placed over the abdomen, and changed frequently.

"The matter of diet is an important factor in the treatment of typhoid fever. The diet should be aseptic, easily digested, and should contain the necessary food elements. Probably no one article of diet meets all these requirements as well as sterilized milk. The patient should take from two to three pints daily. The milk is best taken four times during the day at intervals of four hours, taking eight to ten ounces at a time. Should the patient become tired of the milk, gluten gruel may be substituted for the milk.

"The diarrhoea and bowel symptoms, when present, may be relieved by the application of hot fomentations to the abdomen, warm or hot enemas and twenty grains of subnitrate of bismuth given every four hours.

"The patient should be kept as quiet as possible, and should be turned in bed at intervals, to prevent hypostatic congestion and the formation of bed-sores. The bony prominences which are apt to become eroded should be sponged frequently with a solution of tannic acid in equal parts of alcohol and water; a dram of the tannic acid to a pint of alcohol and water, is about the proper strength to use.

"By the methods briefly outlined above--that is by the free use of water internally and externally, by keeping the intestines thoroughly emptied of poisonous material by the free and frequent use of enemas, by proper feeding and the careful attention of a good nurse to the patient and his surroundings--the duration of the fever may be shortened and the severity of the disease lessened; heart failure, and other complications will seldom occur, and the patient will in nearly every instance make a good recovery. The best method to pursue to prevent heart failure is to keep the poisons which are generated in the bowels and absorbed into the body, and which are the direct cause of the heart failure, eliminated from the body. Should the heart become weak, it may be effectually stimulated by giving hot water to drink, applying heat to the heart in the form of a fomentation, and the application of fomentations to the upper spine.

"In the treatment of a large number of cases of typhoid fever, extending over several years' practice, the writer has never made use of alcohol internally to support the action of the heart, or for any other purpose.

"The number of cases of death from typhoid fever coming under the writer's observation, where the method of treatment pursued has been similar to that briefly indicated above, have been very few, a much smaller per cent. than in practice where alcohol has been used as a 'cardiac stimulant.' I believe that the use of alcohol in the treatment of typhoid fever is not only useless, but absolutely harmful."

Dr. Kate Lindsay, of Battle Creek Sanitarium and Hospital, contributed an article upon Typhoid Fever to the Bulletin of the A. M. T. A. for January, 1896, from which a few notes are here taken:--

"The chief toxic centre is evidently the intestinal tract, especially the termination of the ileum. The ulcerations, necroses, perforations and hemorrhages are most frequently found in the last twelve inches of the small intestine, and may extend into the large intestine. The ulcerated surface and open vessels increase the facility with which the poison finds entrance into the circulation. The microbes, blood clots, necrosed tissue and pus, furnish abundant supplies of toxic matter, which, saturating the system, over-power and stop the activity of the functions of all the organs of the body, causing degeneration of tissues. Death is said to take place from heart, lung or brain failure, but the failure involves every other organ as well.

"Regarding the intestinal tract as any other abscess at this time, the physician should seek for methods of treatment or remedies which will remove the morbid matters, and destroy, or at least inhibit their action, thus decreasing the fever and stimulating the circulation. Secondary toxic centres often develop in the course of this disease, notably in the glands, lungs and dependent organs, the hypostatic congestion resulting from lying in one position, causing stasis of blood, death and necrosis of tissue, both of the external and internal organs. All vessels connected with the dying tissues carry toxins to other parts of the body. Suppurating glands, and phlebitis of the femoral veins are examples of this secondary infection, and are accountable for the heart failure and collapse so often fatal during the second, third and fourth weeks of typhoid fever. * * * * *

"The old idea that in peristaltic action lay the great danger of increase of the hemorrhage and perforation of the bowels, is giving way to the more rational view that gaseous distention and septic absorption, are what bring about fatal results from these complications, and that the moderate peristalsis of the intestinal walls lessens these dangers by closing the gaping ends of the injured vessels, and expelling the septic matter and foul gases. To meet these indications I have found lavage of the bowels, even during hemorrhage, with water of 105?to 110?F. or even hotter, given in moderate quantity of from one pint to three, to give great relief by freeing the large intestines of blood clots, fecal matter and other morbid matter. It also increases peristaltic action in the small intestines, thus favoring the expulsion of gas. The heat stimulates the circulation in the peripheral vessels of the intestines, and overcomes the tendency to blood stasis.

"In the cases cited, ice-bags, alternated with fomentations, were used over the abdomen externally, and heat, or hot and cold, to spine. The extremities were kept warm. From ten to thirty minims of turpentine, in an ounce of gum acacia or starch water, increased the efficiency of the enemata, and aided in expelling the gas and checking hemorrhage.

"The tendency to hypostatic congestion and bed-sores, was prevented by frequent change of position, and the use of hot and cold to the spine by fomentations and compresses, or better still, hot fine spraying, or the alternate hot and cold spray. In one grave case, spraying was kept up for about twelve hours, with only short intermissions. The heart was stimulated by heat applied over it, whenever depression and collapse threatened, and by hot and cold sponging of the spine."

Dr. Noble said some time ago in the London Times:--

"Although it is true that alcohol is an antipyretic, yet its exhibition neither shortens nor modifies (favorably) the diseases of which the fever is but a symptom. The paralysis of the brain which is so frequent a cause of death in typhoid fever, is more often brought about by alcohol than any other cause, and more than one woman suffering from puerperal fever has been done to death by the administration of this substance, which, not being convenienter natur? is contra naturam."

J. S. Cain, M. D., in an able paper, read at the Nashville Academy of Medicine, on "Rational Suggestions in the Treatment of Typhoid Fever," dissents from the practice, which still obtains largely in the medical profession, of administering alcoholic liquors, in the belief that they are "stimulants, conservators of force and even nutrients," and says:--

"After a careful and thoughtful study of this subject, I have reluctantly, and against firm early convictions, been forced to the conclusion that these theories with regard to the beneficial effects of alcohol in disease are wholly fallacious. The only rational conclusion at which I can arrive is that the agent is ever, and under all circumstances, a depressor of temperature; that it arrests the physiological interchange of carbonic acid gas and oxygen in the tissues, as well as in the air vesicles of the lungs; that it impedes the elimination of tissue waste, and causes the accumulation of this refuse in the system; that it is lethal an æsthetic in all quantities; that it is not stimulant in the true sense, and never exerts that influence; and that it supplies no element to the diseased and vitiated system calculated to antagonize disease, repair waste, or invigorate lowered vital forces, and therefore for these purposes is not called for in the rational treatment of typhoid fever."

At the annual meeting of the American Medical Association held in Atlanta, Georgia, in 1896, Dr. G. B. Garber, of Dunkirk, Ind., read a paper upon "Alcohol in Typhoid Fever" from which a few points are here taken:--

"The fact that the mortality from typhoid fever seems to be gradually lowering is no doubt due in great measure to the non-use of alcohol in the treatment of the disease. Hardly a week passes that some of our journals do not report a series of cases treated without the aid of alcohol in any form. I used alcohol in the treatment of the disease until two years ago, when I became alarmed at the mortality; so I changed my plan, and in 1894 I treated thirty-seven well marked cases of varying degrees of intensity. I had two fatal cases, and in both of them I had used alcohol. In 1895 I treated thirty cases of about the same type, with no death. I only used alcohol in one of them, and it caused me more trouble than any of the others. As this case was in the family of a saloon-keeper, I could not control the matter, as they would give it during my absence. On my return I would find the face flushed, the temperature high, the pulse rapid and the patient nervous. By close inquiry I would find that some of the family had given 'just a little good whisky' which had been in the house for twenty years.

"In closing, I wish to state that I am well convinced that in the treatment of typhoid fever our patients will do better and stand a greater chance of recovery, if we abstain entirely from the use of alcohol in the treatment of the disease."

Prof. J. Burney Yeo, of London, in a paper read before the International

Medical Congress held at Rome, Italy, said:--

"In order to maintain the intestinal antisepsis which forms an essential part of this method of treatment, I insist on the necessity of scrupulous attention and caution in feeding patients suffering from enteric fever, great danger arising from a failure to note the extremely limited digestive and absorptive capacity exhibited by such patients.

"In conclusion, the use of alcoholic stimulants, and the common employment of depressing antipyretic agents, must be condemned."

In a report of the treatment of typhoid fever by seventy-two physicians of Connecticut, thirty-eight declared that they did not use alcohol in any stage of this disease. The remainder used it sparingly in the last stages, and only two considered it valuable from the beginning of the disease.

In a discussion of typhoid fever by a medical society meeting in Rochester, N. Y., recently, sixty physicians being present, only three spoke in favor of using alcohol in this disease.

Hygienic physicians all insist upon a rigid fast as long as the high temperature continues, or until the patient is sufficiently hungry to eat a piece of plain, stale, graham bread, "dry upon the tongue." Dr. Charles E. Page of Boston says there would be very few relapses if this plan were carefully carried out. He contends that the whisky and milk diet, together with the not over-fresh air of the average sick room is enough to produce fever in a healthy person, hence is not likely to be conducive to recovery in one already infected with the disease.

In an article in the Arena of September, 1892, Dr. Page says:--

"In my fever practice I have frequently observed the effect of fasts of six, eight, ten and twelve days to be in the highest degree productive of the health and comfort of patients, as, on the other hand I have, during the past twenty years observed the deplorable effects of the almost universal plan of constant feeding. In some of the most distressing cases that have happened to be thrown in my way, when all hope in the minds of friends had been abandoned, I have found that withdrawal of food, drugs and stimulants, and the substitution of simple, fresh, soft water, has produced results that seemed almost miraculous."

Fruit juices are now permitted by many physicians in fever, a few drops of lemon or orange juice, being a grateful addition to the water. Grape juice, unfermented, is highly recommended by some.

A young minister of great promise died recently of typhoid fever. His young wife, only one year married, is in settled melancholy, because she cannot understand why "God took her husband." Inquiry developed the fact that the physician in attendance was a believer in alcohol as a remedy, and used it in this case. In view of the better chances of recovery under non-alcoholic treatment shown by comparative death-rates, may it not be that the alcohol was responsible for the young man's death, instead of its being "God's will to take him?" The Author of all good has too frequently been held responsible for the errors of physicians, and the carelessness of nurses.

VOMITING:--"If the vomiting is due to undigested food, and the sickness can be traced to excess, or to improper diet, draughts of hot water should be taken in order to be rid of offending matter in the stomach. After the stomach is empty bits of ice may be sucked, or cold water sipped. A quarter of a Seidlitz powder may be taken. A flannel, folded to four thicknesses, dipped in hot water, and wrung dry in a towel, may be applied to the pit of the stomach. Cover the flannel with a hot plate, being careful to have the flannel large enough to prevent the plate's burning the skin. Pin a dry towel over all, around the body. This may be renewed every half-hour or hour, as required. Sometimes a cold wet compress on the pit of the stomach, covered with a dry towel is more efficacious, heat developing by reaction. Fluid magnesia is often helpful."--DR. RIDGE.

CHAPTER IX.

ALCOHOL AND NURSING MOTHERS.

It frequently happens that the nursing mother is unable by reason of defective digestive apparatus, or imperfect assimilative powers, to supply sufficient nourishment for her babe. In such case she is often advised to drink ale or beer. It is true that these liquors will excite the secretions of the mammary gland, but it is increase in quantity, not in quality, for the milk is impoverished by the added water and alcohol, taken in the beer. Milkmen sometimes salt cows heavily so that they will drink largely of water, and thus give more milk, but one quart of good, rich milk is worth three quarts of the poor, thin stuff resulting from such method. It is proper feeding, and care, that ensure good milk.

When women complain that they are unable to nurse their babies the cause is often an error in diet. Too great reliance is put upon meat as strength-giving. While meat, used in moderation, may be valuable to many persons, the nursing mother should not depend upon it to any great extent. She will find farinaceous foods, with plenty of warm milk, what she most requires. At bedtime she should have a bowl of well-cooked oatmeal gruel, diluted with rich milk, and sweetened, if she prefer it so. The milk should be added to the gruel while it is boiling, as it digests more readily if scalded. People who cannot, or think they cannot, take milk of itself, often find it easy to digest it, after it is scalded in the gruel. Anything that a mother can do in the way of nourishing her babe will be done upon such a diet, that is, farinaceous foods and milk. Sweet fruits are of course valuable also, as tending to keep the system in good order.

It is well to bear in mind that it is not the quantity of food eaten, but that which is digested, and assimilated, that goes to build up the tissues of the body. So the habit of eating between meals is pernicious, as it disturbs the digestive processes, and robs the stomach of much-needed rest. This habit is the cause, in many cases, of the falling off in the milk after the first month or two.

As nourishment for both mother and babe can come from food only, good appetite, and good digestion are essential to health and strength. The very best help towards gaining a good appetite is exercise in the open air. All mothers recognize the need of keeping their little ones out of doors a while every day, but all do not see the necessity of the same mode of life for themselves. Dr. Nathan S. Davis has said: "I have persuaded thousands of mothers to try fresh air, instead of wine or beer, with gratifying results." The mother who takes her babe out, herself, for its daily airing, is laying up stores of health and vitality, to aid her in providing for the needs of the little one, dependent upon her.

Good digestion is as essential as good appetite. Alcohol, whether in beer, wine, whisky, or any other form, is injurious to the stomach, and a hinderer of digestion, hence must do harm, rather than good, to the mother in search of added nourishment for her babe.

Dr. Condi says:--

"The only drink of the nurse should be water or milk. All fermented and distilled liquors, as well as strong tea and coffee, she should strictly abstain from. Never was there a more absurd or pernicious notion than that wine, ale or porter is necessary to a nursing mother in order to keep up her strength, or to increase the quantity, and improve the properties of her milk. So far from producing these effects, such drinks, when taken in any quantity, invariably disturb more or less the health of the stomach, and tend to impair the quality, and diminish the quantity, of nourishment furnished by her to her infant."

Dr. William Hargreaves says:--

"Every farmer knows that all a healthy cow requires to give good milk and butter is, to give her good feed, and pure water; and he also knows that the way to make a cow give poor watery milk, which they might churn until doomsday without obtaining butter, is to feed her on distillery slops, or grains from the brewery. It is also well known that cheese cannot be made from such milk, it being deficient in curd, or casein.

"Alcohol is not only useless but injurious; for children whose mothers try to keep themselves upon beer, etc., very frequently suffer from vomiting and diarrhoea, and often from convulsions. Sometimes a single glass of whisky, taken by the mother, will produce sickness and indigestion in the child, for twenty-four hours after.

"In the milk of a healthy woman the water ranges from 879 to 905 parts in 1,000. The oily substance ranges from 25 to 42; casein from 15 to 39; sugar of milk from 31 to 45, and the salts from 1 to 4 parts in 1,000.

"Alcoholic drinks materially alter these proportions, for, on the analysis of the milk of the same woman, a few hours before and after the use of a pint of beer, it was found that the alcohol increases the proportion of the water, and diminishes that of casein; and that alcohol is very perceptible in it."

"The only rational way to be adopted by mothers to increase the supply of nutrition for their infants, is to secure plenty of suitable nutritious food, prepared in the way that will most fit it for digestion, while they at the same time, avoid as far as possible all fatigue, and mental excitement. It is impossible that alcoholic beverages can add anything to the nutrition of either the infant or mother."--Dr. Bussey, in Stimulants for Nursing Mothers.

Dr. E. G. Figg, in The Physiological Operation of Alcohol, gives the analyses of the milk of a temperate woman in good health, and of a drinking woman as follows:--

Milk of temperate mother. Milk of drinking mother.

Salts, " " 8.50 Salts, " " 5.50 Casein, " " 3.0 Casein, " " 2.0 Oil, " " 7.50 Oil, " " 6.5 Water, " " 81.0 Water, " " 84.0 Alcohol, " " 2.0 ------ ------ 100.00

Dr. Edward Smith says in his Practical Dietary:--

"Alcoholics are largely used by many women in the belief that they support the system, and maintain the supply of milk for the infant; but I am convinced that this is a serious error, and is not an infrequent cause of fits and emaciation in the child."

Dr. James Edmunds, of the Lying-In Hospital, London, Eng., says in Diet for Nursing Mothers:--

"The nursing mother is peculiarly placed, in that she has to provide a supply of nutriment for the child which is dependent upon her, as well as for the ordinary requirements of her own system. The nutrition of the child is to be provided for upon the same principles, and by the same food-elements, as is the nutrition of the mother, the only difference being that the young child is possessed of less perfect masticatory and digestive powers, and therefore requires food to be presented to it in a state more simple, uniform, and readily assimilable than the adult, who is furnished with strong teeth, and possessed of a fully-grown stomach. The mastication, digestion, and primary assimilation of the nursing infant's food is thrown upon the mother's organs; but the tissues of the child are nourished precisely as are the tissues of the mother, and a nursing mother requires simply to digest a larger supply of wholesome, and appropriate food. As a matter of course mothers with imperfect teeth, or weak stomachs, cannot perform the digestion of extra food for the infant so well as those mothers who have an abundance of reserve power in their digestive apparatus; and with such patients, the question arises, how are they to make up for the deficiency which they soon experience in the supply of milk? Such mothers appeal to their medical advisers to prescribe some stimulant which will enable them to overcome the difficulty which they experience, and often are greatly dissatisfied if informed that there is no drug in the materia medica which will make up for structural weakness in the organs which masticate, digest or assimilate the food. The proper course for such women to adopt is a simple and rational one. They should assist their digestive apparatus as much as possible by securing an abundance of suitable and nutritious food, prepared in the best way, and as is most digestible, while they should lessen the demands of their own system by the avoidance of bodily fatigue, and mental excitement. These means, aided by that philosophical hygiene which is at all times essential to the preservation of pure and perfect health, will enable them to supply a maximum quantity of pure and wholesome milk; and further calls by the child require proper artificial food. Unfortunately such advice fails to satisfy many anxious mothers who refuse to admit, or believe, that they are less robust, or less capable, than other ladies of their acquaintance, and such mothers fall easy victims to circulars vaunting the nourishing properties of 'Hoare's Stout,' 'Tanqueray's Gin,' or Gilbey's 'strengthening Port,' circulars which are always backed up by the example, and advice, of lady friends, who themselves have acquired the habit of using these liquors, and who view as a reproach to themselves the practice of any other lady who may not keep them in countenance, as the perfection of all moral and physical propriety. Unfortunately the pressure of such lady friends is often so persistent as to paralyse the influence of a conscientious and thoughtful medical adviser, while the appetites and beliefs of such friends often throw them into active antagonism to any medical adviser, who may not endorse the habits in which, as they believe, and no doubt conscientiously, duty to their child requires them to indulge. The only course that a medical practitioner, whose family is dependent upon his practice, can safely take with veteran mothers on this question, is to let them have their own way without reiterated admonition. When once they have acquired the habit of depending upon large quantities of beer for nursing their children, they become perfectly infatuated, and are practically incapable of passing through the probationary fortnight which takes place before the digestive apparatus can work under its natural, but to them strange, conditions, while the temporary longing for beer, and the sudden lessening of the quantity of milk afforded by their strained and impoverished systems, are at once set down as clear proofs that their medical adviser is a crochetty, and dangerous person, who must be superseded at the first convenient opportunity. Facts and arguments have no more influence on such mothers than they have upon opium-eaters, drunkards, or inveterate consumers of tobacco; while the extreme propriety of conduct which these ladies manifest, and the encouragement they receive from other medical men, make the convictions based upon their own personal sensations incontrovertible, and their position practically unassailable. I think I might fairly say that among the comfortable middle classes of society the views at present held on this question are so deplorable that a large proportion of children are never sober from the first moment of their existence until they have been weaned; while often after a few years the use of alcohol is again introduced to the children as a 'medical comfort,' as a part of their regular diet, or as an invariable accompaniment of all their juvenile visitation, and company-keeping. Under such circumstances, it is not surprising that temperance reformers appeal in vain on this question, and that their facts and arguments are viewed with plausible indifference, or insidious opposition, by persons whose appetites and instincts have been undergoing debasement, and perversion from the very dawn of their lives. My own deliberate conviction is that nothing but harm comes to nursing mothers, and to the infants who are dependent upon them, by the ordinary use of alcoholic beverages of any kind.

"Infants nursed by mothers who drink much beer also become fatter than usual, and to an untrained eye sometimes appear as 'magnificent children.' But the fatness of such children is not a recommendation to the more knowing observer; they are extremely prone to die of inflammation of the chest (bronchitis) after a few days' illness from an ordinary cold. They die, very much more frequently than other children, of convulsions and diarrhoea, while cutting their teeth, and they are very liable to die of scrofulous inflammation of the membranes of the brain, commonly called 'water on the brain,' while their childhood often presents a painful contrast--in the way of crooked legs, and stunted or ill-shapen figure--to the 'magnificent,' and promising appearance of their infancy.

"Those ladies who adopt the general views I have thus expressed in relation to the nursing of their children, will want to know what is the 'proper artificial food' with which to supplement their milk when it is deficient in quantity. With some patients the milk will fall off in quantity at the end of two or three months. With others, although the quantity may not fall off, the child seems unsatisfied; and there is a third class with whom a profusion of milk is supplied, and the child thrives exceedingly, but the mother gets flabby, weak, nervous, pale and exhausted. In the last case, the mother is simply goaded on by susceptibility of her nervous system, or by inordinate activity of the breasts to yield an amount of milk which her digestive powers are not equal to providing for. The treatment of such cases should be simply repressive. The mother should separate herself somewhat more from the child, and make a rule of only nursing it from five to eight times in the twenty-four hours, while the neck of the mother should be kept cool in regard to dress, and cold sponging may be practiced carefully night and morning. Her attention should be diverted by outdoor exercise on foot, and additionally in a carriage if necessary. When the mother's milk, though apparently not deficient in quantity, proves unsatisfying to the child, great attention should be paid to varying the diet of the mother, while such staple foods should be taken as are most easily and thoroughly assimilated into milk. The unsatisfying quality of the milk will generally be remedied by taking a more varied diet, together with three or four half pints of milk in the course of the day, accompanied with farinaceous matter, as in the shape of well-made milk gruel; and in case these measures fail, the only alternative is to supplement the mother's milk by obtaining a wet-nurse to suckle the child three or four times a day alternately with the mother, or by feeding the child with proper artificial food. The same measures may be resorted to where the milk, though satisfying in character, is deficient in quantity; and in preparing artificial food for the child it must always be remembered that the food requires to be adapted to the stage of development which is manifested by a young infant's digestive organs. The infant's digestive apparatus is, in fact, designed to digest milk, and to digest nothing else, but when the teeth are cut farinaceous matter of a more or less solid character should be gradually mixed with the milk. Almost all the illnesses of infants under twelve months of age are caused by some gross impropriety of diet, or otherwise, on the part of the mother, for which the child suffers through the medium of the milk, or they are caused by feeding the child with improper artificial food. Thick sop, and many other articles often given as food are as indigestible to an infant of three months old as beefsteaks would be to a horse; and, until the child has cut its teeth, it should have nothing but food resembling the mother's milk as closely as possible.

"The proper way to feed an infant of three months old, whose mother is only able to partially support it, is as follows: When the child wakes in the morning it should not go to the mother, but should be taken away by the nurse, and immediately fed from the bottle, sucking its milk through a suitable teat. After the mother has breakfasted the child may go to the breast, and during the day it should be alternately fed from the bottle, and nursed by the mother. At six o'clock the baby should invariably be placed in its crib, by the side of the mother's bed, and fed just before going to sleep, and the habit of going to bed at six o'clock should be strictly and invariably enforced. If once the child be allowed to come down to the family circle after dark, the habit of going to sleep will be broken, and the child will continuously cry to come down. In the course of the evening the mother may nurse the child once, and at ten or eleven o'clock, when the mother goes to bed, the child should be again fed from the bottle, and the mother should have a basin of well-made milk-gruel; and by her bedside should be placed, at the last moment, as much gruel as she is likely to drink with relish during the night. Whenever the child is restless it should be taken out of its crib, gently, by the mother, and nursed, say two or three times during the night, and put back again into its crib, the child never being allowed to sleep with the mother. When the night is fairly over, and the child awakens, it should be fetched by the nurse, and have its first morning meal from the bottle. This plan of feeding should be persisted in continuously until the child has cut its teeth; and it is only when every means have been taken to ensure the sweetness, freshness and niceness, not only of the milk and water, but of the bottle and of the teat, and the child still fails to get on, that, in rare cases, I advise the admixture of a little farinaceous matter, in the way of food containing one part milk, and two parts of properly sweetened barley-water. As the milk teeth come through, other farinaceous matter may be gradually blended with the milk, and there is nothing better than to begin at about eight months with a teaspoonful of baked flour, well boiled in a pint of milk and water, or in the water, to be afterwards cooled with milk. Oftentimes a little salt, as well as sugar, will materially help its digestion. The child will do well on that food--the quantity being duly increased--until it has cut almost all its milk teeth, when it may eat bread and butter, rice, and egg puddings, and occasionally eat a boiled egg once a day. I believe that it is a great mistake to give red flesh meat to children in their early years, unless there be some very special reason for it, and then it should only be temporarily used; but nice potatoes, flavored with fresh gravy from a joint, may be given at dinner, as the child becomes able to feed itself. * * * * *

"Bear in mind that when you take wine, beer or brandy, you are distilling that wine, beer or brandy into your child's body. Probably nothing could be worse than to have the very fabric of the child's tissues laid down from alcoholized blood."

Another English physician deplores "the pernicious habit of drinking large quantities of ale or stout by nursing mothers, under the idea that they thereby increase and improve the secretion of milk, whereas they are in reality deteriorating the quality of that upon which the infant must depend for health and life."

Dr. Edis says:--

"Infant mortality is mainly due to two causes, the substitution of farinaceous food for milk, and the delusion that ale or beer is necessary as an article of diet for nursing mothers. * * * * * Countless disorders among infants are due simply and solely to the popular fallacy, that the nursing mother cannot properly fulfil her duties, unless she resorts to the aid of alcoholics."

Dr. N. S. Davis says:--

"The opinion prevails quite extensively among certain classes of people, and with some physicians, that a liberal use of beer is beneficial to women while nursing their children. They drink it under the impression that it will both strengthen them and make their milk more abundant. But I have never seen a case in which it had been used regularly for any considerable period of time, where it did not result in more or less indigestion from gastric irritation and disordered secretions, and an early failure in the secretion of milk. It probably never increases the flow of milk any more than would the drinking of the same quantity of pure water; while the alcohol it contains, by daily repetition, induces congestion of the gastric mucous membrane, with disordered gastric and hepatic secretions.

"A case strikingly illustrating these results was examined by me to-day. The patient was a young married woman who was nursing her first child, now nine months old. At the time of her confinement she was in fair health, rather nervous temperament, weight 120 pounds. During the first few days her milk did not flow very freely, and she says her physician advised her to drink beer. Consequently she commenced to drink a glass of beer at each mealtime, and a bottle during the night. During the first six months she had sufficient milk for her baby; but before the end of that time she had begun to suffer from flatulency, constipation, gaseous and acid eructations, what she calls 'heart-burn,' and sometimes vomiting. During the last three months she has suffered, in addition to the preceding symptoms, one or two attacks each week of extreme pain, from the lower point of the sternum to the back between the scapula, accompanied by retching, or severe efforts to vomit. To relieve these attacks she has taken liberal doses of gin, in addition to her regular supply of beer. Now at the end of nine months, her milk has nearly ceased to flow, her bowels are costive, her stomach tolerates only small quantities of the simplest nourishment, her flesh and strength are very much reduced, her weight being only 96 pounds; and yet she thinks both the beer and gin make her feel better every time she takes them. Such is the delusive power of the an鋥thetic effect of alcohol. A persistence in the same management would probably terminate fatally in from six to twelve months more, from chronic gastritis, and inanition. But if she will rigidly abstain from all alcoholic remedies, and take only the most bland, unirritating nourishment, aided by mildly soothing and antiseptic remedies, and fresh air, she will slowly recover."

In a clinical lecture delivered before the Senior Class in the Northwestern University Medical School, Dr. Davis told of a case similar to the preceding:--

"The flow of milk in her breasts has also diminished to such a degree that she does not have half enough for her baby. Yet she says the beer makes her feel better after each drink, and that the gin helps to relieve the severe attacks of pain, and consequently she thinks she could not do without them. It is undoubtedly true that the patient feels temporary relief from the an鋥thetic effect of the alcohol in her beer and gin, just as she would from any an鋥thetic or narcotic. And it is equally true that so long as the alcohol is present in her blood it so modifies the hemoglobin and albuminous constituents, as to diminish the reception and internal distribution of oxygen, and thereby retards metabolic changes. But the combined influence of the alcohol in retarding the internal distribution of oxygen and the drain upon the nutritive elements of her blood, in furnishing milk for her baby, led to rapid impoverishment of the blood and tissues, and the early establishment of a sufficient grade of gastritis to cause indigestion, frequent vomiting, and, later, paroxysms of severe gastralgia, with general emaciation, and loss of strength.

"In accordance with the present popular ideas, both in and out of the profession, this patient tells me she has tried a great variety of foods, peptonized, sterilized, and predigested, but all to no purpose. And why?-- Simply because her troubles are not in the kind of food she takes, but in the morbid condition of her blood, and of the mucous membrane and nerves of her stomach. Consequently the rational indications for treatment are: (a) to get her stomach and blood free from the alcohol of beer and gin; (b) to encourage the reception and internal distribution of oxygen by plenty of fresh air; (c) to give her the most bland, or unirritating food in small, and frequently repeated doses, of which good milk with lime-water, and milk and wheat-flour gruel are the best; (d) such medicines as possess sufficient antiseptic, and anodyne properties to allay the irritability of the gastric mucous membrane, and lessen fermentation."

CHAPTER X.

COMPARATIVE DEATH-RATES WITH AND WITHOUT THE USE OF ALCOHOL AS A REMEDY.

A study of statistics relating to the difference in results of the treatment of disease with and without the use of alcohol, cannot but be of great interest to all students of the alcohol question. The appended statistics are culled mainly from the Medical Pioneer of England, now, Medical Temperance Review, the journal of the British Medical Temperance Association, and from the Bulletin of the American Medical Temperance Association.

A paragraph in the British Medical Journal, for Dec. 2, 1893, says:--

"An interesting fact has been noted by Dr. Claye Shaw, at the London County Asylum, Banstead, for the Insane. Since the withdrawal of beer from the dietary, the rate of recovery has gone up. During the past year, for example, the recoveries reached 46.97 per cent. Nearly one half of the patients had thus recovered during the period stated. The inmates take their food better without the liquor, and they are thus taught that intoxicants are not a necessity of ordinary health."

In the Medical Pioneer for January, 1894, Dr. John Mois, medical superintendent of West Haven Infectious Diseases Hospital, states that prior to 1885 he had treated 2,148 cases of smallpox "in the usual routine method, with the use of alcohol when the heart's action seemed to indicate it;" resulting in a mortality of 17 per cent. But since 1885 he has treated 700 additional cases under similar circumstances except that the use of alcoholic preparations was entirely omitted, and the resulting mortality was only 11 per cent.

In the same journal, Dr. J. J. Ridge states that he had treated the 200 cases of scarlet fever admitted into the Enfield Isolation Hospital during the years 1892 and 1893, without alcohol in any form, with a mortality of only 2.5 per cent.; while the mortality in the hospitals under the Metropolitan Asylums Board in 1893, in which alcohol was used in accordance with the usual practice in scarlet fever, was 6.3 per cent.

Dr. J. J. Ridge says later:--

"In January, 1894, I published the result of the treatment of the first 200 cases of scarlatina admitted into the temporary wards of the Enfield Isolation Hospital during 1892 and 1893. I stated that there had been five fatal cases, but that one was dying when admitted and only lived a few hours. The mortality was 2 per cent., or 2.5 if the later case is included.

"Since then 300 more cases have been admitted and discharged and among these there have been 7 fatal. Hence there have been 14 deaths in 500 consecutive cases extending over a period of a little more than four years. One of these ought to be excluded, no time having been given for treatment. Hence the mortality has been just 2.6 per cent. This, I think it will be admitted, is a low mortality, although it is possible it may be even lower when the cases are treated in a permanent hospital about to be erected.

"It may be interesting to state that 4 of the cases died on the third day after admission; 1 on the fourth; 1 on the sixth; 1 on the tenth, with pneumonia; 1 on the thirteenth; 1 on the fifteenth; 1 on the sixteenth; 1 on the eighteenth; 1 on the thirty-sixth, with nephritis and pleuropneumonia; and 1 on the forty-sixth, with otitis and meningitis.

"All the cases have been treated without alcohol either as food or drug, although many have been of great severity with various complications. It is certain that the absence of alcohol has not been detrimental, since the mortality is less than three-fourths of that of the mortality among all notified cases in England and Wales. I am bound to say that it is my firm conviction that had alcohol been given in the usual fashion, the death-rate would have been higher. Cases have been admitted to which alcohol has been given previous to admission, apparently with harm, as they have improved without it. One case was particularly noticeable in this respect. A child, aged 6, had had a good deal of whisky, and was supposed to be dying when admitted on the fourth day of the disease, so that the doctor who had seen it was surprised, when he called the following day to inquire, to find it was still alive. Without a drop of alcohol it began to improve and made a good recovery. I may say that delirium is very rare, even in the worst cases treated non-alcoholically."

Dr. Norman Kerr says:--

"In my paper on 'The Medical Administration of Alcohol,' read to the section of medicine at the Sheffield meeting in 1876, I cited several medical testimonies in favor of non-alcoholic treatment of fevers, notably that of my friend, the late Dr. Simon Nicolls, who had a mortality of less than 5 per cent. in 230 cases.

"The record of the results of a greatly lessened administration of alcohol in the treatment of smallpox in the London hospital ships, is of deep interest. Having been requested to inquire into the effects of this diminished alcoholic stimulation on mortality and convalescence, Dr. Birdwood stated that though the gravity of the cases had increased, with a mortality of 15 per 100 in the metropolis, the ship's death-rate had remained at less than 7 per 100. Convalescence had been more rapid, and there had been fewer and less serious complications from abscesses and inflammatory boils. Other causes had contributed to this improvement, but the medical officers attributed a considerable share in the amelioration to a greatly diminished prescription of alcohol."

The Medical Pioneer says:--

"In 1872 there appeared in the Saturday Review an article in which the medical practitioners of this country were accused of inciting their patients to free drinking, and in the discussion which this article called forth, Dr. Gairdner, of Glasgow, said that fever patients in that city, when treated with milk and without alcohol, did much better than those reported as having been treated by Dr. Todd with large doses of alcohol; the latter resulting in a mortality of about 25 per cent., while those treated by Dr. Gairdner with milk had had a death-rate of only 12 per cent. About this time the British Medical Temperance Association was founded, owing to the exertions of Dr. Ridge, of Enfield, and in 1876 it was enrolled, under the presidency of Sir B. W. Richardson. It now contains 269 members in England and Wales, 53 in Scotland and 80 in Ireland, or more than 400 altogether, all professional men and women. This, I think, is but a sign of the change of opinion on the use of alcoholic fluids in medical practice, for all who remember what medical practice was in London thirty years ago know that the use of wine and brandy in hospital practice was so common that it was quite a rarity in some hospitals to find a patient who was not ordered, by some of the staff, from three to four ounces of brandy or six to eight fluid ounces of wine. The expense caused to the hospitals by this practice was, of course, great, and increased notably between 1852 and 1872, owing to the prevalence of the views of Liebig and his follower, Dr. Todd. The writings of Parkes, Gairdner, Dr. Norman Kerr and of Sir B. Ward Richardson, Dr. Morton and others, gradually lessened this predilection for treating diseases by alcohol, and accordingly between 1872 and 1882 a great change came over the practice of London hospitals. Thus the sum paid for milk in 1852 in Saint Bartholomew's Hospital was ?84, and in 1882 it was ?,012; whilst alcohol in that hospital cost in 1852, ?06; in 1862, ?,446; in 1872, ?,446; and in 1882 only ?53. Westminster Hospital in 1882 spent ?37 on alcohol and ?00 on milk. One hospital, St. George's, long continued to use large quantities of alcohol. That hospital in 1872 had the high mortality among its typhoid fever patients of 24 per cent., which was twice as high as that noted by Dr. Gairdner as occurring in Glasgow, when alcohol was abandoned and milk used instead. Dr. Meyer, who reported these cases of typhoid treated in Saint

George's Hospital at that time, mentioned that alcohol in large doses was given to 87 per cent. of the patients. Three-fifths of these patients took daily eight ounces of brandy when there was danger of sinking from failure of the heart's action. One-fourth of the number took sixteen fluid ounces of brandy in the 24 hours."

"In 230 typhoid cases in St. Mary's Hospital, Dr. Chambers reduced the ratio of deaths from 1 in 5 with alcohol to 1 in 40 without it. Dr. Perry, of Glasgow, found that of 534 cases treated with alcohol, 138 died, while of 491 treated without alcohol, only 9 died."

In a recent text-book on medicine occurs the following:--

"English physicians use spirits in fevers, and all experience sustains the conviction that no substitute has been found for them."

In a late number of the Temperance Record, Dr. Smith gives a different view of the experience of English physicians:--

"When Bentley Todd was at King's College, and leading his profession, brandy was the rule in febrile cases. Then the mortality varied from twenty-five to thirty-five per cent. That the treatment was as fatal as the disease, experience demonstrates:--

"1. Professor W. T. Gairdner, of Glasgow, writing to the Lancet (1864), gave his experience as follows:--

Fever cases Average of treated. wine and spirits. Mortality.

1,829 34 oz. to each 17.69 per cent. 595 2-1/2 oz. to each 11.93 per cent. 212 none 1 death only. (young lives)

"These were mostly typhus cases, but the rationale, so far as alcohol is concerned, is the same as in typhoid.

"2. At the British Medical Association in 1879, Professor H. MacNaughton Jones gave particulars of 340 cases of typhus, typhoid and simple fever. I append a summary:--

Cases. Deaths. Mortality per cent.

Given brandy 58 19 32.7 Given claret 51 2 3.8 Given no alcohol 231 4 1.7

"3. Dr. J. C. Pearson writes to the Lancet (Dec. 5 and 26, 1891), giving his experience of typhoid. He had treated several hundreds of cases without a single death, and never prescribed stimulants in any shape or form in the disease.

"4. Dr. Knox Bond writes to the Lancet (Nov. 25, 1893), giving his experience of typhoid at the Liverpool Fever Hospital. He says: 'As a resident for some years in the fever hospitals, my views of the value of alcohol in fever underwent, solely as a result of the experience there gained, entire modification. The conviction became forced upon my mind that in no case in which it was used did benefit to the patient ensue; that in a proportion of cases its use was distinctly hurtful; and that in a small but appreciable number of cases the resultant harm was sufficient to tilt the balance as against the recovery of the patient.'

"In plain terms, alcohol tended to the destruction of the patients. Dr. Bond's figures are:--

No. of cases. No. of deaths.

Given alcohol 71 18 Given no alcohol 309 15 --- --- 380 33

In May, 1890, Dr. Nathan S. Davis, read a paper before the American

Medical Association upon the use of certain drugs in disease. Among the drugs mentioned was alcohol, and comparative death-rates were given in typhoid fever and pneumonia, between Mercy Hospital, Chicago, during a term of years when no alcohol was used in the medical wards, Dr. Davis being in charge of them, and some of the large metropolitan hospitals using alcohol. In Mercy Hospital without alcohol, the death-rate in typhoid fever was only five per cent.; in pneumonia only twelve per cent.

"Of 161 cases of typhoid fever treated in Cook County Hospital during 1889, 27 died, or one in six--nearly 17 per cent.

"According to the annual report of the Cincinnati Hospital for 1886, 47 cases of typhoid fever were treated during that year, with seven deaths, a mortality rate of 16 per cent.

"The Garfield Memorial Hospital, at Washington, reported for the year 1889, 22 cases of typhoid fever, with 5 deaths--or 22 per cent.

"In the Pennsylvania Hospital the mortality rate in pneumonia for the years 1884-1886, was 34 per cent.

"The mortality of pneumonia in the Massachusetts General Hospital, between the years 1822 and 1889, comprising 1,000 cases, was 25 per cent.; but a gradual increase in mortality had been noted from 10 per cent. in the first decade of the seventy years represented by this report, to 28 per cent. in the last decade.

"According to the report of the Supervising Surgeon General of the U.S. Marine Hospital Service for 1888, the number of cases of pneumonia treated between 1880 and 1887 was 1,649, with 311 deaths--nearly 19 per cent.

"The Cincinnati Hospital reported for 1886 a mortality rate in pneumonia of 38 per cent.

"The mortality rate in the Cook County Hospital, Chicago, for 1889, according to Dr. Heltoin, relating to 80 cases of pneumonia, was 36 per cent."

Only a five per cent. death-rate in typhoid fever without alcohol, and from sixteen to twenty-two per cent. with alcohol; only a twelve per cent. death-rate in pneumonia without alcohol, and from 19 to as high as 38 per cent. with alcohol. Such are the comparative death-rates given by Dr. Davis. They should be committed to memory by every opposer of the use of alcohol, as they show clearly that people have many more chances for recovery, other things being equal, in the diseases mentioned, if alcohol is not used than if it is.

It is worthy of mention in this connection that Cook County Hospital contains in its report for 1897 the following items: Number of patients 19,536; cost of liquors $80.00; per cent. of deaths from all causes, 5.7. The cost of liquors is only .004 for each patient. This shows a decided advance in the disuse of alcohol, when so very little is used in a great hospital, with so large a number of patients.

Dr. A. L. Loomis, in the treatment of 600 typhus fever cases on Blackwell's Island in 1864, excluded alcoholics, with the result of reducing the mortality rate to only six per cent. whereas it had previously been twenty-two per cent., in Bellevue Hospital from which the patients had been removed.

In Battle Creek Sanitarium no alcohol is used in any disease, simply because the management believe better results are obtained by the use of other agencies. In the October, (1893) number of the American Medical Temperance Quarterly now Bulletin of the A. M. T. A., Dr. J. H. Kellogg gives statistics of deaths from various diseases in the Battle Creek Sanitarium. The total of these statistics is as follows: la grippe, 827 cases, 4 deaths--or two per cent.; scarlet fever, 83 cases, 2 deaths--less than three per cent.; 333 cases of typhoid fever, 9 deaths--or 2.7 per cent.; 82 cases of pneumonia, 4 deaths--or 4.9 per cent. These exceptional results are not attributed solely to the non-use of alcohol. The nursing and surroundings were of the best. But these results certainly show that the use of alcohol as a remedy in acute diseases is not necessary, and that patients have a much better chance for life, other things being equal, where alcohol is not used than where it is.

Dr. Kellogg says of the surgical cases:--

"In a hospital of 100 beds, connected with the institution, more than 3,000 surgical cases have been treated, to whom alcohol has never been administered except in connection with chloroform an 鋥 thesia; my uniform custom being to administer an ounce of brandy or whisky five minutes before beginning the administration of the an 鋥 thetic, when chloroform is used.

"The surgical cases include more than 300 cases of ovariotomy, and over 300 other cases involving the peritoneal cavity, such as operations for strangulated hernia, the radical cure of hernia, etc. The statistics of death and recoveries are certainly as good as can be produced by any hospital in the world, dealing with the same class of cases. The total mortality from the operation of ovariotomy, including nearly 300 cases, is less than three per cent., and for the last few years, in which the antiseptic measures have been perfected, the record is still better, showing a succession of 172 cases of laparotomy for the removal of ovarian tumors, or diseased uterus and ovaries, without a death. These cases include a number of hysterectomies, and many cases so desperate that those who trust in alcohol as a heart stimulant, and as a means of supporting the vital energies, would certainly have considered it necessary to resort to the use of this drug. Nevertheless, it was not administered in a single case, and I have seen no reason to regret its non-use in a single instance."

Dr. T. D. Crothers, of Hartford, Conn., tells the following:--

"In a large hospital a study of the mortality of pneumonia indicated a greater fatality at intervals of six months. There were five per cent. more deaths during periods of two months at a time, twice during the year. This extended back for two years, and was finally narrowed down to the service of an eminent physician who gave spirits freely in all cases of pneumonia from their entrance to the hospital. The other visiting physicians gave very little spirits, and only in the later stages. The physician was skeptical of these statistics, but finally consented to test them by giving up spirits practically in all cases of pneumonia. This was continued for a year, and the mortality went back to the average statistics. That physician has abandoned alcohol as a food and a medicine, only in very limited degree. He writes, 'My stupidity in accepting theories and statements of others, concerning spirits, which I could have tested personally, is a source of deep sorrow, and I do not know but it could be called criminal. I certainly feel that punishment would be just.'"

Brandy has been considered the great necessity in cholera, yet the use of it and other alcoholics are known to expose people to greater danger when this disease prevails.

The Bulletin of the A. M. T. A. is authority for the following:--

"During the epidemic of 1832, Dr. Bronson said: 'In Montreal 1,000 persons have died of cholera, only two of whom were teetotalers.' A Montreal paper said: 'Not a drunkard who has been attacked has recovered from the disease, and almost all the victims have been at least moderate drinkers.'

"In Albany, N. Y., the same year, cholera carried off 366 persons above sixteen years of age, all but four of whom belonged to the drinking classes. Packer, Prentice & Co., large furriers in Albany, employed 400 persons, none of whom used ardent spirits, and there were only two cases of cholera among them. Mr. Delevan, a contractor, said: 'I was engaged at the time in erecting a large block of buildings. The laborers were much alarmed, and were on the point of abandoning the work. They were advised to stay and give up strong drink. They all remained, and all quit the use of strong drink except one, and he fell a victim to the disease.' He says also: 'I had a gang of diggers in a clay bank, to whom the same proposition was made; they all agreed to it, and not one died. On the opposite side of the same clay bank were other diggers who continued their regular rations of whisky, and one third of them died.'

"In New York City there were 204 cases in the park, only six of whom were temperate, and these recovered, while 122 of the others died. In many parts of the city the saloon keepers saw and acknowledged the terrible connection between their business and the spread of the disease, and, becoming alarmed for their own safety, shut up their saloons and fled, saying: 'The way from the saloon to hell is too short.'

"In Washington the Board of Health was so impressed with the terrible facts that they declared the grog shops nuisances, ordered them closed, and they remained closed for three months.

"A prominent physician of Glasgow reported: 'Only nineteen per cent. of the temperate perished, while ninety-one and two-tenths per cent. of the intemperate died.' One extensive liquor dealer of Glasgow, said, 'Cholera has carried off half of my customers.'

"In Warsaw ninety per cent. of those who died from cholera were wine drinkers.

"At Tifels, Prussia, a town of 20,000 inhabitants, every drunkard died of cholera."

The St. Paul Medical Journal, of September, 1899, gives the following report of a railway surgeon, Dr. Kane:--

"From June 1, 1898, to June 1, 1899, the author performed a few more than four hundred operations. Forty-nine abdominal sections, fifty odd more operations of a graver sort, one hundred miscellaneous of less gravity than above, over one hundred operations upon female perineum and uterus. Of the four hundred, more than three hundred demanded an ꞏ thesia. There were but three deaths, making the mortality a little less than one per cent.

"The author does not claim a phenomenally low mortality, nor does he claim specially brilliant results. He has to contend with unreasoning fear on the part of the patients for hospital surgeons, and also most of his cases had been in the hands of quacks, and had subjected themselves to remedies prescribed by old women. Many cases came after the family physician had exhausted his resources. He thinks his results are considerably better than the average in hospitals and in country districts. Alcohol medication was dispensed with entirely after the patients came under his care, and to this he attributes much of his success. He does not believe that alcohol is a stimulant, or a tonic. On the contrary, he believes that it retards digestion, arrests secretion, and hinders excretion. The courage and fortitude of his patients were lessened instead of increased by the use of alcoholic medication.

"Pain is better borne, endured longer and more patiently when alcohol is not used.

"He urges the practical surgeon to carefully weigh the subject of alcohol, and verify for himself the expediency of its use."

Dr. B. W. Richardson in the report of his practice for 1895 in the London Temperance Hospital refers to non-alcoholic treatment of rheumatism. He said:--

"Out of seventy-one cases of acute or subacute rheumatism--the large majority acute, and attended with temperatures moving up to 104?F.--sixty-nine recovered, and two, although they were discharged without being put on the recovery list, were so far relieved that a few days' change in country air seemed all that was required to induce full restoration. Comparing the experience of the treatment of acute rheumatic disease without alcohol with that which I have previously observed with alcohol, I can have no hesitation in declaring that it is of the greatest advantage to follow total abstinence absolutely in this disease. The pain and swelling of joints is more quickly relieved under abstinence, the fever falls more rapidly, there is less frequent relapse, and there is quicker recovery. In brief, the experience of treatment of rheumatic fever minus alcohol, presents to me as much novelty as it does pleasure, and I am convinced that if any candid member of the profession could have witnessed what I have witnessed in this matter, he would agree with me that alcohol in rheumatic fever, however acute, is altogether out of place. I am also under the conviction, though I express it with great reserve, that in acute rheumatism, treated without alcohol, the cardiac complications, endocardial and pericardial, are much less frequently developed than where alcohol is supplied."

Dr. Pechuman in Alcohol--Is It a Medicine, published in 1891, says:--

"There is no disputing that many deaths occur each day as the result of the administration of alcohol in acute diseases, to say nothing of the deaths caused by its habitual use; and those who give it ignore the very fundamental principles of physiology and the many published statistics. The Boston Hospital report tells a sad story in this connection; it shows that out of 1,042 cases treated with alcoholics 386 died, while out of the same number treated without alcohol only 81 died. Using plain English 305 were actually killed by it."

Dr. T. D. Crothers, in the January, 1899, Bulletin of the American Medical Temperance Association, gave the following Hospital Statistics, showing a decline in the use of spirits in hospitals:--

"Evidently a great change is going on in the use of alcohol as a remedy in large hospitals. The annual reports of ten hospitals in the New England and the Middle States show the following widely varying figures. The spirits used include beers, wines, whiskies and brandies, and vary from eleven to sixty-one cents a person for all the cases treated. These hospitals treat from eighty to seven hundred cases a year, both surgical and medical, and the medical staff are the leading physicians of the towns and cities where they are located. The hospital where the largest amount of spirits was used is not different from others, nor is the one where the lowest amount is reported. The conclusion is that this difference is due entirely to the judgment of the medical men. The lowest rate (eleven cents each) was in a hospital where one hundred and twenty-one cases had been under treatment. The highest rate (sixty-one cents) was in a hospital of five hundred and forty cases. The mortality from typhoid fever and pneumonia was eight per cent. higher in this hospital than in the one where only eleven cents a head had been expended for spirits. The general mortality did not vary greatly in any of these hospitals, and the records of one year could not be expected to show this. In the remaining hospitals the mortality of the fever and the septic cases was about the same. The free use of spirits did not show any improvement, but rather an increase of the death-rate, while the same amount of spirits used showed but little change, and that in the line of improvement of death-rate. These are only the figures of one year, but they indicate a change of practice, and show the passing of alcohol as a remedy."

CHAPTER XI.

REASONS WHY ALCOHOL IS DANGEROUS AS MEDICINE.

In the chapter upon "The Effects of Alcohol upon the Human Body" are cited some of the reasons assigned by scientific investigators for their disuse of alcohol as a remedy in disease. In this chapter the same may be briefly hinted at, while others, some the results of quite recent research, will be added.

In the Bulletin of the A. M. T. A., for January 1898, Dr. N. S. Davis says:--

"The supposed effects of alcohol as a medicine were originally based solely on the sensations and actions of the patients taking it. The first appreciable effect of the alcohol after entering the blood is that of an an æsthetic; that is, it diminishes the sensibility of the brain and nerve structures, in the same direction as ether and chloroform. And, as the brain is the material seat of man's consciousness, the alcohol renders him less conscious of cold or heat, of weariness or pain, and less conscious of his own weight or of any external resistance. Consequently, when under the influence of small doses, he feels lighter and less conscious of any external impressions, and thinks he could do more than without it. It was these effects that led both the patient and his physician to regard the alcohol as a general stimulant or tonic, notwithstanding the fact that by simply increasing the doses of alcohol the sensibility soon became entirely suspended, and the patient helpless and altogether unconscious. * * * * *

"Simple increased frequency of the heart action is no evidence of either increased force or efficiency in promoting the circulation of the blood. Indeed, it may be stated as a physiological law, that the more frequent the heart action above the normal standard, the less efficiently does it promote the circulation and strength of the living system. But the effect of a moderate dose of alcohol in increasing the frequency of the heart-beat and of blood pressure is so temporary that the doses must be repeated so often that the alcohol accumulates in the blood and tissues, and extends its paralyzing effects to all the vasomotor, cardiac and respiratory nerves. Indeed, all the investigators agree that alcohol in any dose capable of producing an appreciable effect, diminishes the function of the lungs in direct proportion to the quantity taken; and as the lungs are the only channel through which free oxygen reaches the blood, and such oxygen is the natural exciter of all vital activities in the living body, it is not possible to explain how alcohol, or any other drug that diminishes the function of the lungs can, at the same time, act as a cardiac, or any other kind of tonic.

"The truth is that all intelligent physicians and writers on therapeutics of the present day agree in stating that alcohol in large doses directly diminishes all the vital processes in the living body, and in still larger doses suspends the life of the individual by paralyzing the cerebral, vasomotor, respiratory and cardiac functions, generally in the order named. If large doses produce such effects, we must logically claim that small doses act in the same direction, but in less degree. In other words, alcohol is as truly and exclusively an an 鎮 thetic as is ether or chloroform, and, like them, is to be used as a medicine only temporarily to relieve pain, or suspend nerve sensibility. But as for these purposes it is less efficient than either ether or chloroform, and other narcotics, there is no necessity for using it as a remedy in the treatment of disease. And in health its use in any dose can be productive of nothing but injury. The only legitimate fields for the uses of alcohol are in chemistry, pharmacy and the arts."

In another issue of the same magazine, Dr. Davis writes of the investigations pursued by M. Robin of France in regard to the chemistry of respiration. These investigations, he says, afford conclusive proof that the acts of oxidation are defensive processes of the organism in its struggle with bacteria, and therefore that the physician should favor in every possible way the absorption of oxygen in every infection, especially when there are typhoid complications.

He then speaks of the researches of other scientists in the same line, concluding thus:--

"If we add to the foregoing investigations the results obtained by Dr. A. C. Abbott, demonstrating that the presence of alcohol directly diminished the vital resistance to infections, we cannot fail to see that the administration of alcohol in diphtheria, typhoid fever, pneumonia and other infectious diseases, is directly contraindicated. If, as shown by M. Robin, 'the acts of oxidation are defensive processes' against bacterial infections, then certainly the administration of alcohol to patients with such infections is in the highest degree illogical and injurious. The oxygen being obtained for oxidation purposes in the blood and tissues, through the respiratory process, it would be equally absurd to administer alcohol in all cases in which it is desirable to increase the processes of oxidation, as a long series of experiments has shown that the presence of alcohol diminishes the efficiency of the respiratory process in direct proportion to the quantity used.

"How much longer will practical writers continue to recommend for the same patient on the same day, fresh air, sponge baths, and vasomotor and respiratory tonics to increase the absorption of oxygen and oxidation processes, and alcohol in the form of wine, whisky and brandy to directly diminish the respiratory function and all the oxidations of the living system?"

In his address before the Medical Congress for the Study of Alcohol, held at Prohibition Park, Staten Island, July 15, 1891, Dr. Davis said:--

"If the foregoing views regarding the effects of alcoholic liquids on the human system in health, are correct, what can we say concerning their value as remedies for the treatment of disease? If it be true that the alcohol they contain acts directly upon the corpuscular elements of the blood, and so far diminishes the metabolic processes of nutrition and disintegration as to lessen nerve sensibility and heat production, and favor tissue degenerations, their rational application in the treatment of any form of disease must be very limited. And yet the same errors and delusions concerning their use in the treatment of diseases and accidents are entertained and daily acted upon by a large majority of medical men as are entertained by the non-professional part of the public. Throughout the greater part of our medical literature they are represented as stimulating and restorative, capable of increasing the force and efficiency of the circulation, and of conserving the normal living tissues by diminishing their waste; and hence they are the first to be resorted to in all cases of sudden exhaustion, faintness or shock; the last to be given to the dying; and the most constant remedies through the most important and protracted acute general diseases. Indeed, it is this position and practice of the profession that constitutes, at the present time, the strongest influence in support of all the popular though erroneous and destructive drinking customs of the people.

"The same an鋰thetic properties of the alcohol that render the laboring man less conscious of the cold or heat or weariness, also render the sick man less conscious of suffering, either mental or physical, and thereby deceive both him and his physician by the appearance, temporarily, of more comfort. But if administered during the progress of fevers or acute general disease, while it thus quiets the patient's restlessness and lessens his consciousness of suffering, it also directly diminishes the vasomotor and excito-motor nerve forces with slight reduction of temperature, and steadily diminishes both the tissue metabolism and the excretory products, thereby favoring the retention in the system of both the specific causes of disease and the natural excretory materials which should have been eliminated through the skin, lungs, kidneys and other glandular organs. Although the immediate effect of the remedy is thus to give the patient an appearance of more comfort, the continued dulling or an 鋥 thetic effect on the nervous centres, the diminished oxygenation of the blood, and the continued retention of morbitic and excretory products, all serve to protract the disease, increase molecular degeneration, and add to the number of fatal results.

"I am well aware that the foregoing views, founded on the results of numerous and varied experimental researches and well-known physiological laws, and corroborated by a wide clinical experience, are in direct conflict with the very generally accepted doctrine that alcohol is a cardiac tonic, capable of increasing the force and efficiency of the circulation, and therefore of great value in the treatment of the lower grades of general fevers. But there have been many generally accepted doctrines in the history of medicine that have been proved fallacious. And the more recent experiments of Professors Martin, Sidney Ringer, and Sainsbury, Reichert, H. C. Wood and others, have clearly demonstrated that the presence of alcohol in the blood as certainly diminishes the sensibility of the vasomotor and cardiac nerves in proportion to its quantity until the heart stops, paralyzed, as that two and two make four.

"After an ample clinical field of observation in both hospital and private practice for more than fifty years, and a continuous study of our medical literature, I am prepared to maintain the position that the ratio of mortality from all the acute general diseases has increased in direct proportion to the quantity of alcoholic remedies administered during their treatment. How can we reasonably expect any other result from the use of an agent that so directly and uniformly diminishes the cerebral respiratory, cardiac and metabolic functions of the living human body?"

The Medical Pioneer of January, 1896, contained a very interesting article by Dr. J. H. Kellogg upon "The Influence of Alcohol upon Urinary Toxicity, and its Relation to the Medical Use of Alcohol." He gives the results of many of his own experiments to determine the effects of alcohol in hindering the elimination of poisonous matter by the kidneys. The subject of one experiment was a healthy man of 30 years, weighing 66 kilos. For fifty days prior to the experiment he had taken a carefully regulated diet, and the urotoxic coefficient had remained very nearly uniform. The urine carefully collected for the first eight hours after the administration of 8 ounces of brandy diluted with water, showed an enormous diminution in the urotoxic coefficient, which was, in fact, scarcely more than half the normal coefficient for the individual in question. The urine collected for the second period of eight hours showed an increase of toxicity, and that for the third period of eight hours showed still further increase of toxicity, the coefficient having nearly returned to its normal standard.

Of this Dr. Kellogg says:--

"The bearing of this experiment upon the use of alcohol in pneumonia, typhoid fever, erysipelas, cholera and other infectious diseases, will be clearly seen. In all the maladies named, and in nearly all other infectious diseases, which include the greater number of acute maladies, the symptoms which give the patient the greatest inconvenience, and those which have a fatal termination, when such is the result, are directly attributable to the influence of the toxic substances generated within the system of the patient as the result of the specific microbes to which the disease owes its origin. The activity of the liver in destroying these poisons, and of the kidneys in eliminating them, are the physiologic processes which stand between the patient and death. In a very grave case of infectious disease, without this destructive and eliminative activity the accumulation of poison within the system would quickly reach a fatal point. The symptoms of the patient vary for better or worse in relation to the augmentation or diminution of the quantity of toxic substances within the body.

"In view of these facts, is it not a pertinent question to ask how alcohol can be of service in the treatment of such disorders as pneumonia, typhoid fever, cholera, erysipelas and other infections, since it acts in such a decided and powerful manner in diminishing urinary toxicity--in other words, in lessening the ability of the kidney to eliminate toxic substances? In infectious diseases of every sort, the body is struggling under the influence of toxic agents, the result of the action of microbes. Alcohol is another toxic agent of precisely the same origin. Like other toxins resulting from like processes of bacterial growth, its influence upon the human organism is unfriendly; it disturbs the vital processes; it disturbs every vital function, and, as we have shown, in a most marked degree diminishes the efficiency of the kidneys in the removal of the toxins which constitute the most active factor in the diseases named, and in others of analogous character. If a patient is struggling under the influence of the pneumococcus, Eberth's bacillus, Koch's cholera microbe or the pus-producing germs which give rise to erysipelatous inflammation, his kidneys laboring to undo, so far as possible, the mischief done by the invading parasites, by eliminating the poisons formed by them, what good could possibly be accomplished by the administration of a drug, one of the characteristic effects of which is to diminish renal activity, thereby diminishing also the quantity of poisons eliminated through this channel? Is not such a course in the highest degree calculated to add fuel to the flame? Is it not placing obstacles in the way of the vital forces which are already hampered in their work by the powerfully toxic agents to the influence of which they are subjected?

"In his address before the American Medical Association at Milwaukee, Dr. Ernest Hart, editor of the British Medical Journal, very aptly suggested in relation to the treatment of cholera, the inutility of alcohol, basing his suggestion upon the fact that in a case of cholera, the system of the patient is combating the specific poison which is the product of the microbe of this disease, and hence is not likely to be aided by the introduction of a poison produced by another microbe; namely, alcohol. This logic seems very sound, and the facts in relation to the influence of alcohol upon urinary toxicity or renal activity, which are elucidated by our experiment, fully sustain this observation of Mr. Hart.

"In a recent number of the British Medical Journal, Dr. Lauder Brunton, the eminent English physiologist and neurologist, in mentioning the fact that death from chloroform an鑵thesia rarely occurs in India, but is not infrequent in England, attributed the fact to the meat-eating habits of the English people, the natives of India being almost strictly vegetarian in diet, partly from force of circumstances doubtless, but largely also, no doubt, as the result of their religious belief, the larger proportion of the population being more or less strict adherents to the doctrines of Buddha, which strictly prohibit the use of flesh foods.

"The theory advanced by Dr. Lauder Brunton in relation to death from chloroform poisoning, is that the patient does not die directly from the influence of chloroform upon the nerve centres, but that death is due to the influence of chloroform upon the kidneys, whereby the elimination of the ptomaines and leucomaines naturally produced within the body, ceases, their destruction by the liver also ceasing, so that the system is suddenly overwhelmed by a great quantity of poison, and succumbs to its influence, its power of resistance being lessened by the inhalation of the chloroform.

"The affinity between alcohol and chloroform is very great. Both are an鑵 thetics. Both chloroform and alcohol are simply different compounds of the same radical, and the results of our experiment certainly suggest the same thought as that expressed by Dr. Brunton. How absurd, then, is the administration of alcohol in conditions in which the highest degree of kidney activity is required for the elimination of toxic agents!

"In a certain proportion of chronic cases there is a tendency to tissue degeneration. Modern investigations have given good ground for the belief that these degenerations are the result of the influence of ptomaines, leucomaines and other poisons produced within the body, upon the tissues. It is well known that many of these toxic agents, even in very small quantity give rise to degenerations of the kidney. It is this fact which explains the occurrence of nephritis in connection with diphtheria, scarlet fever and other infectious maladies. Dana has called attention to the probable role played by ptomaines produced in the alimentary canal in the development of organic disease of the central nervous system.

"It is thus apparent that the integrity of the renal functions is a matter of as great importance in chronic as in acute disease, hence any agent which diminishes the efficiency of these organs in ridding the system of poisons, either those normally and regularly produced, or those of an accidental or unusual character, must be pernicious and dangerous in use."

Among the more recent findings of science in regard to the effects of alcohol are the action of this drug upon the leucocytes or "guardian cells" of the body. Leucocytes are defined to be "minute, nucleated, colorless masses of protoplasm, capable of ameboid movements, found swimming freely in blood and lymph, in the reticulum of lymphatic glands, and in bone-marrow and other connective tissue." The white corpuscles of the blood are leucocytes. "The work of these cells is to prey upon and take into their substance bacteria and other micro-organisms within the blood and tissues. This destruction of bacteria, and other noxious organisms, has the biological name of phagocytosis."

Dr. Alonzo Brown in Physician and Surgeon says of phagocytosis:--

"Recently a brilliant theory has been projected into the histological world. It is the principle of phagocytosis. The beauty of it is so great that we are attracted by it, and its reasonings have riveted general attention. It is said that certain cells have the power to absorb and so destroy other cells. This is phagocytosis. It is said that 'the cells which are known to possess phagocytocic properties are the leucocytes, mucous corpuscles, connective tissue cells, endothelia of blood vessels and lymphatic vessels, alveolar eypithelium of the lungs, and the cells of the spleen, bone, marrow and lymphatic glands.' (Senn). This is a very significant array of colloid matter; and it has been repeatedly affirmed by the highest authorities that alcohol is poisonous to the colloid element.

"Now, among the most important of the phagocytes just enumerated are the leucocytes. They embrace and enfold the pathogenic germs with which they come in contact by what is known as an ameboid force. They enclose, disintegrate and absorb the enemy. It is well known that the moment the leucocytes are submitted to an alcoholic solution, their ameboid movements cease, and their function is arrested. It is plain that their phagocytocic power is immediately destroyed. It is possible, also, that the fixed tissue-cells are likewise impaired or killed by alcoholic imbibition. How deleterious, and even deadly, must the internal administration of alcoholic liquors then be in the treatment of diphtheria, and of other diseases having a germinal origin? It therefore follows, to my mind, that all the diseases which are the result of germinal infection, are most badly treated when alcohol is used in their therapy.

"With extreme brevity I advert to another view in the field. It is that of adynamic disease. It has been conclusively proven that alcohol decreases the muscular power. It decreases (from the minimum dose to the maximum) the power of the heart as well as that of all other muscles. I say this has been absolutely demonstrated by Richardson and others. In death from adynamia it is through failure of muscle, that is, of the heart, of the scaleni and intercostals, of the diaphragm, and of the laryngeal muscles, et cetera. All of the muscles may gradually fail, become wearied unto death. How pernicious then must alcohol be in adding its influence to bring about the tragic end!

"It is my belief that it is in diphtheria that the most dire results are to be observed. In that disease the vast majority of cases die by asthenia, or else by sudden failure of the heart. To what is this sudden cardiac paralysis due? The elucidation is as follows. In the grave cases there is almost invariably a subnormal temperature, together with great muscular prostration. Also it is a physiological fact that a decrease of the temperature slows nervous conduction. As the system is made colder, the nervous force flows slower and slower. In diphtheria the heart muscle is very weak, the temperature falls, the lessened nervous energy but feebly animates the muscular fibres, and so actual paralysis ensues, death closing the scene almost instantaneously. Now, in such a state of imminent danger, brought about by such causes, what could be worse than to administer an agent which notably reduces temperature, and at the same time enfeebles muscular power? May I add, what could be the remedy in such a condition? and I answer, External heat freely applied to the whole surface of the body. This will prevent the cardiac paralysis whenever it is preventable."

The Medical Pioneer of Dec., 1892, contained an editorial article upon "The Toxine Alcohol," which deals with leucocytes and their functions. The following is the article:--

"Dr. Broadbent's introductory address at the opening of the session at Owen's College, Manchester, deserves more attention than most of these formal deliveries. He dwelt on the intellectual interest which attaches to the study of medical science, and illustrated it, among other ways, by the interest excited by recent observations on the action of bacilli and the combat which goes on between these invading hosts and the guardian cells or leucocytes of the living body. Inflammation surrounding a wound is regarded as caused by the influx and multiplication of leucocytes to engulf and destroy septic bacilli which have gained entrance from the air, a 'local war' of defence. The issue of this pitched battle will depend on the relative number and activity of the respective hosts. Inflammation round a poisoned wound is an evidence of vital power and a means of protecting the system at large from invasion and devastation. If this first line of defence is broken through, the bacilli pass through the lymphatic spaces and ducts to the glands, and another battle ensues which produces glandular swelling and inflammation and possibly abscess. This second line of defence may be insufficient and then we get general septic 鎚 ia. It is now well proven that the injury is done, not by the bacilli themselves but by the toxines which they secrete or excrete. Dr. Broadbent very properly points out that the action of the bacilli of fever in the body is strictly comparable to the action of yeast in a fermentable liquid. The yeast cells grow and multiply at the expense of the sugar, in destroying which they produce alcohol, carbonic dioxide and other substances. When the alcohol amounts to some 17 per cent. of the liquid the process is stopped by the poisonous action of the alcohol on the yeast cells. In just the same way the toxines produced by the bacilli at length stop their further multiplication and put an end to the disease. Alcohol is in fact, the toxine produced by yeast, and, like many other toxines, it is not only poisonous to cells which produce it, but to any animal into whose veins it may happen to get.

"There can be little doubt that the state of immunity which one attack of certain fevers confers against future attacks depends partly upon what is called the phagocytic action of leucocytes. These have been actually observed to draw into their interior and destroy bacilli which would otherwise have multiplied and produced their special effects. There can be little doubt, either, that we are continually taking into our systems bacilli of all sorts, and that, again, disease is averted by the activity of the germ-devouring leucocytes. Dr. Broadbent describes an experiment which proves that power of resisting disease is largely dependent on the activity of these cells. A rabbit, having had a certain quantity of bacilli injected under its skin, suffers from inflammation at the spot, and perhaps abscess, but recovers. At the same time, another rabbit is treated in precisely the same way, but, simultaneously, a dose of chloral is injected into another part of the body. The chloral, circulating in the blood, is known to paralyze leucocytes, and, as a result of this, they do not collect and wage war on the bacilli injected under the skin; there is very little local reaction, the bacilli get free course into the lymph and blood, and the animal dies. But, in the words of Dr. Broadbent, 'alcohol in excess has a similar action on the leucocytes, and this, as well as the deteriorating influence of chronic alcoholism on the tissues, predisposes to septic infection. A single debauch, therefore, may open the door to fever or erysipelas.' A similar experiment of Doyen confirms this. He found that guinea pigs can be killed by the cholera microbe, when introduced by the mouth, if a dose of alcohol has been previously administered. It has been the general testimony of observers in cholera epidemics that those addicted to much alcohol are far more liable to fatal attacks. But while large doses of alcohol are, of course, more obviously injurious, it would be absurd to imagine that lesser quantities are entirely without influence in the same direction. It has, indeed, been shown by Dr. Ridge, that even infinitesimal quantities of alcohol, such as one part in 5,000, cause a more rapid multiplication of the bacillus subtilis and other bacilli of decomposition, while, by the same quantities, the growth of both animal and vegetable protoplasm is retarded. Hence there can be no longer any question that alcohol renders the body more liable to conquest by invading microbes, less able to resist and destroy them. Alcohol, a toxine injurious to living cells, is destroyed or removed from the body as fast as nature can effect it, but while it remains, and while able to affect the cells at all, its action is detrimental to healthy growth and healthy life, and the less we take of such an agent the better for us. This is a dictum which it becomes the profession to enunciate far and wide. 'The less, the better' is a watchword which all may use, and the wise will interpret it in a way which will infallibly preserve them altogether from all possible danger from such a source."

On the sixteenth of December, 1897, Dr. Sims Woodhead, president of the British Medical Temperance Association, gave a masterly address in London upon "Recent Researches on the Action of Alcohol." The lecture was illustrated by lantern slides. From the report given in The Medical Temperance Review of Jan., 1898, the following is culled:--

"In a series of drawings of kidney you will notice first that there is a condition known as cloudy swelling; this is one of the first changes that can be observed. Notice the characteristic features of this cloudy swelling in the cells of all these specimens. The large swollen cells are granular, and very frequently there is a granular mass in the lumen of the tubule. In some cases the cells are so much swollen that the lumen of the tubule is represented merely by a 'star-shaped' radiating chink. The nucleus is usually somewhat obscured, that this alcoholic cloudy swelling (similar to that met with as the result of the administration of certain poisons) is the first change observed in the parenchymatous cells of the organs of animals that have died of acute alcoholic poisoning. This condition, unless the cause is removed, goes on to a condition of fatty-degeneration, as shown in the next specimen in which we have, in addition to the granular appearance of the protoplasm of the cell, a deposition of masses of fat in and at the expense of this protoplasm.

"There is another series of changes to which I wish to draw your attention. In the tubules of the kidney we have, in addition to the granular appearance of the protoplasm of the cells, an increase in the number of leucocytes, and connective tissue cells between the tubules around the glomeruli and along the course of the blood-vessels. This condition of small cell infiltration, we know, is constantly associated with inflammatory conditions of the kidney as in other organs. Here then are the changes in the epithelium plus increase in the number of leucocytes.

"I show you too a specimen of heart muscle, in which the granular degeneration, or cloudy swelling is well marked whilst here and there the process is going on to fatty degeneration, similar to that seen in the kidney. Here again, then, the active elements of the organ are becoming broken down, or, at any rate, losing their normal structure and affording evidence of fundamental changes in these cells. Such changes are set up, not by any one poison alone, or by any single disease toxin, but by members of many groups of poisons, by alcohols, ethers, etc. indeed by very various poisons-- animal, vegetable and mineral.

"Now, it is a peculiar fact, as shown by Massart, Bordet and others, in researches on chemiotaxis, that nearly all these poisons have the power of repelling leucocytes, and of seriously interfering with them in the performance of their functions, and this power assumes a special significance in connection with our subject this afternoon.

"Now, two of the great functions of leucocytes under ordinary conditions are those of policing and scavenging. Massart and Bordet showed, under the action of certain substances, alcohol amongst others, these functions are lost, but following up Metchnikoff and others they observed that after a time these same leucocytes became accustomed to the presence of these poisons, gradually becoming 'acclimatized' as it were. At first paralyzed or repelled, they after a time pluck up courage to attack the invading substances and carry on or renew their accustomed work of scavenging; they try to get rid of both poisons and poison-producers, and even acquire the power of forming substances (anti-toxins) which can neutralize the poison and allow the cells to devote their energy to doing their own proper work.

"Here are drawings of minute abscesses that have formed in the wall of the heart. We see at once the part that the leucocytes play in attacking micro-organisms, and of localizing their action. Look at the blood-vessel in the wall of the heart with its plug of micro-organism (staphylococci) in the centre of a clear space; here the leucocytes are not numerous, indeed they are very sparsely scattered, and appear to have been driven back by the organisms or their toxics. Then a little distance away from the toxin and toxin-forming organisms, the leucocytes are coming up in large numbers, forming a sort of protecting army, as it were. This is known as leucocytosis. In the small patent vessels around this commencing abscess numerous leucocytes, far in excess of the usual proportion, may be seen--the nearer the abscess, the more numerous they become. Thus the leucocytes make their way to what is to become the wall of the abscess, and form a layer around a mass of micro-organisms, localizing, or attempting to localize, such mass. So long as the leucocytes can make their way to this mass, and shut it off from the surrounding tissue, so long we shall have no extension of the abscess.

"Now, if you add something--alcohol in the case we are considering--which not only exerts a negative chemiotaxic action--i. e., which drives the leucocyte away--but which, as we have seen, also causes degeneration of nerve, muscle and epithelial cells, shall we not injure the infected patient both directly and indirectly by interfering with the return of the leucocytes driven away, by diminishing or altering the functional activity of these cells, and indirectly by interfering with the excretion of the poisons (owing, as we have seen, to a degenerated condition of the secretory epithelium)? Have we not, in fact, a cumulative action of two substances, either of which alone would do damage, but not in the same proportion as do the two when acting together.

"Now let us see what we may learn from a series of experiments carried out by Dr. Abbott, working in the Laboratory of Hygiene of the University of Pennsylvania, under the auspices of the committee of fifty, to investigate the Alcohol Question.

"These are his conclusions:--

1. "That the normal vital resistance of rabbits to infection by streptococcus pyogenes is markedly diminished through the influence of alcohol when given daily to the stage of acute intoxication. 2. That a similar, though by no means so conspicuous, diminution of resistance to infection and intoxication by the bacillus coli communis also occurs in rabbits subjected to the same influences.

"Throughout these experiments, with few exceptions, it will be seen that the alcoholized animals not only showed the effects of the inoculations earlier than did the non-alcoholized rabbits, but in the case of the streptococcus inoculations, the lesions produced (formation of miliary abscesses) were much more pronounced than are those that usually follow inoculations with this organism.

"With regard to the predisposing influence of the alcohol, one is constrained to believe that it is in most cases the result of structural alterations consequent upon its direct action on the tissues, though in a number of animals no such alterations could be made out by microscopic examinations. I am inclined, however, to the belief, in the light of the work of Berkley and Friedenwald, done under the direction of Professor Welch, in the pathological laboratory of the Johns Hopkins University, that a closer study of the tissues of these animals would have revealed in all of them structural changes of such a nature as to indicate disturbances of important vital functions of sufficient gravity fully to account for the loss of normal resistance.

"Following up Dr. Abbott's experiments, Dr. Del 閉 rde, working in Calmette's laboratory in the Institut Pasteur at Lille, made a series of observations which are, from many points of view, of very great interest and importance as he attacks it from an entirely new standpoint, one that will, I hope, ere long, be taken up by those working in this country. It has already been demonstrated that 'alcoholics' suffer far more seriously from microbic affections than do those of sober life, and it is now accepted that amongst them the mortality from this class of disease is higher than amongst those who are not accustomed to take alcohol regularly or to excess.

"It is pointed out, as most of us have from time to time had the opportunity of observing, that, taking pneumonia as an example of this class of disease, there can be no doubt that the alcoholic patient has not merely an appreciably smaller chance for recovery, but an apparently slight attack becomes one in which the chances of recovery come to be against the patient rather than in his favor. I well remember when I was House Physician in the Royal Infirmary at Edinburgh that Dr. Muirhead, who almost invariably treated his pneumonic patients without alcohol, used to say that an ordinary case of acute pneumonia should always recover under careful treatment, but that cases of pneumonia in 'alcoholics' were always most anxious cases and in every way unsatisfactory. (Slides were shown on screen to illustrate the changes taking place in pneumonia, the conditions of leucocytosis, and the very important part which leucocytes play in the process of 'clearing up' during the course of the patient's recovery). Dr. Del 閉 rde in an admirable summary gives the principal features of pneumonia in alcoholics. He describes it as running a comparatively prolonged course, as being often accompanied by a violent delirium, following which is a period of prostration or of coma; even in those who recover, abscesses frequently occur in the liver, or in other organs. He also points out that there may be a similar chain of events in other infective conditions such as erysipelas and typhoid fever, but as he insists that, until Abbott's experiments on the streptococcus,[A] staphylococcus[A] and bacterium coli,[A] in alcoholized and non-alcoholized animals, little attempt has been made to indicate the mechanism, or, at any rate, the process by which alcoholized individuals are rendered more susceptible to the invasion and action of micro-organisms.

[Footnote A: Microbes or bacteria of different kinds.]

"As we have already seen, Abbott's experiments prove beyond doubt that attenuated disease-producing organisms, which in healthy animals do not kill immediately, bring about a fatal result when the animal has previously been treated with alcohol. In order to determine which was the most important factor in the destruction or weakening of the resisting agents in the body, Dr. Del閱rde conceived the idea of experimenting with those diseases in which it has been found possible to produce, artificially, as it were, and under controlled conditions, an immunity or insusceptibility in healthy animals. He carried out a series of experiments on rabbits, immunizing against and infecting with the virus of hydrophobia, tetanus and anthrax.[B] To these rabbits he first administered a quantity of alcohol, from 6 to 8 c.c. at first, and gradually rises to 10 c.c. doses per diem.

[Footnote B: Carbuncle.]

"There is in the first instance a slight falling off in weight of the animal, but after a time this ceases, and the animal may again become heavier, until the original weight is reached. He then took a series of animals and vaccinated them against hydrophobia. In one set the animals were afterwards alcoholized and then injected with a considerable quantity of virulent rabic cord. It was here found that immunity against rabies had not been lost.

"In a second set the vaccination and alcoholization were carried on simultaneously, a fatal dose (as proved by control experiment) of rabic cord was then injected, when it was found that little or no immunity had been acquired. In a third series the alcohol was stopped before the immunizing process was commenced. In this case marked immunity was acquired.

"As regards rabies, then, acute alcoholism, especially when continued for comparatively short periods, simply has the effect of preventing the acquisition of immunity when alcohol is administered during the period when the immunizing process ought to be going on. This indicates that the action of the alcohol in acute alcoholism is direct, and that although its administration prevents the acquisition of immunity it does not alter the cells so materially that they cannot regain some of their original powers, whilst once the immunity has been gained by the cells, alcohol cannot, immediately, so fundamentally alter them that they lose the immunity they have already acquired. When we come to the consideration of the case of tetanus, however, we are carried a step further. Dr. Del閙rde repeating his immunizing and alcoholizing experiments, but now working with tetanus virus in place of rabic virus, found--and, perhaps, here it may be as well to give his own words:--

(1) "'That animals vaccinated against tetanus and afterwards alcoholized lose their immunity against tetanus;

(2) "'That animals vaccinated against tetanus and at the same time alcoholized do not readily acquire immunity;

(3) "'That animals first alcoholized and then vaccinated may acquire immunity against tetanus if alcohol is suppressed from the commencement of the process of vaccination.'

"In the case of anthrax too, as we gather from another series of experiments, it is almost impossible to confer immunity, if the animal is alcoholized during the time that it is being vaccinated, and although the animals, first alcoholized and then vaccinated, may acquire a certain amount of immunity, they rapidly lose condition and are certainly more ill than non-alcoholized animals vaccinated simultaneously.

"We have already mentioned that Massart and Bordet some years ago pointed out that alcohol, even in very dilute solutions, exerts a very active negative chemiotaxis, i. e., it appears to have properties by which leucocytes are repelled or driven away from its neighborhood and actions. Alcohol thus prevents the cells from attacking invading bodies or of reacting in the presence of the toxins which also, as is well known, exert a more or less marked negative chemiotaxis, i.e., the cells appear to be paralyzed. In all diseases, then, in which the leucocytes help to remove an invading organism or in which they have the power of reacting or of carrying on their functions in the presence of a toxin, we should expect that alcohol would to a certain extent deprive them of this power or interfere with their capacity for acquiring a greater resisting power or of reinforcing the powers of resistance. It appears indeed to reinforce the poison formed by pathogenic organisms. Dr. Del 閔 rde maintains moreover that chronic alcoholism increases enormously the difficulty of rendering an animal immune to anthrax, whilst as those who have had any experience of cases of anthrax know full well alcoholics, whether acute or chronic, manifest a remarkable susceptibility both as regards attacks of anthrax and the fatality of the disease when once contracted. Further as clinical proof of the correctness of another of these sets of experiments, Dr. Del 閔 rde instances two cases of rabies which have come under observation in the Institut Pasteur--one, a man of 30 years of age, of intemperate habits who after a complete treatment of 18 days after a bite in the hand died of hydrophobia; the other, a child of 13 years who was bitten on the face by the same dog that had attacked the other patient, and on the same day--who underwent the same treatment remained perfectly well. In this case the more severe bite (the face being the most serious position in which a person can be bitten) was received by the child; indeed the intemperate habits of the man, who even took alcohol during treatment, appear to have been the only more serious factor in his case as compared with that of the child.

"From all this Dr. Del 閖 rde draws the practical conclusion that patients who have been bitten by a mad dog should as far as possible abstain from the use of alcohol not only during the process of treatment, but also for some time afterwards, even for a period of eight months, during which period, apparently, increase of immunity may be going on. Beyond this he maintains that doctors often commit a grave error in administering strong doses of alcohol to patients suffering from certain infectious diseases such as pneumonia, or from certain intoxications such as those produced by snake-bite, during which an increase in the number of leucocytes appear to be a necessary part of any process that leads to the cure of the patient. Finally, he points out how necessary it is that we should respect the integrity of the leucocytes in the presence of microbic infections or intoxications. We may accept these statements all the more readily as Dr. Del 閖 rde states that 'although we must recognize that small doses of dilute alcoholic beverages are indicated in certain cases where it is necessary to stimulate the nervous system, one must guard oneself against an abuse which may certainly be prejudicial to the putting into operation of the mechanism of defence against the organisms of disease.'

"In so far as these conclusions rest on a series of exact experiments we are justified in accepting them as being a most valuable contribution to the question; where there is no experimental basis, we must exercise our own judgment. To show the very strong impression that exists that there is some connection between severe cases of pneumonia and alcohol I may mention that the other day I heard a gentleman (not a medical man) say, 'It is well known that most men (of a certain profession) die from alcoholism.' When asked to explain he said, 'They all die from cirrhosis or pneumonia, and if those conditions are not due to alcoholism, what is?'

"There can be no doubt that in addition to its specific action, alcohol has a general action--the mal-nutrition, which is usually associated with the use of alcohol, especially as a result of its action on the mucous membranes of the stomach, etc."

That the "guardian cells" of the body play a part in a considerable number of diseases was illustrated by Dr. Woodhead by drawings and photographs, shown on the lantern screen. The photographs included cells containing anthrax, typhoid and tubercle bacilli, the spirilla of relapsing fever, specimens from cases of anthrax. Specimens were shown in which the cells were actually ingesting and digesting the specific micro-organisms. In a case of typhoid, showing large masses of typhoid bacilli in one of Peyer's patches, there were seen certain of the cells which contained the typhoid bacilli, some of them undergoing degenerative changes, and showing unequal standing.

Of the researches made by Dr. Abbott referred to in the foregoing lecture Dr. N. S. Davis says:--

"Thus we have another and direct positive demonstration of the fact that the presence of alcohol in living bodies not only impairs all the physiological processes, but also impairs their vital resistance to the effects of all other poisons. It was hardly necessary, however, to trouble the rabbits to obtain proof of this; for such evidence may be found in abundance by examining the vital statistics of every civilized country. The late Frank H. Hamilton, in his valuable work on military hygiene, gives an interesting account of an experiment executed, not on a few rabbits, but on whole regiments of human beings, who were being exposed to the inhibition, not of the streptococcus pyogenes, but to the infections of malarial and typho-malaria fever. And, as many were attacked with sickness, it was thought by some of those in authority that if the soldiers were given a specified ration of alcoholic liquor two or three times a day, it might enable them to resist the morbid influences to which they were exposed. The proposed ration was accordingly ordered, and Dr. Hamilton informs us that the soldiers taking the liquor ration succumbed to the morbific influences surrounding them so much more rapidly than before, that in less than sixty days the order was countermanded, and the liquor ration stopped. And that eminent surgeon and sanitarian added, with peculiar emphasis, that he wished never to see the same experiment tried again."

Dr. J. J. Ridge, of London, has learned through his experiments that alcohol not only hinders the leucocytes in their war upon disease germs, but also tends to the multiplication of germs. Of this he says:--

"The antagonism of alcohol to the fundamental functions of life is further exhibited by its action on the cellular elements of living tissues and the free cells or leucocytes of the blood. Dr. Lionel Beale long ago pointed out how it affected the protoplasm of cells, and diminished the movements of amoebae, to which leucocytes are apparently analogous.

"But while alcohol is thus injurious to living protoplasm, or constructive protoplasm as it may be called, that which builds up, and forms all kinds of structures, and living beings of all higher types, I accidentally discovered that in minute quantities, under about one per cent., and even in such almost incredible amounts as 1 part in 100,000, (1/10 millilitre in 10 litres) it favors the growth and multiplication of many microbes whose function is antagonistic to the protoplasm of organized beings, and which may therefore be called destructive protoplasm. We know that these microbes are kept at bay by the vitality of the tissues; if this vitality is lowered they may prevail: as soon as life departs they set to work, and decomposition is the result. It is, therefore, not very surprising that an agent, like alcohol, which, we have seen, lowers the vitality of constructive protoplasm, should, on the other hand increase the vitality of destructive protoplasm. At any rate such is the fact. In the presence of these minute quantities of alcohol, decomposition goes on more rapidly, and the micrococci and bacilli, thrive and swarm more abundantly. This is easily demonstrable by the more rapid, and thicker, cloudiness of any clear decomposable liquor in the course of a day or two, or in a few days, according to circumstances. But I have demonstrated the more rapid multiplication of some forms by means of plate cultivations, of which I show specimens. It is true of the bacteria of decomposition, of the streptococci, and staphylococci of pus, and of diphtheria. Time alone has been wanting to demonstrate this in other cases, which I hope to do."

The Medical Week some time ago contained this paragraph:--

"Dr. Viala, in collaboration with Dr. Charrin, says: 'I have carried out a series of researches on the toxicity of various alcoholic beverages in common use, such as wines and brandies of all brands, from those which are reputed the best to those of very inferior quality. All these products have been analyzed with the greatest care. Our experiments were carried out on fifty animals. Intravenous injections confirm Dr. Daremberg's statement that liquors considered as the best are the most toxic, more particularly as regards their immediate effects.'"

Although the foregoing statement directs the reader's attention to the comparative effects of different alcoholic liquors, it also plainly implies several facts of great importance. The first is, that all alcoholic liquors, fermented or distilled, are toxic or poisonous; and the more pure alcohol they contain, the more poisonous are they, the qualities of liquor differing only in the rapidity of their injurious effects.

In the same number of the Medical Week, Professor Gr 閃 ant states that after injecting a quantity of alcohol into the venous circulation of a dog equal to one twenty-fifth, or four per cent., of the estimated weight of the blood of the animal, he found by several analyses at different times that it required "a little over twenty-three hours for complete elimination of the alcohol from the blood." If we consider these results obtained by Viala, Charrin, Daremberg and Gr 閃 ant, with those obtained by Dr. A. C. Abbott, showing the direct effect of alcohol in diminishing the normal vital resistance of the living body to infection, we see excellent reasons why the liberal use of alcohol in the treatment of such infectious diseases as diphtheria, typhoid fever and pneumonia, under the supposition that it was a cardiac tonic, has resulted in so great a mortality as from thirty to sixty per cent.

Dr. A. Pearce Gould, a London hospital surgeon of the first rank, has made special study of the surgery of the blood-vessels, and of the chest. He was one of the earliest to practice and advocate the careful removal of the axillary glands in all operations for cancer of the breast.

He is a strong believer in the value of total abstinence as promoting robust health of body and mind. He regards the value of alcohol in disease as exceedingly small, and prescribes it only very rarely. He thinks that alcohol increases the activity of cancer and other malignant growths, an opinion which is of great importance from one with such exceptional opportunities for observation in these complaints.

Dr. N. S. Davis in the American Medical Temperance Quarterly of January, 1895, gives reports of cases which came under his observation as a consulting physician, where the use of alcoholics throughout an extended illness favored the continuance of delirium, or mild mental disorder, after convalescence was established. In each case the withdrawal of the alcohol was followed by a cessation of the mental delusion.

One of these cases may be taken as an example:--

"The third case was that of a woman over sixty years of age, who had suffered from a mild grade of fever and protracted diarrhoea, somewhat resembling a mild grade of enteric typhoid fever.

"As she became much reduced in strength during the latter part of her diarrhoea, her friends began to give her wine, and sometimes stronger alcoholic drink, under the popular delusion that these could strengthen her. Her mind soon became wandering, and she was troubled with illusions, which were attributed to her weakness, and the so-called stimulants were increased. But the mental disorder increased also, and continued after the fever and diarrhoea had ceased, until the question was raised concerning the propriety of her removal to an asylum for the insane.

"Being consulted at that time, and listening to an accurate history of the case, I suggested that the an 鋥 thetic effect of the alcohol on the cerebral hemispheres, in connection with its effect on the hemoglobin, and other elements of the blood, in lessening the reception and internal distribution of oxygen, might be the cause of both the perpetuation of her weakness, and her mental disorder. I advised a trial of its entire omission, and the giving of only simple nourishment, and moderate doses of strychnine and digitalis, as nerve tonics. My advice was followed, though not without much hesitation on the part of her friends. The result, however, was entire recovery from the mental disorder, and some improvement in her general health."

Puerperal mania resulted in one case cited, from the use of a moderate amount of wine at mealtimes; when the wine was abandoned the mania subsided.

CHAPTER XII.

WHY DOCTORS STILL PRESCRIBE ALCOHOLICS.

Workers in the department of Medical Temperance of the Woman's Christian Temperance Union are told repeatedly by the better class of physicians that they would be glad often not to prescribe alcohol if patients and their friends would not insist upon its use. There is a deep-rooted prejudice in favor of alcohol as a remedy in the minds of the great multitude of people, and they are ready to distrust as fanatical, or incompetent, any physician who does not use it. Dr. Norman Kerr, a well-known physician of England, says, that during a ten years' residence in America, he found people unwilling to pay him as much for his services as they were willing to pay one who prescribed alcoholics. Even those who were abstainers from liquors as beverages distrusted him for not using these things as medicines. Indeed, this prejudice goes so far with many that they will refuse to employ a non-alcoholic physician, if they know him to be such. In consequence of this latter fact, there are great numbers of skilful physicians who say nothing about alcohol lest they be considered "faddists," and lose practice, but who never prescribe it unless it is asked for by the patient or his friends.

Again, consulting physicians will sometimes insist upon the use of alcohol, and thus seeds of distrust of the non-alcoholic physician will be sown.

Dr. J. J. Ridge says of medical prescriptions:--

"Hundreds of medical men order alcoholic liquors from habit, from ignorance of their real effect, from fashion, or from a desire to please, or not to offend, their patients. Port-wine is constantly being ordered when persons are recovering from various diseases; day by day they regain their strength, and the port-wine gets all the credit of it, especially since each glass seems to diffuse a comfortable glow over the whole body. They forget that the process of recovery would have gone on without the port, and that hundreds and thousands of people do get well without it. They often ignore the fact that they are taking real tonics in addition. They are misled by the sensations which the alcohol causes; they do not know that it relaxes the blood-vessels instead of improving their tone; that it exhausts the heart by making it beat away more rapidly to no profit. Hence the convalescence is actually more prolonged than it would otherwise be. Gentle exercise, regulated baths, good food, balmy sleep, these are the true restoratives of the exhausted system, and no jugglery with sedatives, such as alcohol, can produce the desired result.

"It is by its sedative action that alcohol has obtained its position in public opinion. It will render persons insensible to various uneasy sensations, and the majority prefer to continue the bad habits which produce the uneasy sensations, and then to take them away by a dose or two of some alcoholic liquor, or, indeed, to take this before the uneasy sensations come on. In this way they do themselves injury and make themselves unconscious of it. Dr. Beaumont, who had the opportunity of examining the interior of Alexis St. Martin's stomach, and of seeing how digestion went on, was astonished to see how inflamed the mucous membrane could be without any consciousness of it. He observed, as a matter of fact, that alcoholic drinks of all kinds hindered the process of digestion, and produced this morbid condition of the mucous membrane. The relief, therefore, which can be obtained by alcohol is delusive and dangerous.

"But some persons say they are afraid to abandon the use of alcohol because they have been in the habit of taking it for a long period. This fear is entirely groundless. The alcohol will be missed for a time, just as a person who has been using crutches would miss them if thrown away; but they will do better without both after a little while. There is no kind of constitution which renders a person unable to do without alcohol. The prisoners in all our jails have to leave off their drink at once, and altogether, on entering there, and no harm ever ensues in consequence. But some say that this is because their diet is so carefully arranged, and the hygienic condition of the prison so perfect. Quite so. This shows us clearly that when total abstainers become ill outside the prison, their illness is to be attributed to some error in diet or hygiene, or to some accidental circumstance. It is absurd to think that the infraction of one law of health can be nullified by breaking another; that if you eat too much, or too fast, or too often, or what is not good for you, you can escape the consequences by injuring yourself with alcohol."

Dr. N. S. Davis was for many years openly sneered at by many of his professional brethren as "a cold-water fanatic." Since his views are now being rapidly adopted by progressive medical men all over the civilized world, it may be that soon those physicians who cling to alcohol will deserve the soubriquet of "alcohol fanatics." Dr. Davis said:--

"If I am asked why the profession continues to prescribe these drinks, I answer; simply from the force of habit and traditional education, coupled with a reluctance to risk the experiment of omitting them while the general popular notions sanction their use. Nothing is easier than self-deception in this matter. A patient is suddenly taken with syncope, or nervous weakness, from which abundant experience has shown that a speedy recovery would take place by simple rest and fresh air. But in the alarm of friends something must be done. A little wine or brandy is given, and as it is not sufficient to positively prevent, the patient in due time revives just as would have been the case if neither wine nor brandy had been used.

"Of course both doctor and friends will regard the so-called stimulant as the cause of the recovery. So, too, when patients are getting weak, in the advanced stage of fever, or some other self-limited disease, an abundance of nourishment is regularly administered, in the greater part of which is mixed some kind of alcoholic drink. The latter will always occupy the chief attention, and if, after a severe run, the fever, or disease, finally disappears, it will be said that the patient was sustained or 'kept alive' for over two or three weeks, as the case may be, 'solely by the stimulants,' when, in fact, if the same nourishment and care had been given without a drop of alcohol, he would have convalesced sooner, and more perfectly, as I have seen demonstrated a thousand times in my experience."

Dr. Casgrau, of Dublin, says that physicians who make personal use of alcohol are not able to give an unbiased opinion about its action, as one of its most marked effects is that of a narcotic to the mental powers; such physicians are not so acute to observe the action of this, or any drug.

Sir B. W. Richardson, M. D., in an address upon the reasons why physicians still prescribe alcoholics, says that the magnetism of public opinion has great weight with professional men.

"All professions are under that subtle influence. All professions whatever their duties, whatever their learning may be, are sensitive and obedient to that influence. In their pride they think they lead public opinion; it is a mistake, they always follow it on every question in which the people, at large, have a voice. They can assist in influencing the public voice, and sometimes, to quote the words of Abb?Purcelle, spoken in the dawn of the great French Revolution, they may prove that 'respect for sovereign power sometimes consists in transgressing its orders,' but as a general rule not merely the orders but the inclinations are obeyed. We have to wait on, and for, public opinion, and in nothing so much as on the subject of alcohol. The use of alcoholic beverages rests not on argument but on habit, custom. To those whom it affects personally it is an absolute monarch. It makes its own empire. By the very action which it has upon the body of those who receive it into themselves it rules and governs. The joke of the inebriate man that when he had taken his potation he was quite another man and that then he felt it his duty to treat that other man, is literally true, a terse and faithful expression of a natural fact. The man or woman born and bred under the influence of alcohol is of the race of alcohol, and as distinct a person as any racial peculiarity can supply. The reason, the judgment, the temper, the senses are attuned by it. It is loved by its lovers like life. The grape to them is no longer a luscious fruit; it is 'the mother of mighty wine,' and he who is bold enough to disown that motherhood must stand apart. How can a profession however strong, march all at once against such an overwhelming influence? Itself born, perchance, under the influence bred under it, how shall it immediately be transformed? Why disobey the influence? It is in the interest of the doctor to obey, in a worldly sense of view; but more--it is in his nature to obey. The strong bands of nature and interest go hand in hand. Is it wonderful that the genius of a professional man so situated should, according to the quality of his genius, uphold, root and branch, the r 鬺 e of his nativity? On the contrary the wonder is that he has ever done anything else. It is most natural that he should be amongst the last to take up what revolutionizes all the manners, and customs, and faiths, of society. A lady will ask her physician the question, May I take wine, Sir? As much as you like Madam; it is very bad for you and I take none, but that is your business entirely. Henceforth that gentleman is said to be one who prescribes alcohol in any quantity. In fact, he never prescribes it, for although when forbidding is hopeless, there is all the difference in the world between prescribing and permitting, permitting goes down as if it were prescribing. Often a patient will try to compromise. On an ocean of whisky and water, brandy and soda, or other poisonous mixture, he is floating into fatal paralysis. You tell him so faithfully, and he says he knows it and will drop down to claret. If you assent, he tells his friends you have changed his brandy or whisky to wine; if you dissent, he says you have left your duty as a doctor undone, in order to become an advocate for abstaining temperance, about which he is as competent a judge as you are, and he won't pay fees for that advice. He pays to be cured of his disease, not to be dragooned into a system peculiar in its tenets. In an alcoholic world there is a strong argument in this decision. It rolls splendidly, especially down hill."

After speaking of non-alcoholic physicians, and their opinions of the harmfulness of alcohol, he adds:--

"On the other side, there are practitioners who, under the magnetism of public opinion, as earnestly believe the opposite in relation to alcohol, who declare they could not, conscientiously, practice their profession if they were debarred the use of alcohol, and who look on the advance and the growth of scientific abstaining principles--which they cannot avoid recognizing--with positive dread. The extremists on this side are indeed extreme in their fanaticism. They shut their eyes to the most obvious facts, and do not hesitate in their blindness to misrepresent the most obvious truths. They affirm that under the influence of total abstinence and, by inference, because of total abstinence, the yearly decreasing death-rate of the population is accompanied by reduction of vitality; that people who live long are more enfeebled than those who live short lives and merry; that under abstinence from alcohol fearful diseases are being developed; that the total abstainers have less power for resisting disease than the moderate temperate; and that under the current system of advance towards total abstinence, a very small advance yet by the way, diseases of a low type have developed and extended their ravages."

It is only physicians of large conscientiousness, or of great independence of character, who will dare to go counter to the prejudices of the people.

Consequently, it is necessary to educate the people in the teachings of those physicians, whose eminence in the profession has permitted them, or whose conscientiousness has driven them, to expose the delusions concerning the medical value of alcoholic beverages. When the people cease to believe in alcoholic remedies, physicians will no longer prescribe them. But while the majority desire the "physicians' prescription" as a cover for indulgence, there will be found physicians willing to give such prescriptions.

That the prescription of alcohol by physicians is largely a matter of routine may be seen from the following two cases, reported to the writer by county superintendents of the department of Medical Temperance.

In the first case, the physician said to the nurse, "If the patient's heart becomes weak, you might give a little brandy or whisky." Seeing reluctance expressed upon the nurse's countenance, he added hastily, "Or coffee, strong coffee will do just as well." The nurse in reporting this to the writer, said, "Why couldn't he have ordered coffee in the first place if he thought it equally good?"

The second case was that of an aged woman whose physician ordered whisky as a tonic. Her granddaughter ventured to ask, "Would not whisky have a narcotic rather than a tonic effect?" He replied thoughtfully, "Well, tell the truth, I suppose it would."

CHAPTER XIII.

ALCOHOLIC PROPRIETARY OR 'PATENT' MEDICINES.

America has been called the Paradise of Quacks, and with good reason. For years patent medicine manufacturers had such complete control of the American press, both secular and religious, that it was almost impossible to reach the public with information as to the real nature of these concoctions. Consequently the people accepted with amazing credulity the startling claims to miraculous cures of various pills and potions as set forth under glaring headlines in the daily papers. The publicity of the last few years has hurt the traffic seriously, but it still has a great hold upon the ignorant and credulous part of the population, and there is still a very large number of these preparations upon the market. Many persons think that the Pure Food Law guarantees every drug preparation now sold to be perfectly safe for use. This is a great error. The guarantee means simply that the manufacturer guarantees that his preparation is as he states upon the label; the government guarantees nothing concerning the matter. That the guarantee of the manufacturer is not always truthful has been shown by analyses of some preparations made by state and national chemists. All the advantage that the public has through the Pure Food Law, so far as drug preparations are concerned, is that the percentage of alcohol must be printed upon the label, and the presence of certain dangerous drugs, such as morphine, cocaine, and acetanilid must be indicated. Thus persons intelligent as to the nature of these drugs will avoid medicines which the label says contains them. The ignorant are not protected. It was difficult to secure even this small restriction upon the sale of proprietary medicines because of the opposition of a large number of newspaper publishers who were sharing the ill-gotten gains of the medical fakirs.

A careful compilation of manufacturers' announcements list 1,806 so-called patent medicines sold in open markets, in which alcohol, opium or other toxic drugs form constituent parts. 675 of the preparations are known as "bitters," stomachics, or cordials, and alcohol enters into their composition in quantities varying from fifteen to fifty per cent.; 390 are recommended for coughs and colds, nearly all of which contain opium. Sixty remedies are sold for the relief of pain, and no other purpose. 120 are for nervous troubles, and of this number, sixty-five have entering into their composition coca leaves, or kola nut, or both, or are represented by their respective active principles, cocaine or caffeine. 129 are offered for headaches, and kindred ailments, and usually with a guarantee to give immediate relief. In these are generally compounded phenacetine, caffeine, antipyrine, acetanilid, or morphine, diluted with soda, or sugar of milk. Dysentery, diarrhoea, cholera morbus, cramp in bowels, etc., have 185 quick reliefs or "cures" to their credit, nearly all of which contain opium, many of them in addition, alcohol, ginger, capsicum or myrrh in various combinations, and there are numerous cases on record where children and adults have been narcotized by their excessive use. Some manufacturers print on the labels covering these goods, words of caution limiting the amount to be taken. Forty-eight compounds for asthma contain caffeine and morphine. Sufferers from toothache have their choice from thirty-eight remedies, and thirty-six soothing, or teething, syrups are provided for infants.

Many people have ignorantly and innocently formed an alcohol, morphine, or cocaine habit through the use of patent medicines. Many deaths have occurred from headache powders of which acetanilid is the chief ingredient. Dr. Harvey W. Wiley, chief of the Bureau of Chemistry, says of these headache powders:--

"A woman has a headache and she uses one of these remedies. It relieves the pain. When she has another attack she uses it again and again with the same result. After a while she finds the usual amount of the remedy does not cure the pain. She uses two portions, and so the habit is formed until absolute danger is confronted. For one thing must not be forgotten: these remedies are powerful, for if they were not they would be of no effect. They are in certain doses deadly; they depress the nervous system; they disturb the digestion; they interfere with natural sleep; they require to be used in increasingly larger quantities as the system becomes accustomed to their use; they are almost without exception excreted by the kidneys, thus adding an additional burden to organs already badly overworked. They produce a habit of gaining relief which becomes an obsession and incapable of being resisted."

It may be asked, "How is it if these mixtures are harmful only, that so many people profess to have received benefit from them?" There are different reasons for this.

1. The nature of such drugs as alcohol, opium and cocaine is to benumb sensation, so that pain is stilled, and the pain, or functional disturbance forgotten for the time, because the nerves are drugged into insensibility. The person feels better while under the influence of the drug, so thinks it is benefiting him.

2. There are people who imagine they have diseases which they do not have; since trained physicians occasionally err in diagnosis, it is not strange

if the laity should do likewise. Such persons are always ready to aver that a certain medicine "cured" them.

A ludicrous example of this is a woman out West, whose picture graces the advertisements of a certain nostrum, accompanied by a testimonial that said nostrum cured her of a "polypus"! Upon being written to as to how such a preparation could effect such a cure, she answered that, after giving the testimonial, she found that she had not had a polypus!

3. Some of the cures attributed to drugs, are doubtless due to Nature. It is estimated that from 30 to 90 per cent. of ailments are cured by Nature, unassisted, and often in spite of, the drugs swallowed. Many of the books advertising these remedies (?) give excellent rules of health, which, if followed, would restore persons to vigor more speedily without the accompanying medicine, than they can be restored while the system has the poisonous drugs to throw off. It may be reasonably assumed that a goodly number of recoveries ascribed to drug treatments are due, in reality, to the resisting force of a good constitution, or to obedience to the laws of health given in the circular.

4. It is not uncommon for people suffering from certain diseases to have temporary remissions in the course of the disease. No doubt, some of the cases reported as cures are such spontaneous remissions, which are followed, after the testimonials have been written, by relapse. The majority of people are ignorant of the natural course of diseases--of what happens when no treatment is taken. They do not know that a great many affections are characterized by periods of apparent recovery. For instance in some varieties of paralysis, as well as in consumption, the sufferer may to appearance recover completely for a few months or longer; if a remedy was being used at the time, it would naturally get the credit of causing the favorable change.

However, all of the glowing testimonials of wonderful benefits accruing from patent medicines are not what they seem to be. Dr. J. H. Kellogg says in his Monitor of Health:--

"The average manufacturer of patent medicines regularly employs a person of some literary attainment whose duty it is to invent vigorous testimonials of sufferings relieved by Dr. Charlatan's universal panacea. In many instances persons are hired to give testimonials, and answer letters of inquiry in such a way as to encourage business. The shameless dishonesty and ingenious villainy exhibited are beyond description."

Recently an advertisement of one of these nostrums stated in the headlines that said nostrum was used in the Frances Willard Temperance Hospital, Chicago. The testimonial appended purported to be from a nurse in that hospital, but the testimonial did not state, as did the headlines, that the preparation was ever used in that hospital. The president of the hospital board of trustees states that the nurse positively denies having given any testimonial to the company thus advertising. She did give one to another patent medicine concern, but not to this, and never said either was used in the hospital, nor have they been. Suit could be brought for damages, but unfortunately the patent medicine people have unlimited money, and the hospital has not.

Early in the present year there appeared in many daily papers a large advertising picture of a man whose name was appended as a professional nurse of a western city.

The following testimonial accompanied the picture:--

"Mr. ---- of ----, who is a professional nurse of experience, writes,--'My friend is improving, thanks to ----, and you. I am called on to nurse the sick of all classes. I recommend ---- to such an extent that I am nicknamed ---- (giving name of nostrum) by nearly everybody.'"

As the writer of this book was acquainted with a physician residing in the small city mentioned in the advertisement, she wrote to him, requesting that he investigate this testimonial.

He replied that he found the chief part of the advertisement, namely, that Mr. ---- was a professional nurse, false; "First, by his own statement as he told me this morning that he never claimed to be a professional nurse. And my personal acquaintance with him, as well as that of a number of other physicians in our little city, and reliable men and women of this community who are acquainted with him, all testify to the same thing, namely; that he is not a professional nurse, neither is he a nurse, or even a reliable man. He is an innocent, ignorant man, very close to the pauper class. He told me when I read the commendation to which his name is affixed, that it was all true except the professional nurse part, and that was entirely false, as stated above."

As the picture was of a fine-looking, intelligent-appearing man it probably was as genuine as the testimonial.

The following was clipped from a copy of Merck's Report, April, 1899, a druggists' paper published in New York city:--

MANY DRUGGISTS INDIGNANT.

A   PATENT-MEDICINE   ADVERTISEMENT   CONTAINS UNAUTHORIZED ENDORSEMENTS.

"Fully a score of East-side druggists are up in arms over the unauthorized use of their names in a full-page newspaper advertisement of a widely-known specific. This advertisement appeared recently in certain New York daily papers, and retail druggists who have made it a rule of their business never to recommend any particular proprietary article, found themselves quoted in unqualified laudation of the article so liberally advertised. The names and addresses of the druggists were given in full, and when several of the men quoted conferred together they found that the most barefaced misrepresentation had been resorted to.

"One of the pharmacists thus misrepresented, happened to be Sidney Faber, the secretary of the Board of Pharmacy. He was not selling this particular specific, and had never said a word for or against it, nevertheless, six or eight lines of endorsement of the article were directly attributed to him. He called on some of his druggist neighbors whose names he saw in the advertisement, and ascertained that they, too, had been falsely and unwarrantably quoted. Mr. Faber promptly wrote to the proprietors of the specific in question, and denounced the published endorsements bearing his name, as a forgery. His indignation was by no means appeased when he received a letter from the proprietary concern, couched in the following language: 'We regret to learn that you have been annoyed by any statements that have appeared in New York city papers. We will forward your letter to them.'

"Within the past few days several of the druggists whose names were used in this advertisement without authority, have been considering the advisability of taking legal proceedings in order to ascertain their rights in the matter. It is contrary to pharmaceutical ethics for a pharmacist to specially endorse any proprietary article, or patent medicine. Some of the offended druggists propose to contribute to a fund for the purpose of publicly, and widely, advertising this unwarranted use of their names."

When patent medicine advertisers would dare to resort to such a wholesale fraud as this, what may they be expected to refrain from?

As an illustration of how commendations from notable persons are sometimes obtained, the following is cited: In the winter of 1899, appeared an advertising picture of the lovely Christian lady from Denmark, the Countess Schimmelmann, who was spending some time in Chicago. Below her picture were the words:--

"Adeline, Countess Schimmelmann, whose portrait is here given, in a recent letter to the ---- company, (mentioning proprietors of nostrum) speaks of friends of hers who have been benefited by ---- (mentioning nostrum), and who first advised her to recommend it to her sick friends.

"The Countess, as is well known, is a prominent member of the Danish court. Her coming to this country has been much talked of. Her real object is one of charity. She is stopping in Chicago, and from there writes her straightforward endorsement of ---- (mentioning nostrum)."

The italics are the writer's. The picture and the testimonial were cut from the paper, and sent to the countess, asking if she had so spoken of this medicine, and, if so, did she, a strong total abstinence woman, know that this mixture contains a large percentage of alcohol.

She responded as follows:--

"Thank you for asking me about the enclosed. A white-ribbon lady came and asked me if I would do her the great kindness to recommend ---- compound (made up of the juice of celery). I said I could not personally recommend it as I neither use, nor want, medicine. But some very reliable friends of mine (temperance people, and true Christians) told me I would do a good thing in recommending it as they used it, and found it excellent. Then I wrote the following: 'I myself cannot recommend ---- compound as I do not suffer from any of the ailments it is said to be good for, but reliable friends of mine tell me that it is excellent, and I would do a good thing in recommending it to my friends. Adeline, Countess Schimmelmann.'

"I will only consent to the publishing of this letter if you publish the whole letter, and no extract from it, as the white-ribbon lady did for the ---- compound."

If a white-ribboner played this mean trick upon this distinguished Christian worker she is unworthy of membership in the Woman's Christian Temperance Union. It is more than likely that the "white-ribbon lady," was a paid advertising agent of the patent medicine manufacturer, and wore a white-ribbon to gain the confidence of the Countess.

Whether patent medicine manufacturers know how to doctor all ills to which human flesh is heir may be doubted, but that their advertising agents are skilful "doctors" of testimonials is very evident to any one acquainted with the facts.

The Department of Public Charities of New York city in a "Report on the use of so-called Proprietary Medicines as Therapeutic Agents," says:--

"In connection with this subject it might be mentioned that, for years past, the name of Bellevue Hospital has been taken in vain by a number of persons and firms, without any authority whatever. It is a common occurrence that samples of proprietary medicines, foods, mineral waters, plasters, etc., etc. are sent to the hospital, or to members of the house-staff for 'trial,' whereupon the subsequent advertisements of the articles in question often assert that the latter are 'used in Bellevue Hospital,' leaving the impression upon the mind of the reader that the article, or articles, have been used with the sanction of some member of the Medical Board. It is probably impossible to find a remedy for this evil, from which many other institutions of repute likewise suffer. To publish a denial of such false assertions would only aggravate the evil. The utmost that can be done appears to be, to caution the medical staff against any entanglements with, or encouragement of, the agents of the interested parties."

This report, which was adopted by the Medical Board of Bellevue Hospital, classifies proprietary preparations as "Objectionable" or "Unobjectionable" according to the following rules:--

"Unobjectionable preparations are those, the origin and composition of which is not kept secret, and which are known to serve a useful and legitimate purpose. Malted Milk is an example. Objectionable proprietary preparations, by far the largest group of the whole class, comprise all those which are aimed at under the medical code of ethics under the term 'secret nostrum,' which term may be more closely defined thus:

"A secret nostrum is a preparation, the origin or composition of which is kept secret, the therapeutic claims for which are unreasonable or unscientific, or which is not intended for a legitimate purpose.

"Examples: The various 'Soothing Syrups,' 'Female Regulators,' 'Blood Purifiers,' and thousands of others."

Dr. A. Emil Hiss, Ph. G., says of the secrecy of these preparations:--

"A secret compound with a meaningless title is presumptively a fraud. Why a secret if not to permit extravagant, or fraudulent, claims as to therapeutic merit? * * * * * The ruling motive of the secret being essentially false and dishonest, its employment in the interest of any remedy is clearly a sufficient cause for its condemnation and ostracism."

Mothers sometimes wonder why their boys take so readily to cigarettes, or their daughters to cocaine, never thinking that the soothing syrup, or cough mixture given freely by themselves to their children developed a craving for something stronger later on. Mrs. Winslow's Soothing Syrup, advertised for years in church as well as secular papers as "invaluable for children," is cited in the report for 1888 of the Massachusetts State Board of Health as containing opium; also Ayer's Cherry Pectoral, Dr. Bull's Cough Syrup, Jayne's Expectorant, Hooker's Cough and Croup Syrup, Moore's Essence of Life, Mother Bailey's Quieting Syrup, and others too numerous to mention. The report says:--

"The sale of soothing syrups, and all medicines designed for the use of children, which contain opium and its preparations should be prohibited. Many would be deterred from using a preparation known to contain opium, who would use without question a soothing syrup recommended for teething children."

Again, on page 149 the following is quoted from a prominent physician:--

"Among infants, and in the early years of life, soothing syrups are the cause of untold misery; for seeds are doubtlessly sown in infancy only to bear the most pernicious fruit in adult life. It is said that one of the best known soothing syrups contains from one to three grains of morphia to the ounce of syrup. I believe that stringent legal measures should immediately be taken to stop the sale of so-called soothing syrups containing opium, morphia or codeine."

The writer has known mothers so ignorant of the nature of these soothing syrups as to deliberately put the baby to sleep upon them in order to insure relief from care for some hours.

Prof. J. Redding, M. D., says on this point:--

"While it may be true that an adult, of his own free will, and without incentive, or predisposing causes, does occasionally become a drunkard, I am convinced that nine hundred and ninety-nine out of every one thousand individuals who become drunkards are made so in embryo, infancy, or childhood, by the use of alcoholic decoctions, soothing syrups, opiates, calomel, etc. which are given as medicines to allay pain, obtund nerve sensibility, to cure the little sufferer of his vital manifestations, of his mental discomforts, but leave the actual disease and its, perhaps, putrid causation to time and debilitated vitality to remove."

Of the danger and harmfulness of patent cough mixtures The American Therapist says:--

"Cough mixtures as a rule, do more harm than good. Nine times out of ten the principal ingredient is opium. It is true that opium may lessen the tendency to cough, but it does great damage by arresting the normal secretions, and the system becomes affected by the poisons from the kidneys, skin, stomach, intestines and the mucous membrane lining the upper air passages. Not only do these mixtures arrest every secretion in the body, but they also show their deteriorating and degrading effect through the stomach. They contain substances which tend to disorder and derange digestion."

Several years ago the Post-Office Department at Washington was led to take an interest in the question of fraudulent "patent" medicines, and an examination of many of these nostrums was undertaken by government chemists. Fraud orders were issued against some of the most flagrant offenders, forbidding them the use of the mails. This has not done away with the evil, however, for they usually move to another city, and begin business again under another name.

The examinations made for the Post Office Department revealed the fact that a great many of the so-called medicines on the market were intoxicating beverages in disguise. The Internal Revenue Department then took up the matter and a long list of these beverage medicines was sent out to internal revenue agents with instructions that these must not be sold henceforth unless by persons paying a special tax for the sale of alcoholic beverages.

Some of the manufacturers of these nostrums availed themselves of opportunity given to add a recognized medicinal agent to their flavored alcohol and water and such preparations were stricken from the list of those requiring a whisky license for their sale. Peruna and Hostetter's Bitters were the best-known of these. Peruna had been up to this time what government chemists called "a cheap cocktail." The report of the pure food commissioner of North Dakota for 1906 gives on page 157 an analysis of it as now upon the market: "Alcohol by volume, 21.25 per cent.; total solids, 3.846 per cent.; ash, .158 per cent." The report says:--

"The only thing of a medicinal nature that we could find in this preparation appeared to be a small amount of senna combined with a bitters of some kind."

Proprietary "Foods" have not escaped attention from chemists. Dr. Charles Harrington, for several years secretary of Massachusetts Board of Health, was the first to publish an analysis of these preparations showing their alcoholic strength and their small nutritive content. He lists "foods" examined by him as follows:--

"Liquid Peptonoids 23.03 alcohol; maximum amount recommended will yield less than one ounce of nutriment per day, and the equivalent of 3.50 oz. of whisky. Hemapeptone 10.60 alcohol; Hemaboloids 15.81 alcohol; the maximum dose recommended yields about 1/4 oz. of nutriment, and the equivalent of about 1-1/2 oz. of whisky daily. Tonic Beef 15.58 alcohol; doses recommended yield about 1/2 oz. nutriment daily, and the equivalent of one ounce of whiskey. Mulford's Predigested Beef 19.72 alcohol; doses recommended yield about 1-1/4 oz. nutriment daily, and the alcoholic equivalent of about 6 oz. of whisky. There were "Foods" for the sick examined which were non-alcoholic, but their nutritive value was about nothing in comparison to their cost."

The Committee on Pharmacy of the American Medical Association reports on the following foods thus:--

Carpanutrine 17.3 alcohol; Liquid Peptones (Lilly & Co.) 22.0; Nutrient Wine of Beef Peptone (Armour) 21.5; Nutritive Liquid Peptone 23.0; Panopepton 18.5; Peptonic Elixir 18.8; Tonic Beef 16.1. The report on these says: "There are no fatty substances present in these products; their food value from this point of view is, therefore, nil."

A prominent physician of Philadelphia said of these "Foods" in the Journal of the A. M. A.:--

"I have long been convinced that many a patient has suffered severely when preparations such as these were being used, and that not a few of them have died, chiefly of starvation. * * * A very important disadvantage of these foods is their alcoholic content. Even in the small doses customarily used, the quantity of alcohol is often irritating to the stomach, and may be disadvantageous in other ways."

The Committee on Pharmacy also reported on cod-liver oil preparations. They said: "A preparation claiming to represent cod-liver oil which does not contain oil in some form is fraudulent. Waterbury's Metabolized Cod-Liver Oil and Hagee's Cordial of Cod-Liver Oil are cited as examples. It is claimed by the manufacturers that the latter represents 33 per cent. of pure Norwegian cod-liver oil, but in neither of these preparations did the tests made by the committee show any oil. Analysis revealed sugar, alcohol, and glycerine, none of which is contained in cod-liver oil."

Vinol is advertised as Wine of Cod-Liver Oil, but is admittedly without oil, and according to analysis contains 18.8 per cent. alcohol. Wampole's Tasteless Preparation of Cod-Liver Oil showed 20.05 per cent. of alcohol.

Cod-Liver Oil is considerably out of date now as a prescribed remedy because physicians have found that it impairs appetite. Cream and fresh butter and olive oil are advised instead.

Australia has been such a harvest field for patent medicine manufacturers that a government commission was appointed to study the subject. This commission presented a voluminous report to the parliament of 1907. This report gives an analysis of most of the extensively advertised medicines. Doan's Backache Kidney Pills are said to be made of oil of juniper 1 drop, hemlock pitch 10 grains, potassium nitrate 5 grains, powdered fenugreek (Greek hay) 4 grains, wheat flour 4 grains, maize starch 2 grains. The report says: "The stuff is the cheapest kind of skin-plaster made up into pills." The seeds of fenugreek are used mainly for poultices. Doan's Dinner Pills contain two drastic purgatives, podophyllin and aloin. Both of these are dangerous drugs. Aloin frequently produces hemorrhoids (piles). The British Medical Journal says that the material in forty of the Kidney Pills and four Dinner Pills would cost one English halfpenny (one cent).

Vitae-Ore is given as consisting of ordinary sulphate of iron (green vitriol) to which a little Epsom salts has been added. Munyon's Kidney Cure, which claims to cure Bright's disease, gravel, and all urinary diseases, is given as composed entirely of sugar. Dr. Williams' Pink Pills are said to be an iron pill much the same as the ordinary Blaud's Pills which are sold in drug-stores for half, or less than half, the price of the proprietary article. (Iron is said by recent investigators to be very injurious to the stomach.)

The Committee on Pharmacy of the American Medical Association has analyzed many proprietary medicines; from their reports the following analyses are taken. "Health Grains," which are claimed to be a remedy for "Dyspepsia, Indigestion, Nervousness, etc.," were found to consist of 87.50 per cent. of coarse quartz sand, and 12.50 per cent. of rock candy and syrup.

"Hoff's Consumption Cure consists essentially of sodium cinnamate and extract of opium, a mixture at one time suggested for the treatment of tuberculosis, but which has been discarded by physicians. A medicine which depends on opium for whatever therapeutic effect it may have is, when sold indiscriminately to the laity, inherently vicious."

Sartoin Skin Food for "sunburn, and all skin blemishes" was made of Epsom salts colored with a pink dye. The government prosecuted the company sending out Epsom salts as a "food," and they were fined $20 for thus seeking to dupe silly women.

Malt extracts are very extensively used at the present time, under the popular notion that they are an aid to starch digestion. That they are a product of the brewery has caused them to be looked upon with suspicion by cautious people, but the multitude has apparently given no thought, or care, as to whether or not they may be alcoholic. Dr. Charles Harrington presented the results of an examination of these preparations at a meeting of the Boston Society of Medical Sciences, held Nov. 17, 1896. The following is quoted from the journal of the society for November, 1896:--

"Twenty-one different brands of liquid malt extract were obtained and analyzed. That they were not true malt extracts is shown by the fact that in no one was there the slightest diastatic power; all were alcoholic, some being stronger than beer, ale, or even porter. In a number of specimens a large amount of salicylic acid was detected."

Dr. J. H. Kellogg, in commenting upon this report, said in the Dec., 1896, Bulletin of the A. M. T. A.:--

"In the light of these facts, it is apparent that ale or lager beer might as well be prescribed for a patient as these so-called malt extracts, which are practically nothing more than concentrated ale or lager."

There are malt extracts, made up like honey, or syrup, in consistency, which are valuable.

The following list of malt extracts, with accompanying letter from Prof. Sharples, is taken from a paper published by Hon. Henry H. Faxon, of Quincy, Mass.:--

"Boston, Mass., March 20, 1897.

"I enclose a list of the malt extracts examined in this office during the past year or two. These samples were all in original packages, obtained by officers in various parts of Eastern Massachusetts. They probably very fairly represent the various malt extracts on the market. I have added two samples of Porter and one of Old Brown Stout for purposes of comparison.

"Yours respectfully, "S. P. SHARPLES. "State Assayer."

Name. Solids. Alcohol.

5193 English Malt Extract 9.70 5.63 5214 Old Grist Mill Malt Extract 10.57 5.54 5418 Old Grist Mill Malt Extract 9.98 5.63 5490 Old Grist Mill Malt Extract 12.28 5.86 5626 Old Grist Mill Malt Extract 9.63 5.00 5207 Liquid Food, a Malt Extract 10.47 4.27 5225 Pure Malt, a Liquid Food, a

Tonic 9.71 5.00 5416 Pure Malt, a Liquid Food, a Tonic 10.76 6.32 5619 King's Pure Malt[C] 9.52 6.60 [Footnote C: The label on King's Malt states that for a strong, healthy person, with a good appetite, a pint with each meal and another on retiring at night will not be too much.] 5421 A Nutritious Tonic, Pure Malt Extract 10.88 6.24 5226 Noris' Extract of Malt 11.57 5.94 5258 Noris' Extract of Malt 9.31 6.55 5397 Noris' Extract of Malt 10.63 6.24 5485 Noris' Extract of Malt 10.50 6.63 5620 Noris' Extract of Malt 12.55 5.90 5229 Pabst Malt Extract, The Best Tonic 10.43 5.16 5230 Hoff's Malt Extract (Tarrant's) 11.33 8.88 5489 Hoff's Malt Extract (Tarrant's) 12.25 7.17 5231 Johann Hoff'sches Malz-Extract, Gesundheit's Beir 11.31 4.34 5491 Johann Hoff'sches Malz-Extract, Gesundheit's Beir 11.02 4.85 5621 Johann Hoff'sches Malz-Extract, Gesundheit's Beir 10.49 4.50 5408 Johann Hoff'sches Malz-Extract, Gesundheit's Beir 11.47 4.78 5340 Haffenreffer & Co. Malt Wine 11.02 6.65 5423 Haffenreffer & Co. Malt Wine 11.71 5.63 Liquid Bread, A Pure Extract of Malt 6.78 6.63 5395 Durgin's Malt, Liquid Extract of Malt 7.12 5.94 5433 Durgin's Liquid Extract of Malt 6.49 5.55 5396 Wyeth's Liquid Malt Extract 14.80 3.35 5488 Wyeth's Liquid Malt Extract 15.50 2.86 5622 Wyeth's Liquid Malt Extract 15.73 2.35 5406 Wampole's Concentrated Extract of Malt 9.84 9.86 5407 Anheuser-Busch's Malt Nutrine 15.98 3.00 5600 Anheuser-Busch's Malt Nutrine 15.82 2.25 5417 Malt Extract (Sterilized), John L. Gleeson 7.97 4.71 5422 Malt Extract (Sterilized), Charles C. Hearn 8.58 5.00 5436 Burkhart Brewing Co.'s Malt Extract 10.73 7.01 5486 Menzel's Extract of Malt 5.90 5.24 5625 Menzel's Extract of Malt 6.75 4.35 5623 King of Malt Tonics, Lion Tonic 10.95 7.05 5624 Teutonic, "A concentrated Extract of Malt and Hops" 9.95 7.45 5409 Van Nostrand's Old Stout Porter, "a pure malt extract" 7.97 6.55 5233 Philadelphia Porter 5.34 6.63 5232 Burke's Guiness Stout 6.66 7.17

The alcohol in the above table represents the cubic centimeters of alcohol in a 100 cubic centimeters of the liquid. The solids are the number of grams of solid extract in each 100 centimeters of the liquid.

S. P. SHARPLES.

The British Medical Journal, and the British Medical Temperance Review have been calling attention to the danger in coca wines. Intemperance among invalids is said to be greatly on the increase from the use of these wines. In every case the basis of these preparations is strongly alcoholic wine, ranging from 18 to 20 per cent. The coca added is either the leaves, or liquid extract of coca, or hydrochlorate of cocaine.

Dr. Frederic Coley says in the British Medical Journal:--

"Coca, and its chief alkaloid, cocaine, are drugs which possess some power of removing the sense of fatigue, just as analgesics remove the consciousness of pain. But they no more remove the physical condition of muscles, and nerve centres, of which the sense of pain gives us warning, than a dose of morphine, which removes the pain of toothache, removes the offending tooth, or even arrests the caries in it. The truth of this will be obvious to any one who remembers enough of physiology to know what fatigue really means. A muscle which is tired out is different chemically from the same muscle in its more normal condition, when it is ready to respond vigorously to ordinary stimuli. It has lost something, and is, besides, overcharged (poisoned, in fact) with the products of its own activity, and it can only be restored by a fresh supply of the material which it requires, and the carrying away of the poisonous waste products. Fatigue of nerve centres is no doubt strictly analogous to fatigue of muscles.

"It is practically impossible for us, by voluntary exertion, to reach the degree of absolute fatigue, which the physiologist produces by electric stimulation of a nerve-muscle preparation. The sense of fatigue becomes so intense that voluntary effort cannot overcome it. So no man can produce asphyxia by simply holding his breath, because the besoin de respirer becomes irresistible; but it is quite possible for a narcotic to so dull the sensory part of the respiratory reflex mechanism as to permit asphyxia to take place.

"The sense of fatigue, and the besoin de respirer are both Nature's danger signals. Drugs which hide such signals from us are a more than doubtful benefit. If it were possible for us to suppose that a fraction of a grain of cocaine could afford to exhausted nerve centres, and muscles, the nutriment which they require for their restoration, and at the same time eliminate the poisonous waste products, then it would be reasonable to prescribe the drug for use by all who are overworked, and perhaps suffering from the malnutrition consequent upon, 'nervous dyspepsia,' as well as mere want of rest.

"In this go-ahead century it is no wonder that many are but too ready to experiment with a drug which professes to be able to remove fatigue, and to enable a man to go on working when, without its aid, weariness had become unendurable. Cocaine claims all this; and it is most dangerous just because, for a time, it seems able to keep its promise. That is how victims to cocainism are made. Let us be honest with our overworked patients, who want us to help them with drugs; let us tell them that rest is the only safe remedy for weariness.

"To combine such a drug as coca, or cocaine, with an alcoholic stimulant, is to multiply the dangers of cocainism by those of alcoholism. It would be impossible to find terms sufficiently severe in which to condemn the recklessness of those who promiscuously recommend such a compound for all who are overworked or debilitated. One firm actually has the assurance to advertise a preparation of this kind as a remedy for dipsomania. Truly this is casting out devils by Beelzebub, with a vengeance. Invoking Beelzebub for such a purpose has never been a success. And I suspect that any form of coca wine will make a great many more dipsomaniacs than it will cure."

Dr. Walter N. Edwards, F. C. S., says of coca wines:--

"These wines are sold as being useful in an immense variety of ailments. The following are a few of the many that are named upon the bottles or in the circulars accompanying them:--

"Weakness after illness, "Nervous disorders, "Sleeplessness, "Influenza, "Whooping cough, "Exhaustion of mind and body, "Allays thirst, "Restores digestive function, "Enables great physical toil to be undergone, "Great value in excesses of all kinds, "General debility, "Prevents colds and chills, "Makes pure, rich blood, "An鎚ia, "Invaluable after pleurisy, pneumonia, etc., "Aid to the vocal organs.

"This is a fairly respectable list of complaints, and the very fact that these preparations of coca wine are put forward as a cure for so wide a range of various complaints is in itself a condemnation of them.

"When any particular remedy is said to be of universal application for a large number of different complaints it may be looked upon with great suspicion.

"It must always be remembered that there is the commercial side to this question. The proprietors have no particular regard for the welfare of the people; their business is to make a profit, and many of them gain enormous fortunes. By skilful and lavish advertisements, and by carefully worded testimonials, they appeal to the credulity of the public, and often deceive even those who regard themselves as belonging to the thinking classes.

"There are two specific dangers in regard to these wines. They are ordinary wines, either port or sherry for the most part, and therefore strongly alcoholic. The user of them is in considerable danger of cultivating a taste for alcohol, and certainly, there is the greatest possible danger to any one having had the appetite, of reviving it.

"The dose is an elastic one, it can be repeated with considerable frequency three or four times a day.

"What would be said of growing girls or youths having recourse three or four times a day to the wine bottle? This is exactly what they are doing when coca, and the so-called food wines are placed in their hands as medicine.

They like the pleasant taste, there is the call of habit and appetite, and so there arises the greatest possible danger of a general liking for alcoholic liquors being set up. The ailing man or woman of set years is in similar danger, for they are having recourse to alcohol when their powers of mind and body are to some extent exhausted, and they are thus less able to resist the fascination for alcohol that may so quickly be brought into existence.

"Another element of danger is that the recourse to coca and kola is an attempt to get more out of the body, and the mind, than nature intended. Overwork, overstrain, worry, all produce exhaustion of physical and nervous power. Nature pulls us up by asserting herself, and we feel run down and seedy, and, perhaps, quite unwell. What is wanted is rest, proper diet, and change. These would quickly be restorative, and once again we should be fit for the duties of life.

"In a busy age there is the strongest possible temptation to seek a restorative by some occult method, rather than to give the rest and refreshment that nature demands. It is upon this that the whole trade in these so-called restoratives depends.

"There is no food quality in alcohol, cocaine or kola, but there is in them all a narcotizing influence that in its lesser stages is hurtful, and in its greater stages disastrous.

"The cocaine habit may be cultivated as easily as the alcohol habit, and the two forms of disease, alcoholism and cocainism, are by no means rare. The great factor in each of them is the loss of will power, and when that is accomplished the descent to complete moral and physical ruin is quite easy.

"A pure and simple life, in accord with the laws of health and hygiene, is the panacea both for the maintenance, and the restoration of health, and that is what we should strive to aim at, rather than having recourse to drugs that are not only ineffective, but positively dangerous."--United Temperance Gazette.

In Dr. Milner Fothergill's Practioners' Hand-book of Treatment, fourth edition, the following statement is made:--

"Coca wine, and other medicated wines are largely sold to people who are considered, and consider themselves, to be total abstainers. It is not uncommon to hear the mother of a family say, 'I never allow my girls to touch stimulants of any kind, but I give them each a glass of coca wine at 11 in the morning, and again at bedtime.' Originally coca wine was made from coca leaves, but it is now commonly a solution of the alkaloid, in a sweet and strongly alcoholic wine. This is really the gist of the whole matter; coca wine is largely consumed by people who fondly believe themselves to be total abstainers, and who are active enough in denouncing those who take a little wine, or a glass of beer at their meals. The sooner their delusion is dispelled the better for themselves, and for the unfortunate children over whom they exercise supervision."

Another physician tells of seeing a distinguished ecclesiastical dignitary, a sworn foe of alcohol and its congeners, giving his young child a generous daily allowance of one of these wines.

The user of coca wines runs a double risk--an alcohol craving may be revived, or created; and, at the same time, cocainism may be set up, and nothing but physical, mental and moral ruin follow.

The British Medical Journal of January 23rd, 1897, says:--

"There can be no doubt that in many parts of the world cocaine inebriety is largely on the increase. The greatest number of victims is to be found among society women, and among women who have adopted literature as a profession; and there is no doubt that a considerable proportion of chronic cocainists have fallen under the dominion of the drug from a desire to stimulate their powers of imagination. Others have acquired that habit quite innocently from taking coca wines. The symptoms experienced by the victims of the cocaine habit are illusions of sight and hearing, neuromuscular irritability, and localized an 鉦 thesia. After a time insomnia supervenes, and the patient displays a curious hesitancy, and an inability to arrive at a decision on even the most trivial subjects."

Dr. F. Coley says later on in the article before referred to:--

"There is another combination which, though utterly absurd from a therapeutical point of view, is not in itself quite so dangerous as coca wine. It will probably do a larger amount of mischief, however, because more people take it. I refer to the various preparations, so largely advertised, which profess to be compounded of port wine, extract of malt, and extract of meat. To the medically uneducated public this doubtless seems a most promising combination: extract of meat for food, extract of malt to aid digestion, port wine to make blood. Surely the very thing to strengthen all who are weak, and to hasten the restoration of convalescents. Unfortunately what the advertisements say--that this stuff is largely prescribed by medical men--is not wholly untrue.

"I do not suppose that any physician of anything like front rank would make such a mistake. But busy general practitioners may be excused if they prove to be a bit oblivious of physiology, and so become attracted by a formula which is more plausible than sound. In the first place, we all know that extract of meat is not food at all. From the manner of its production, it cannot contain an appreciable quantity of proteid material. It consists mainly of creatin, and creatinin, and salts. These are, it is needless to say, incapable of acting as food. Extract of meat, and similar preparations, have their uses however; made into 'beef-tea,' their meaty flavor often enables patients to take a quantity of bread, which would otherwise be refused; or lentil flour, or some other matter may be added. In this way, though not food itself, it becomes a most useful aid to feeding. It is besides, a harmless stimulant, especially when taken, as it always should be, hot. It should be needless to add that to combine extract of meat with port wine is simply to ignore its real use. The only intelligible basis for such an invention must be the wholly erroneous notion that extract of meat is a food."

The prices asked for "secret nostrums" are said by chemists to be ofttimes far beyond the value of the materials. Of one article the New Idea, a druggists' paper, says:--

"It retails at $1.50 per bottle. Such an article could be put up for less than fifteen cents, including bottle, leaving by no means a small margin for the profit of its manufacturers."

The same paper says of a cure for catarrh, neuralgia, etc. sold in the form of a small ball:--

"This cure costs $2.50 per ball. A handsome profit could be made upon it at 5 cents a ball."

Some proprietary preparations are not harmful, but are positively inert. The Mass. State Board of Health in report of 1896 gives Kaskine as an example of these. Although sold at a dollar an ounce it was found to consist of nothing but granulated sugar of the fine grade used in homeopathic pharmacy, without any medication or flavoring whatever.

Dr. Edward Von Adelung in an article in Life and Health, Dec., 1897, tells of a well advertised cure for consumption, the analysis of which showed it to be composed of water, slightly colored by the addition of a very small quantity of red wine, and two mineral acids, muriatic and impure sulphuric, in quantities just sufficient to lend it a taste! He says:--

"Fortuitously I had the opportunity of observing the influence of this remedy on a consumptive who took it regularly, and who was so enamored of its favorable action that he gave up his business to conduct an agency for its sale. It was not long after he had entered upon his new vocation that I received word of his death, due to pulmonary hemorrhage."

The "returned missionary" fraud has been exposed by different druggists' papers, among them the New Idea. The "missionary" would advertise a "free cure," if people would send to him. The "cure" would be in the form of a prescription. There being no drugs in any drugstore bearing the names given in the prescription, the dupe was expected to pay an exorbitant price for them to the philanthropic "missionary." In one case of this kind the "medicinal plants brought from South America, the only place where they grew," were upon examination by chemists of the New Idea found to be ordinary drugs, not one of which comes from South America.

The same paper tells of another "South American" fraud, 60,000 bottles of which were said to be sold in Detroit in a few weeks, by an itinerating vendor.

A certain liver, and kidney, and constipation cure, sold in the form of herbs, is said by New Idea to be chiefly couch grass, and senna leaves. Yet it sells for 25 cents for a small package.

To this paper the public is also indebted for the information that a kind of wafer advertised to "cure in a few days all coughs, colds, irritation of the uvula and tonsils, influenza, bronchitis, asthma, sore throat, consumption, and all diseases of the lungs and chest" was found to consist wholly of sugar and corn starch!

Medical World recently told of the investigation of "H----" by Prof. John Uri Lloyd of Cincinnati. It was advertised as a plant discovered by a doctor traveling in Florida. Its juices were said to be antidotal to snake poisoning, and would also cure the opium habit. Prof. Lloyd found it to be a liquid consisting of a solution of sulphate of morphine and salicylic acid, in alcohol and glycerine, with suitable coloring matter.

Another fraud exposed by New Idea was a "cure" for the peculiar ills of women. The cure is put up in the form of little oblong blocks about a half inch in length.

"A circular accompanies them, and is well calculated to produce alarm in the young. It is another sample of the demoralizing documents which unscrupulous quacks are continually circulating among the laity, in order to create alarm, and profit by this alarm."

After giving a description of the diseases peculiar to the sex it is stated that all of these are curable by using eight dollars worth of this wonderful medicine.

New Idea continues:--

"The cure consists, according to our examination, of nothing but flour, made into a paste and allowed to harden in the form of small oblong blocks. Evidently the quack relied upon the faith-cure principle, and his auxiliary treatment, as set forth in the rules of living given in the circular."

While these inert preparations are of the nature of frauds, they will not injure the health, nor make drunkards, or opium fiends, as the disguised preparations of whisky and morphine are likely to do.

That the use of patent medicines has made many drunkards is a fact well attested. The American Association for the Study of Inebriety appointed a committee several years ago to investigate the various nostrums advertised especially for the benefit of alcohol and opium inebriates. The report of this committee, prepared by Dr. N. Roe Bradner, late of the Pennsylvania Hospital for the Insane, in speaking of the marvelous cures advertised in connection with the use of these mixtures, calls them "volumes of gilded falsehood, designed for an innocent, unsuspecting public," and adds:--

"The use of such nostrums would do more toward confirming than eradicating the habit, if it existed, and would invite and create addiction to an almost hopeless fatality, where the habit had not previously existed. Insanity, palsy, idiocy, and many forms of physical, moral and mental ruin have followed the sale of these nostrums throughout our land."

Dr. E. A. Craighill, President of the Virginia State Pharmaceutical Association, is quoted in the July (1897) Journal of Inebriety, as saying:--

"In my experience I have known of men filling drunkards' graves who learned to drink taking some advertised bitters as legitimate medicine. It would be hard to estimate the number of young brains ruined, and the maturer opium wrecks from nostrums of this nature. I could write a volume on the mischief that is being done every day to body, mind and soul, all over the land, by the thousands of miserable frauds that are being poured down the throats of not only ignorant people, but, alas, intelligent ones, too."

A lady informed the writer recently that her brother had taken forty bottles of one of these preparations, and had become a drunkard through it.

Many seem unaware that the ethics of the medical profession restrain reputable physicians from advertising themselves or their remedies, so that these much-lauded patent medicines are put upon the market by quacks, never by physicians of good standing. It is purely a money-making enterprise, without consideration of the health or destruction of the people. It is popularly supposed that physicians decry these things from fear that their sale will injure regular practice. This is another error as they increase work for the doctor by aggravating existing trouble, as well as causing disease where there was only slight disturbance.

Dr. F. E. Stewart, Ph. G., of Detroit, Mich., says in the October, 1897, Life and Health:--

"Taking all these facts into consideration, it is apparent that the patent, trade-mark and copyright laws should be so interpreted and administered by the court that they will secure the greatest good to the greatest number, and aid in attaining the end of government, viz., 'moral, intellectual and physical perfection.' It is not the object of these laws to create odious monopolies, to throw a mantle of protection over fraud, to enable quacks and charlatans to encroach on the domain of legitimate medical and pharmacal practice, or to support an advertising business designed to mislead the public in regard to the nature and value of medicines as curative agents. The morals of the community are injured by some of this advertising, intellectual vigor is impaired by the use of many things advertised, and physical, as well as moral, degradation frequently results. Crime is often inculcated--even the crime of murder, that the nostrum manufacturer may profit thereby. Cures for incurable diseases are promised, and guaranteed. Every scheme that human and devilish ingenuity can devise to wring money from its victim is resorted to, which can be employed without actually bringing the advertisers into court. All this wicked quackery parades under the guise of 'patent' medicines, and asks the protection of our courts. It is time for the medical and pharmaceutic professions to unite, and unmask this monster, and show the public its true nature. And this can be accomplished in no better way than through a study of the object of the laws which the secret nostrum manufacturers are now endeavoring to prostitute for their own advantage, and the teaching of the public what these laws were enacted for.

"The secret nostrum business in some of its phases has assiduously found its way into the medical arts, and physicians, pharmacists, and manufacturing houses, seem to have forgotten, to a certain extent, the obligations which they owe to the public. Medicine, in all its departments, must be practiced in accord with scientific, and professional requirement, or it will sink to the level of a commercial business. The end of medical practice is service to suffering humanity, not the acquisition of money. Money making is a necessary part of the practice of medical arts, not, however, its chief object. This fact must be kept in view always. Once lost sight of, and trade competition substituted for competition in serving the interests of the sick, medical and pharmacal practice will become an ignoble scrabble for wealth, in which the sick become victims of avarice and greed. Better set free a pack of ravening wolves in a community than to change the end of medical practice to a commercial one, for physicians and pharmacists would soon degenerate into quacks and charlatans, and take shameful advantage of the community for gain."

Where Dr. Stewart speaks of murder he probably refers to the sale of abortofacients.

Dr. Roe Bradner, of Philadelphia, in his report upon alleged cures for drunkenness before the Society for the Study of Inebriety several years ago, said:--

"There is a certain other class of so-called remedies, prepared sometimes by physicians and pharmacists, that do a great deal of harm. I allude to the 'non-secret proprietaries' that claim to publish their formulas, but do not. One in particular has made thousands, and likely tens of thousands, of chloral drunkards, dethroned the reason of as many more, besides having killed outright very many. It is impossible for any one to estimate the mischief that is being done by such remedies, and the physicians who recommend them."

Advertising is still the great hindrance in protecting the people from medical imposters. Professor E. W. Ladd, Pure Food Commissioner of North Dakota, says on this point:--

"These patent medicines, some of which are of merit, and others are only 'dopes,' or preparations intended to defraud the public, have been altogether too generally advertised and sold to the public. In many ways it seems a deplorable fact that by an unfair method of advertising the American people have come to be consumers to such an extent of a class of medicines, which, at times, are positively detrimental to health. In other instances the continued use of the product is liable to result in the formation of a drug habit which may lead to serious consequences.

"It should not be understood that this department condemns the use of legitimate proprietary or patent medicines, but it insists that there is a need for wiping out of existence about half of the products now generally sold, and with regard to the others the public have a right to know what is contained in them, and not be misled by false statements, or by statements so cunningly worded as to positively mislead the unwary reader. * * * In view of the fact that about 90 per cent. of the nostrums on the market are sold by newspaper and magazine advertising and not by the customer seeing the package, it would seem advisable to amend the law so as to cover this point."

There is no doubt that it is the advertising which makes the patent medicine business so tremendously profitable. One firm boasted, prior to the exposure of the fraud nature of their preparation, that they spent $5,000 a day in advertising. What must have been made on the nostrum to allow such expenditure? It is said on good authority that the cost of these nostrums does not exceed fifteen to sixteen cents a bottle, and they sell for a dollar a bottle. Such profits make it easy to buy up newspapers that are conscienceless as to the robbery of the unfortunate sick.

The only effectual way of putting an end to the sale of nostrums is to make illegal the advertising of such preparations in the public press. Norway has safeguarded her people thus. The difficulty in gaining such a law in America will be the opposition of the newspapers, the large majority of which still cling to this selfish method of adding to their gains. Even the so-called religious press is not all clean yet in this respect. Once they could be excused because of lack of knowledge. Now there is no excuse.

During the debate in Congress upon the patent-medicine clause of the Pure Food Bill, Senator Heyburn said:--

"I have always been aggressively against the advertisements of nostrums. Some time ago a friend of mine, a very old fellow, that I had taken a special interest in securing a pension for, had reached the age and condition of dependency. I succeeded in getting him a comfortable pension that would pay his bills for household provisions. Once, when I found he was very poor, I said to his wife, 'What are you doing with your pension?' She said, 'Don't you know, Mr. Heyburn, that it takes at least one-half of that pension for patent medicine?' Then she enumerated the patent medicines they were taking. It was being suggested to them through advertisements that they were the victims of ills that they were not troubled with, and that they could find relief through these different medicines.

"I am in favor of stopping the advertisements of these nostrums in every paper in the country."

It may well be asked, Would any one of these well-to-do newspaper owners entrust himself, or any of his family, in time of sickness to the cure-all imposters whose nostrums they advertise? If one of their children had an 鎚 ia would they rely on Pink Pills for a cure? If they had a genuine catarrh would they expect it to be cured by Peruna? Never! They would seek the very best medical advice obtainable. Yet, for the ignorant, credulous, sick and suffering poor they allow traps to be laid to rob of both money and such chances of recovery as might come from proper medical attendance.

CHAPTER XIV.

"DRUGGING."

The main reason why so many people use patent medicines is the popular supposition that drugs cure disease. This is a great error. Drugs never cure disease. Nature alone has power to heal. There are agents, which in the hands of a trained and painstaking physician may assist nature, but the physician needs to understand something of the idiosyncrasies of his patient's system, or the use of these agents may do great harm instead of good. Those medical men who have made the most diligent study of health and disease assert as their deliberate opinion that excessive professional drugging has been decidedly destructive of human life.

Dr. Jacob Bigelow, professor in the medical department of Harvard University, in a work published a few years ago stated as his belief that the unbiased opinion of most medical men of sound judgment, and long experience, is that the amount of death and disaster in the world would be less, if all diseases were left to themselves, than it now is under the multiform, reckless, and contradictory modes of practice, with which practitioners of diverse denominations carry on their differences, at the expense of the patient.

Sir John Forbes, M. D., F. R. S., said:--

"Some patients get well with the aid of medicine, more without it, and still more in spite of it."

Dr. Bostwick, author of The History of Medicine, said:--

"Every dose of medicine given is a blind experiment upon the vitality of the patient."

Dr. James Johnson, editor of the Medico-Chirurgical Review, says:--

"I declare as my conscientious conviction founded on long experience and reflection, that if there were not a single physician, surgeon, man-midwife, chemist, apothecary, druggist nor drug on the face of the earth, there would be less sickness and less mortality than now prevail."

Prof. J. W. Carson, of the New York College of Physicians and Surgeons, says:--

"We do not know whether our patients recover because we give them medicine, or because nature cures them. Perhaps bread-pills would cure as many as medicine."

Prof. Alonzo Clark, of the same college, has said:--

"In their zeal to do good physicians have done much harm; they have hurried many to the grave who would have recovered if left to nature."

Prof. Martin Paine, of the New York University Medical College, said:--

"Drug medicines do but cure one disease by producing another."

Dr. Marshall Hall, F. R. S.:--

"Thousands are annually slaughtered in the quiet sick-room."

Dr. Adam Smith:--

"The chief cause of quackery outside the profession is the real quackery in the profession."

Prof. Gilman:--

"The things that are administered for the cure of scarlet fever and measles kill far more than those diseases kill."

Prof. Barker, of New York Medical College:--

"The drugs that are administered for the cure of scarlet fever kill far more patients than the disease does."

Prof. Parker:--

"As we place more confidence in nature, and less in preparations of the apothecary, mortality diminishes."

The examining physician of a large insurance company in New York said to a Mercury reporter:--

"The primary cause of so many cases of la grippe in this and other cities is the almost universal habit of drug taking from the milder tonics to patent medicines. Whenever the average man or woman feels depressed or slightly ill, resort is made at once to medicine, more or less strong. If they would try to find out the cause of the trouble, and seek to obviate it by regulating their mode of living, the general health of the community would be better. The drug habit tends continually to lower the tone of the system. The more it is indulged in the more apparent becomes the necessity of continuing the downhill course. The majority of persons do not look beyond the fact that they seem to feel better after the use of a stimulating drug, or patent medicine. This feeling comes from a benumbing action of the drug, because it has no uplifting action. With the system in such a weakened state, the microbes of the disease find excellent ground to grow."

Dr. J. H. Kellogg says in the April, 1899, Bulletin of the A. M. T. A.:--

"Every drug capable of producing an artificial exhilaration of spirits, a pleasure which is not the result of the natural play of the vital functions, is necessarily mischievous in its tendencies, and its use is intemperance, whether its name be alcohol, tobacco, opium, cocaine, coca, kola, hashish, Siberian mushroom, caffeine, betel-nuts, mat?or any other of the score or more enslaving drugs known to pharmacology. As the result of the depression which follows the unnatural elevation of sensation resulting from the use of one of these drugs, the second application finds the subject on a little lower level than the first, so that an increased dose is necessary to produce the same intensity of pleasure or the same degree of artificial felicity as the first. The larger dose is followed by still greater depression which demands a still larger dose as its antidote, and thus there is started a series of ever-increasing doses, and ever-increasing baneful after-affects, which work the ultimate ruin of the drug victim. All drugs which enslave are alike in this regard, however much they may differ otherwise in their physiological effects. Alcohol is universally recognized as only one member of a large family of intoxicating drugs, each of which is capable of producing specific functional and organic mischief, besides the vital deterioration common to the use of so-called felicity-producing drugs.

"Is it not evident, then, that in combating the use of alcohol we are attacking only one member of a numerous family of enemies to human life and happiness, every one of which must be exterminated before the evil of intemperance will be up-rooted?"

Among the most popular drugs for self-prescription at the present time are the coal-tar products. Of these Dr. N. S. Davis has said:--

"Only a few years since, the profession were taught to regard the degree of pyrexia, or heat, as the chief element of danger in all the acute general diseases. Consequently, to control the pyrexia became the leading object of treatment; and whatever would do this promptly, and at the same time allay pain and promote rest, found favor at the bedside of the patient.

"It was soon ascertained that antipyrin, antifebrin, phenacetin and other analogous products, if given in sufficient doses, would reduce the heat, and allay the pains with great certainty and promptness, not only in continued fevers, but also in rheumatism, influenza, or la grippe, etc.; and thus their use soon became popular with both the profession and the public. No one, however, undertook to first ascertain by strictly scientific appliances the actual pathological processes causing the pyrexia in each form of disease, or even to determine whether in any given case the increased heat was the result of increased heat production, or diminished heat dissipation. Neither were any of the remedies subjected to such experimental investigation as to determine their influence on the elements of the blood, the internal distribution of oxygen, the metabolism of the tissues, or on the activity of the eliminations. Consequently their exhibition was wholly empirical, and the one that subdued the pyrexia most promptly was given the preference. Yet we all know that the pyrexia invariably returned as soon as the effects of each dose were exhausted, and in a few years the results showed that while the antipyretics served to keep down the pyrexia, and give each case the appearance of doing well, the average duration of the cases, and their mortality, were both increased.

"Step by step experimental therapeutic investigations have proved that the whole class of coal-tar antipyretics reduce animal heat by impairing the capacity of the hemoglobin and corpuscular elements of the blood to receive and distribute free oxygen, and thereby reduce temperature by diminishing heat production, nerve sensibility and tissue metabolism. Therefore, while each dose temporarily reduces the fever, it retards the most important physiological processes on which the living system depends for resisting the effects of toxic agents; namely, oxidation and elimination. This not only encourages the retention of toxic agents and natural excretory materials by which specific fevers are protracted, but it greatly increases the number of cases of pneumonia that complicate the epidemic influenza, or la grippe, as it has occurred since 1888-89.

"The bad work that people make in dosing themselves with patent medicines, without a physician's prescription is not unfrequently punctuated with a sudden death from overdosing with antipyrin, sulphonal, or some other coal-tar preparation."

Dr. C. H. Shepard, Brooklyn, N. Y., says:--

"Quinine is a most fatal drug. Of course, it is the orthodox treatment for malarial conditions, but quinine never did nor never can cure malaria or any other disease. The action brought about by its use is simply to benumb the nervous activity and interfere with the natural action of the system to throw off the poison, which is expressed by the chill. Because of this interference with the manifestation or symptom of the disease, many imagine that the disease is being cured, but there never was a greater mistake. A drug disease is added to the original disease. This is shown by the invariable depression that follows the administration of the drug, and the length of time required to recuperate, which imperils restoration, and sometimes hastens the final results. This is ordinarily met by the use of what are called stimulants, that is, more drugs, and the last state is worst than the first; the poor patient is thus made the victim of a triple wrong, which only a most vigorous constitution can pass through and live, and even then he is crippled and made more liable to whatever disease may come along ever afterward.

"Disease is not entity to be killed by a shot from a professional gun, but a condition, an effort of outraged nature to free itself from an incumbrance, and should be aided rather than hindered by the administration of any nerve irritant. There never will come a time when the laws of health can be evaded. Nor is there any vicarious atonement. The full penalty of disobedience will invariably be exacted. The hunt for a panacea is as sure to be disappointing in the future as it has been in the past."

A writer in the Brooklyn Citizen says:--

"Few people are aware of the extent of a peculiar kind of dissipation known as ginger-drinking. The article used is the essence of ginger, such as is put up in the several proprietary preparations known to the trade, or the alcohol extract ordinarily sold over the druggist's counter. Having once acquired a liking for it, the victim becomes as much a slave to his appetite as the opium eater or the votary of cocaine. In its effect it is much the most injurious of all such practices, for in the course of time it destroys the coating of the stomach, and dooms its victim to a slow and agonizing death.

"The druggist who told me about the thing says that as ginger essence contains about one hundred per cent. alcohol, and whisky less than fifty per cent., the former is therefore twice as intoxicating. In fact, this is the reason why it is used by hardened old topers whose stomachs are no longer capable of intoxicating stimulation from whisky. They need the more powerful agency of the pure alcohol in the ginger extract. He told me that he had two regular customers, one a woman, who had ginger on several occasions for stomachic pains. The relief it afforded her was so grateful that she took it upon any recurrence of her trouble. She found, too, that the slight exhilaration of the alcohol banished mental depression. In this way she got to using it regularly, and finally to such excess that she was often grossly intoxicated. Large doses produce a quiet stupor; additional doses induce a profound lethargic slumber, which lasts in some cases for twenty-four hours. His other customer was a peddler, who came at a certain hour every morning, bought a four-ounce bottle and drank its contents by noon. The man craved the stuff so ardently that he was unable to go about his business until he set the machinery of his stomach in operation, and started the circulation of the blood by means of the fiery draught. He says that the habit is well known to the drug trade."

"The morphia habit, the cocaine habit, the chloral habit, and other poison habits which are prevalent in this and other countries, are only different manifestations of a wide-spread and apparently increasing love for drugs which benumb or excite the nerves, which seems to characterize our modern civilization. Indeed, there appears to be, at the present time, almost a mania for the discovery of some new nerve-tickle, or some novel means of fuddling the senses. It is indeed high time that the medical profession raised, with one accord, its voice in solemn protest against the use of all nerve-obtunding and felicity-producing drugs, which are all, without exception, toxic agents, working mischief and only mischief in the human body."--DR. J. H. KELLOGG.

Much discussion upon careless drug-taking has resulted from remarks made recently in London by Sir Frederick Treves, the King's surgeon, at the opening of a hospital. He said that the time is fast approaching when physicians will give very little medicine, but will instead teach the people right methods of living so that sickness may be avoided.

Although there are some physicians who appear to enjoy the old routine of giving heroic doses of ill-tasting liquids, there are others who agree with Sir Frederick, and admit that they would often be glad to give no medicine if their patients would be satisfied without it. But the great mass of people are unwilling to take a physician's advice as to proper clothing, suitable diet, and regular habits of living. They do not seek his advice upon those points; what they want is a drug that will benumb uneasy sensations while they live as they please.

Not long ago a business man of intelligence was heard to complain because he had tried several physicians and all had failed to cure his sciatica. He said they all told him he must live differently; several said he must quit smoking and lay aside wine and beer or he could not be cured. With scorn he said, "What are physicians good for if they don't know a drug that will cure as simple a thing as rheumatism?" He could not and would not believe that rheumatism might be the result of his wrong habits.

Akin to him in thought is a woman, much above the average in intelligence, who a few months ago had an operation performed upon her stomach. The stomach was enlarged so that the food did not pass through the pylorus, the opening into the intestines. The operation consisted in making a new opening and connecting it with an intestine. This bright woman now complains that the operation was not a success, because she still has times of great distress with indigestion. Upon being asked what she eats, she laughed and said, "Everything, peanuts, mince-pie, sauer-kraut, frankforts; whatever is going. I have a vigorous appetite, and keep peanuts and figs in my room, for I often have to eat in the night."

Until multitudes of people like that business man, and that bright woman, are educated in matters of health, it will not be easy for physicians to bring Sir Frederick's prediction to fulfilment.

The popular supposition is that drugs cure disease, and all that the medical adviser is for is to choose the drug that will produce the desired effect with the greatest speed. Consequently the physician is in many cases driven to prescribe drugs that simply allay pain without removing the cause of the pain. He cannot remove the cause without the patient's co-operation, and as that would require the abandonment of wrong habits few are willing to accept health at such a price. What man will abandon beer to escape rheumatism, or smoking to save his eyesight if he has weakness there? Or, what woman will cease tea-drinking if she has neuralgia?

The Journal of the American Medical Association for November 16, 1907, contained an editorial article in which, after reference to drugs necessary in the practice of a physician or surgeon, this is said:--

"The remark of Holmes years ago that it would be better for the patients, but worse for the fish, if most of the drugs were thrown into the sea, is probably even more true to-day. The vast majority of these drugs have not the slightest excuse for existence."

Dr. T. D. Crothers, in his valuable book upon Morphinism and other drug addictions, reports a case of murder where it was shown that the assailant was delirious from large doses of quinine. He says assaults are often clearly traced to the drug taking of the assailant. A surgeon from a New York hospital, in speaking of drug habits before an audience at Chautauqua, New York, said that some of the ovarian difficulties which demand operations are the result of over-dosing with quinine.

There are people who keep morphine in the house all the time lest some little pain or ache should find them unprepared.

Dr. Crothers, who has perhaps made more of a study of the evil results of drug taking than any other man in America, says of this:--

"Morphine as a common remedy, taken for pains and aches, may suddenly develop into an incurable craze for its continuous use. * * * The early relief which morphine brings to the sufferer is often the beginning of an unknown journey ending in disease and death."

Cases are on record where morphine given to mothers soon after the birth of children to allay pain, has resulted in the death of the infant, the morphine having poisoned the milk.

Cocaine is possibly the most insidious of all drugs yet known. Few of those who become enslaved to it ever are able to lay it aside. It leads to hallucinations of sight and hearing. Many persons have become enslaved to cocaine unwittingly through its use in catarrh snuffs, asthma "cures," and other proprietary preparations, the composition of which was secret. Some states now have strict laws regulating the sale of this dangerous drug.

It is not only the enslaving drugs which are injurious to the body, but even such apparently simple agents as liver pills and pills for the relief of constipation may do more harm than good if resorted to frequently. Some of the ingredients used in the pills for the relief of constipation are said to be injurious to the liver.

Dr. Nathan S. Davis, late dean of the Northwestern University Medical School, Chicago, said of the coal-tar remedies, such as phenacetin and antipyrin, in the treatment of influenza and la grippe:--"While each dose temporarily reduces the fever it retards the most important physiological processes on which the living system depends for resisting the effects of toxic agents, namely, oxidation and elimination. This not only encourages the retention of poisonous agents by which fevers are protracted, but it greatly increases the number of cases of pneumonia that complicate la grippe. The bad work that people make in dosing themselves with patent medicines is not infrequently punctuated with a sudden death from overdosing with antipyrin, sulphonal, or some other coal-tar preparation."

Deaths from acetanilid are becoming more and more frequent. The presence of acetanilid in headache powders "guaranteed to be harmless" and thrown upon the door-steps as samples has led many persons into grave danger, and not a few to death. Bromo-Seltzer, Orangeine, Antikamnia, Taylor's Headache Powders, and various other preparations have all contained this drug.

The use of cocaine is advancing rapidly in this country.[TN: see Errata at end of text] The following article is taken from The Banner of Gold, of Feb., 1899:--

"Value of cocaine leaves imported at the port of New York in 1894 $14,284 Imported in 1897 54,122 Indicated value of imports for 1898 75,000

"In these simple figures are contained the elements of a warning sermon that would startle all America. We seem to be rapidly becoming a nation of cocaine fiends. If the number of those addicted to the use of the dreadful drug continues to increase at the present rate, the importation of what was originally regarded as a blessed alleviation of pain, will have to be classed with opium, and its use prohibited by law, except for medicinal purposes.

"At present the cocaine fiend can purchase the drug without trouble, and the ease with which it is taken is a fatal recommendation to those who crave a nerve-deadener. No laborious cooking of pills over a lamp, cleaning of implements, or troublesome necessity for secrecy, as with the use of opium. Cocaine can be taken at any time, with scarcely any trouble, and without a soul besides the user being aware of his being in the toils.

"At first, that is. It will not be long before every intimate friend will observe a change, a gradual and scarcely perceptible change, come over the appearance and general conduct of the cocaine fiend.

"Begun in many cases in a legitimate way, as an an鎧thetic, the surprisingly pleasant effect is sought for again by the one who has had a glimpse at the portals of the elysium. This is the beginning of the terrible habit. The effect is a sense of exhilaration followed by a quiet, dreamy state that causes the worried man to forget his troubles, and the sufferer his pain. Once this freedom from physical and mental sickness has been experienced, the cocaine fiend will rob or kill to get the drug. Enforced non-use of it will not cure the victim. Sentence him to a term of imprisonment, and he will go straight from the jail door to the nearest drug store to secure cocaine before he eats or sleeps.

"From an occasional use of the drug to insatiable craving is the rational course of the cocaine fiend. From thence to the insane asylum and the grave is a swift and easy descent.

"In his fall from health to physical and mental disintegration, the cocaine fiend undergoes a terrible experience. When not in the temporary heaven that the drug provides, the victim is in the lowest depths of an inferno. He suffers from insomnia, anorexia, and gastralgic pains, dyspepsia, chronic palpitations, and will-paresis. He is a terror both to himself and others. The life of the man is a living death. He knows it, and with this knowledge staring him in the face, he rushes for the drug, and is happy for a brief period under its influence.

"It is time something was done to keep from this high-strung nation a drug so deadly. Clear-minded medical men have recommended its exclusion from the country, believing that its use medicinally should be foregone rather than that such a cursed temptation should be placed in the way of weak humanity.

"What the real action of the drug is, and how to counteract its influence, are at present puzzling questions to the medical fraternity. A leading member of the profession to whom these questions were put replied after careful consideration as follows: 'Its physiological action is practically unknown. As an analgesic, it is uniform in its action, and this is due to the suspension of the physiological functions of the sensory cells which it comes in contact with. Beyond this, it is an excitant of the cerebro-spinal axis, later it has a peculiar action on the encephalon, manifest in a wide range of psychical phenomena. Beyond this a great variety of widely variable symptoms appear. In some cases all the intellectual faculties are excited to the highest degree. In others a profound lowering of the senses and functional activities occur. Morphine-takers can use large quantities of cocaine without any bad symptoms. Alcoholics are also able to bear large doses. Not unfrequently the excitement caused by cocaine goes on to convulsions, and death. Sometimes its action is localized to one part of the cerebro-spinal axis, and then to another. In some cases well-marked cerebral an 鎚 ia appears, and for a time is alarming, but soon passes away.

"Small doses frequently given are more readily absorbed than large doses. Habitues always use weak solutions, the effects being more pleasing with less excitation. Morphine and alcoholic inebriates very soon acquire certain tolerance to large doses taken at once. The cocaine user takes large quantities, but in small doses frequently repeated. He becomes frightened at the effects of large doses, and when he cannot get the effects from small (to him safe) doses, he resorts to alcohol, morphine, or chloral. In many cases memories of the delusions and hallucinations are so vivid and distressing that other narcotics are used to prevent their recurrence. In other cases the recollection is very confused and vague, and strong suspicions fill the mind that the real condition is grossly exaggerated by the friends for some deterring effect. In common with opium and alcoholics, there is moral paralysis, untruthfulness, and low cunning in order to conceal and explain the condition by other than the real causes."

Hoffman Drops are used considerably as a heart stimulant. They are much more intoxicating than whisky, and, used as a beverage, make the drinker crazy while under their influence. According to Dr. F. E. Jones, of Mass. Board of Health, they consist of 325 parts ether, 650 parts alcohol, and 25 parts ether oil. They are said to have a very bad effect upon the kidneys.

The Banner of Gold for Oct., 1898, contained a lengthy article upon the dangers of drugging, from which an extract is given here:--

"Philanthropists, when trying to stay the hand of rum, do not overlook the victims of drugs. If you will go, under the protecting 鎔 is of an officer, to an opium den, such as are to be found in every large city, and as a visitor view for yourself the degradation of hopeless opium users, then train your batteries towards removal of the cause. Do not depend upon preaching, or the writing of essays, or the delivery of an address before some society whose mission ends in telling others what to do, but put on the armor of earnestness, go into the nursery, and demand of the mother to know why, when little lumps of human clay are placed in her keeping for the sacred purpose of moulding them into men and women, she deliberately feeds the prattling babe with soothing syrups, sleeping drops, paregoric, and opiates in various other forms, rather than with the healthful food, and simple remedies, that nature only requires. With such commercial nostrums the thoughtless mother too often paves the way for her offspring to a life of toxic-slavery by creating a systemic condition, which, in maturer years, develops an abnormal craving, or appetite, for narcotics and stimulants. Follow this little victim of nursery malpractice through the imitative age, and you will discover in him the cigarette smoker, the tippler, the self-abased youth, and later, the man whose life is shadowed with the curse of baneful appetite.

"Ask the druggist, and the saloon keeper, why they dispense deadly poisons so freely to old and young, and they will tell you the law permits it; a sad commentary!

"Converted men relapse into evil ways through coquetting with sin; and cured inebriates relapse to drink, and drugs, through the use of proprietary medicines, with which the domestic market is flooded. Tonics, compounds, nerve remedies, bitters, vitalizers, appetizers, balsams, pectorals and kindred nostrums contain, with few exceptions, from 7 to 50 per cent. of alcohol, or opium in varying quantities, each preponderating in kind, as the effect is designed to be stimulating, or sedative. The active principle of some of the best known catarrh remedies is cocaine, and a few manufacturers are honest enough to so announce on the labels covering their goods; more do not, and leave the victims to discover the truth after they have paid the penalty of ignorance, and developed the cocaine habit. Wholesale legislation, as well as vigorous education, is needed along these lines, and while considering means of betterment, the reputable citizen, the clergyman, and others of good moral repute, whose names are so generally used to herald the efficacy of so-called remedial inventions, should not be overlooked for ethical attention.

"For the information of those of our readers, who are not familiar with the nature and use of toxic drugs, we here refer briefly to the prominent characteristics of a few most dangerously potent for evil, and seductive in kind.

OPIUM AND MORPHINE:--"Gum opium, the dried milky exudate from the green capsules of the white poppy, and its product--morphine--are the most reliable drugs known for the relief of pain. The dose of gum opium in medicine is from 1/4 to 1 grain. It contains from 8 to 14 per cent. of morphine, which is its principal alkaloid. Opium is a much more stable, and stronger, sedative than morphine. The cumulative effect of repeated medicinal doses is frequently observed, and is followed by dangerous symptoms. It is both a sedative and hypnotic, and, if given in large doses, quiets the brain, and excites the spinal cord. Small doses have little perceptible effect upon the circulation, but, under the influence of large doses, the pulse is retarded, and the respiration becomes fuller, deeper, and slower. In poisonous doses the pulse may become rapid, and great depression follow, the respiratory centres are paralyzed, thus causing death. If taken in from 2 to 4 grain doses it produces deep comatose sleep, full breathing, full pulse, dry skin, and contracted pupils. If the dose is sufficiently large, the sleep will be more profound, the patient can hardly be roused, and if awakened quickly, he sinks back into slumber. The face may be swollen, and reddened, and the lips deeply tinged with blue. At this stage the breathing may be characterized as puffing. Respiration may be from 8 to 10 per minute, perhaps be reduced to 4, 2 or 1, and as the toxic effect is more marked, it becomes shallow, the pupils are contracted, and the patient is so thoroughly narcotized that nothing will arouse him, the heart ceases to beat, and he dies by respiratory failure, or paralysis of the pneumogastric nerve.

"Morphine, extracted from gum opium by a slow and expensive process, is used much less in proprietary medicines than is tincture of opium, which is more easily manufactured.

"A medicinal dose of sulphate of morphine is from 1/8 to 1/4 of a grain. One grain is a dangerous dose, and 2 grains are liable to prove fatal.

Morphine is a true narcotic. It is a sedative, lessens tissue change, and weakens every function of the body.

TINCTURE OF OPIUM, OR LAUDANUM:--"Laudanum, or the tincture of opium, is a mixture of gum opium with alcohol and water, the solution consisting of equal parts of alcohol and water. Each ounce contains 5-1/2 grains of powdered gum opium and half an ounce of alcohol, and is equal in alcoholic strength to one ounce of strong whisky. The ordinary medical dose is from 12 to 15 minims, or from 25 to 30 drops. It is much used as a domestic remedy for pain from any cause, such as ear or toothache, indigestion, insomnia, summer complaints with children or adults, and is often used in poultices over painful sores or swellings. It is also used in many medicines for throat and lung troubles, in nearly all medicines for painful chronic diseases, and in many of the well advertised spring tonics, as well as in nearly all the compounds that are offered for sale for blood troubles, or as alteratives. The opium in laudanum acts the same as morphine, or any other of the thirty preparations of opium, officially recognized by the medical profession.

PAREGORIC:--"Paregoric of standard grade is half alcohol, which is as strong of alcohol as high proof whisky. It contains a little opium, some benzoic acid, oil of anise, and camphor. The dose is from 15 to 60 drops.

COCAINE:--"Cocaine is an alkaloid of coca leaves, and is used in medicine in the form of hydro-chlorate. It is used locally in powder or solution to relieve pain. It is a strong local an鋥 thetic. The ordinary dose when used as medicine is from 1/4 to 1/2 grain, and is very unstable and treacherous in its effects. Some patients will tolerate large doses while in others small doses produce unpleasant effects. Deaths are recorded from the use of 1-7 to 1 grain.

CHLOROFORM:--"Chloroform is an an鋥 thetic, and death is often caused by a few inhalations. The dose internally is from 3 to 20 minims. It is not much used in medicine, except to control pain, and produce sleep. It is inhaled to produce mild slumber, or complete insensibility in surgical operations. Death may come suddenly, and without warning, at any time during its administration.

CHLORAL:--"Chloral, or hydrate of chloral, is an hypnotic. It is of but little value in medicine, except to control nervousness, and produce sleep. The dose is from 15 to 30 grains. It should be administered with caution, and only by the physician. It is made by passing chlorine gas through pure alcohol, and gets its name from the first syllables of the two words, chlorine and alcohol. It produces death by inhibition of the heart's action, and by paralyzing the pneumogastric nerve.

BROMIDIA:--"Bromidia is the trademark of an hypnotic, the manufacturers of which give out to the public that each fluid drachm contains 15 grains of chloral hydrate, or 1 ounce to every 4 ounces of bromidia.

SULPHONAL:--"Sulphonal is a coal tar preparation, and is valuable in medicine as an hypnotic only. An ordinary dose to produce sleep is from 10 to 40 grains. If it is given in these doses for several days in succession it produces great weariness, an unsteady gait, and may involve paralysis of the lower limbs, with great disturbance of digestion, and scanty secretion of urine of about the color of port wine. There are a number of cases of death reported as resulting from acute, or chronic poisoning, by sulphonal.

PHENACETINE:--"Phenacetine is a product of coal tar, and an antipyretic, a drug that lessens the temperature in high fevers, and rapidly disintegrates the blood.

ANTIFEBRIN:--"Antifebrin, another of the coal tar preparations, is the registered name for acetanelid. Its effects are very similar to the effects of phenacetine, and it is used in fevers for lessening the temperature, and for neuralgic pains. The medicinal dose is from 3 to 10 grains. Unpleasant effects follow its continued use, such as great exhaustion, blueness of the lips, and a slow, labored pulse.

HEADACHE REMEDIES:--"The indiscriminate use of the many coal tar products and other hypnotics, such as sulphonal, phenacetine, antifebrin, chloral, bromidia, etc., under the guise of headache remedies is productive of much disaster, all being nerve paralyzants."

The public owe a debt of gratitude to those physicians, and chemists, who give freely such valuable information as to the real nature and effects of dangerous drugs. While it is true that the popular belief in drugging is due to professional practice, yet it is also true that what the people know of the preservation of health, and of the danger of alcohol and other drugs is largely owing to the medical profession. There is as much difference among the members of the medical profession as there is among the members of any profession; some are careless, selfish, unprincipled, unobservant of the effects of various medicines; while others are anxious to teach the people how to avoid sickness, and gain strength. It is the latter class who warn against the self prescription of drugs, especially those of the dangerously seductive, narcotic class.

Yet, with all the warnings, few pay heed. Even highly educated, intelligent people seem possessed of a blind faith in the power of drugs. Every little ache or pain must have its sedative, be the future penalty what it may.

Were people to quit drugging themselves, avoid indigestible viands, eat at regular hours, chew well, stop eating when they have had enough, take a sufficiency of exercise, sleep and fresh air, with a hot bath once a week, and a cold "towel bath" each morning, laying aside all alcoholic beverages, tea and coffee, and tobacco, there would be very little sickness in the world. Over-eating leads to the drug habit for relief from uneasy sensations, so does improper food, or poorly cooked food.

It should be remembered that it is not possible to violate the laws which relate to the physical well-being, and then escape the natural penalty of transgression by swallowing a few doses of medicine. Remedies may postpone the results of physical transgression, and may even seem to prevent them altogether, but careful observation will show that the escape from punishment is only apparent. Sometimes a parent escapes, while his child pays the penalty of his transgression, in a weakly nervous system, which may lead to insanity, or other trouble.

CHAPTER XV.

TESTIMONIES OF PHYSICIANS AGAINST ALCOHOLIC MEDICATION.

"In abandoning the use of alcohol it should be clearly understood that we abandon an injurious influence, and escape from a source of disease, as we do when we get into a purer atmosphere. There is not the slightest occasion to do anything, or to take anything to make up for the loss of a strengthening or supporting agent. No loss has been incurred save the loss of a cause of disease and death."--DR. J. J. RIDGE, of London Temperance Hospital.

Sir. B. W. Richardson, M. D., said of the London Temperance Hospital:--

"No alcohol is administered, and no substitute for it. Any drug with similar action would be bad; warmth and suitable nourishment are relied on to keep up the system. We know that people who take alcohol often feel better; this is from the narcotic action. The pain may be stilled, and the disease forgotten, but it has not been removed; its symptom has been narcotized."

Another writer says:--

"I am asked for a substitute for brandy, and frankly and gladly I tell you there is no substitute, for I have no knowledge of any agent equally pleasing to the palate, and yet so destructive of life."

Dr. Norman Kerr, President of the Society for the Study of Inebriety,

England, says:--

"My own experience of thirty-four years in the practice of my profession has taught me that in nearly all cases and kinds of disease the medical use of alcohol is unnecessary, and in a large number of instances is prejudicial and even dangerous. Having given an intoxicant, in strictly definite and guarded doses, probably on the whole only about once in 3,000 cases (then usually when nothing else was available in an emergency), and having had most varieties of disease to contend with, my death-rate and duration of illness have been quite as low as my neighbors. The experience of the London Temperance Hospital and other similar institutions, the current reports of that hospital being now reliable scientific records, amply support this experience.

"The chief peril of narcotic drugs has always appeared to me to lie in their disguising the real state of the patient from himself as well as from his doctor and his friends. If there is any serious ailment, such as cholera or fever, the sufferer may seem to be and may feel better. He is not better. He is actually worse--made worse by the alcohol, and not unseldom, after the evanescent alcoholic disguise and deceptive improvement has faded, it is found that the malady itself has been progressing, unseen and unsuspected from the delusive aspect of the alcohol, steadily toward a fatal termination, which might, in many cases, have been averted but for the true state of the patient having been completely masked.

"Wherever the blame really has lain, one thing is now clear, that alcoholic intoxicants are very rarely useful as a medicine; are at the best dangerous remedies; and that, other things being equal, the less they are resorted to the better for the chances of the patient's recovery, the better for body and brain, the better for physical, intellectual and moral well-being. Alcohol does not nourish, but pulls down; does not stimulate, but depresses; does not strengthen, but excites and exhausts. Alcohol is the pathological fraud of frauds, degenerating while it claims to be reconstructing, enfeebling while it appears to be invigorating, destroying vitality while it professes to infuse new life."

A medical writer in the Toledo, O., Blade holds up in clear light the relation of the materia medica and alcohol, and the opportunity of the physician to become a benefactor, and active temperance worker. His remarks follow:--

"One of the signs of the times in the temperance movement is the steady growth among physicians of a sentiment against the administration of liquor of any kind as a medicine. The accepted scientific view of alcohol is that it is a poison, and its administration should be as guarded as that of any other poison used as a medicine. Perhaps the hardest thing a physician finds in his effort to restore his patients to health without the use of liquors is the common, but erroneous, belief that they are 'strengthening,' and that the convalescent, by their use, reaches recovery more quickly. The error is in supposing that any alcoholic liquor is nourishing, or strengthening. They are neither. Alcohol does not nourish, but it pulls down; it does not strengthen, but excites and exhausts, for every stimulation is necessarily followed by a period of depression, and this is inevitably unfavorable to the patient.

"There is a grave responsibility resting on the physician who prescribes alcoholic liquor. It may arouse in a susceptible patient a dormant, inherited tendency to drink. He may, by authorizing its use during the period of convalescence, fix a habit upon a patient of feeble will, which the latter will never be able to shake off. No physician who realizes this great moral responsibility will be willing to accept it habitually. He certainly knows that the best medical authorities agree that alcoholic intoxicants are rarely useful as a medicine; that at best they are dangerous remedies, and that the less they are resorted to, the better for both brain and body.

"In point of fact the physician who does his duty to his patient teaches him the error of the prevalent belief in the virtues of liquor in restoring the sick to health. He becomes an active temperance worker in effect. And he can do a noble and useful work in the rescue of those who are under the control of the drink habit. * * * * *

"Furthermore, every physician owes it to his profession to teach his patients the utter fallacy of the common belief that alcohol is an article of food value. It has no such value. The use of intoxicants in any quantity whatever, or at any time, is entirely useless and unnecessary. The continued use of them gradually induces structural degradations and functional derangements of the great bodily organs, thus leading to the gravest physical disorders."

"I have demonstrated by actual experience that no form of alcoholic drink is necessary, or desirable, for internal use, either in health, or any of the varied forms of disease; but that health can be better preserved, and disease more successfully treated, without the use of such drinks.* * * * * Simple truth compels me to say that I have never yet seen a case in which the use of alcoholic drinks either increased the force of the heart's action, or strengthened the patient. But I could detail very many cases in which the administration of alcoholics was quieting the patient's restlessness, enfeebling the capillary circulation, and steadily favoring increased engorgement of the lungs and other internal viscera, and thereby hastening a fatal result, where both attending physician and friends thought they were the only agents that were keeping the patient alive.

"I have found no case of disease and no emergency arising from accident, that I could not treat more successfully without any form of fermented or distilled liquors than with. It is easy to see that the an鋞thetic properties of alcohol can be made available by an intelligent and skillful physician to meet a very limited number of indications in the treatment of some cases that will come before him. But the same intelligence and skill will enable him to select other remedies capable of meeting the same indications more perfectly, and, with less tendency to secondary bad effects. I have no hesitation, therefore, in stating that for the attainment of the highest degree of success in the management of all forms of disease, whether acute or chronic, we need no form of fermented, or distilled, alcoholic drinks. And whoever will boldly make the trial, will find that his patients, of every kind, will make better progress, on good air and simple nourishment, without any admixture of alcoholic liquids, than they will with such addition. In other words he will find that the supposed benefits of this class of agents in medicine, are as illusory as they are in general society, and that the words of the wise man are worthy of careful consideration when he says: 'Wine is a mocker and strong drink is raging, and whosoever is deceived thereby is not wise.'"--DR. N. S. DAVIS, Chicago, Ill.

"Dr. Hirschfeld, a well-known physician of Magdeburg, Germany, was recently arrested on a charge of malpractice. The specific charge was that he had refused to give alcohol to one of his patients who was supposed to need it. The doctor, like the more advanced German physicians, is discarding liquor from his practice, and made such a hot defence to the charge that the court not only discharged the physician, but assessed the cost of the defense against the prosecution."--Bulletin of A. M. T. A.

Dr. Greene, of Boston, when addressing his brethren and sisters of the medical association in that city, upon alcohol, said in closing:--

"It needs no argument to convince you that it is upon the medical profession, to a very great extent, that the rum-seller depends to maintain the respectability of the traffic. It requires only your own experience, and observations, to convince you that it is upon the medical profession, upon their prescriptions and recommendations for its use upon many occasions, that the habitual dram-drinker depends for the seeming respectability of his drinking habits. It is upon the members of the medical profession, and the exceptional laws which it has always demanded, that the whole liquor fraternity depends, more than upon anything else, to screen it from opprobrium, and just punishment for the evils which the traffic entails upon society; and it is because the rum-seller, and the rum-drinker, hide under this cloak of seeming respectability that they are so difficult to reach either by moral suasion, or by law. Physicians generally have only to overcome the force of habit, and the prevailing fashion in medicine, to find an excellent way, when they will all look back with wonder and surprise, that they, as individuals, and members of an honored profession, should have been so far compromised."

"It will be asked, Was there no evidence of any good service rendered by the agent in the midst of so much obvious bad service? I answer to that question THAT THERE WAS NO SUCH EVIDENCE WHATEVER, AND IS NONE."--SIR B. W. RICHARDSON.

"A prominent general practitioner expressed surprise that any one could do without alcohol in general medicine. He was persuaded to make a trial, by abandoning the internal use of spirits as medicine. A year afterward he wrote that his success in the treatment of disease had been equal to that of any year in the past, and that his cases recovered as well without alcohol as with it. In a recent medical meeting he remarked, 'I thought for many years that I could not do without spirits as medicine. I was mistaken. I am constantly treating cases of all degrees of severity without alcohol, and my success is fully equal to the average.'"--Quarterly of A. M. T. A.

"Happily, the belief in alcohol is passing away."--DR. C. R. FRANCIS, late Professor of Medicine, Calcutta Medical College.

Dr. Moor, the distinguished editor of the Pacific Record, says:--

"While the use of alcohol is always injudicious and injurious, it is particularly so in summer, when the system is predisposed to disturbances of the gastro-intestinal tract.

"Alcohol flushes the capillaries of the mucous membranes just as it does the capillaries of the skin, and where there is already a smouldering congestion, it will take but little to light the fire of acute inflammation, which will rage with greatly increased intensity.

"It is wiser to habitually avoid even the medicinal use of alcohol, as there are plenty of other stimulants which will give the desired results without entailing any disastrous after effects."

"All the pleasant sensations of increased mental and physical power, which the use of alcohol produces, are deceptive and arise from the paralysis of the judgment and the momentary benumbing of the sense of fatigue which afterwards returns so imperiously with perhaps even greater intensity."-- PROF. ADOLF FICK, of Wurzburg.

Dr. Frank Payne, vice-president of the London Pathological Society, says:--

"Alcohol is a functional and tissue poison, and there is no proper or necessary use for it as a medicine."

"When I first heard that there was going to be a total abstinence hospital, I thought it would be a complete failure. That was because I had been taught as a student to regard alcohol as absolutely necessary in the treatment of disease. Nevertheless I was an abstainer myself. When I was asked to join as physician, I did not consent without a good deal of consideration, and then only on the understanding that if I thought a person needed it, I should be allowed to administer alcohol. I remember the first case of severe typhoid fever I had. He was hovering between life and death, and I was anxiously watching to see whether it would be necessary to give alcohol, but the man made a good recovery without it. After watching many cases to whom I should have given alcohol if I had been treating them elsewhere, I came to the conclusion that I had been completely deluded. I gave it at one time to a woman in the Hospital who was in a dying condition, but it did not save her. I do not think I am likely to administer alcohol again. We have had progress and efficiency in the Hospital. It has been like an experiment for the profession, and our success shows that this giving of alcohol is certainly a matter for re-consideration for the medical profession. I believe that they are mistaken. There is no doubt that the amount of alcohol used in other hospitals has diminished greatly, compared with what was used in the past. To the outside public also this Hospital is an example. I believe that an immense number of the public have been teetotalers some time in their lives, but a great many of them have gone back to the drink in time of illness, because they have been advised to do so. This Hospital is a standing witness that disease and surgical injuries can be treated without alcoholic liquors."--DR. J. J. RIDGE, of London Temperance Hospital.

"I find very little use for alcohol in the practice of medicine. Where there is one element of good in alcohol there are thousands that are bad."--DR. ALFRED MERCER, Syracuse, N. Y., Professor of Medicine in Syracuse Medical School.

"Alcohol is rarely necessary. Other remedies are much more efficacious. In my department of the University of Buffalo I follow Cushny, who claims that alcohol is a poison, a depressant in direct proportion to the amount ingested, and a so-called false food."--DR. DE WITT H. SHERMAN, Adjunct Professor of Therapeutics, University of Buffalo Medical Department.

"I believe that alcohol is the greatest foe to the human race to-day. I feel that it would not be a serious harm if its use as a medicine were totally discontinued."--DR. WALTER E. FERNALD, Professor in Tufts Medical School, Boston, Mass.

"I rarely or never prescribe alcohol as a medicament or a food, or sanction its use as a beverage. Physiologically I look upon alcohol as a narcotic, with perhaps a primary stimulating effect, but I believe that such desired action as it is capable of producing can be equally well brought about by other agents. As a beverage the use of alcohol, particularly in excess, is attended with definite and well-known dangers."--DR. A. A. ESHNER, Professor of Clinical Medicine, Philadelphia Polyclinic and College for Graduates in Medicine.

"I agree with you altogether in your agitation against the use of alcohol in any form. I believe that wine is a mocker, and belief in wine as a benefit, mockery."--DR. MATTHEW WOODS, Philadelphia, Pa.

"It is extremely seldom that I ever advise the use of alcohol in any form for my patients."--ELLIOTT P. JOSLIN, M. D., Professor in Harvard Medical School, Boston, Mass.

"My belief is that there is very little need of the medical use of alcohol. I almost never use it in my practice, and think that its use by practitioners generally is far less than it was a few years ago."--DR. E. G. CUTLER, Professor in Harvard Medical School, Boston, Mass.

"I believe that the trend of teaching in the Harvard Medical School has been growing less favorable, of late years, to the use of alcohol in the treatment of disease, and in fact it is far less used than it was a generation ago."--DR. JAMES J. PUTNAM, Professor in Harvard Medical School.

"My personal opinion in regard to the use of alcoholic drinks is very decidedly averse to such use. I have long been of the opinion that while the use of alcohol may restrain tissue metamorphosis, it cannot legitimately be considered a food."--DR. WILLIAM O. STILLMAN, Albany Medical College, Albany, N. Y.

"I do not think you will meet with very many physicians who favor alcohol and its use. I believe the trend of the teaching in the Albany Medical College is that alcohol is not a food or stimulant."--DR. A. VANDER VEER, Albany, N. Y., Medical School.

"I think the medical profession could get along perfectly well without the use of alcohol, except as it is needed in the manufacture of drugs. As a therapeutic agent, it has very little value. I do not suppose I have used a pint of alcohol in the last ten years. I think the tendency of the medical profession throughout the country is to give up alcohol in the treatment of disease."-- DR. MATTHEW D. MANN, Dean of the Medical Department of the University of Buffalo, N. Y.

"I very seldom prescribe alcohol as a medicine, and think its effects are positively harmful in the vast majority of medical cases."--DR. ALLEN A. JONES, Adjunct Professor of Medicine, Buffalo, N. Y.

"At the Baptist Hospital I have not ordered alcohol for a patient in several years. At the Massachusetts General Hospital, in the out-patient department, I never prescribe it."--DR. RICHARD BADGER, of Harvard Medical School, Boston.

"Alcohol is used much too freely in the treatment of the sick, especially in such conditions as mild typhoid fever, neurasthenia and early tuberculosis. It should be prescribed only when there is definite indication for it, and then in definite dose for a limited period in the same manner as any other powerful and potentially harmful drug."--DR. S. S. COHEN, Jefferson Medical College, Philadelphia.

"It is seldom necessary to prescribe alcohol as a medicine."--DR. JAMES B. HERRICK, Professor of Medicine in Rush Medical College, Chicago.

"As I have said but little about the use of medicine in the treatment of typhoid fever, save for one symptom, I may add, for the purpose of definiteness, that I use none except for special symptoms. The rare exceptions are stimulants such as strychnia, in less marked indications coffee. Alcohol as a routine drug I have entirely abandoned, having found that the doses formerly given before or after the bath are altogether unnecessary. Hot milk internally, or hot water bags externally, more than replace spirits according to my experience."--DR. GEORGE DOCK, New Orleans.

"I have no use for alcohol, either personally, or in my practice. Yet I cannot say that I have entirely abolished it. Alcohol is used in compounding most of our tinctures, but in remedies proper my experience has been that other stimulants, such as ammonia, strychnine, caffeine, kolafra, etc., answer the same purpose without alcohol's dangerous effects. In my practice, which is confined to surgery, I find very, very little use for it. During the past year, in extreme cases, I used it in hypodermic injections, and afterwards felt that ether, or ammonia would have answered the same purpose. I think, in general practice, physicians are dispensing with alcohol more and more, but perhaps unconsciously."--D. W. B. DE GARMO, Professor of surgery in Post-Graduate Hospital, New York City.

"Medicine, to-day, would be in a more satisfactory condition if the use of alcohol as a medicine had been interdicted a hundred years ago, and the interdict had remained to the present day. The benefits derived from its use are so small (even when they can be proved, which is much more rarely the case than most people imagine), and the advantages gained are so slight, that they are completely outweighed when we set against them the evil that has been wrought by the abuse of alcohol, and that has arisen out of the loose methods of prescription that have obtained, and even still obtain, in regard to this drug."--DR. G. SIMS WOODHEAD, F. R. C. P., F. R. S., Director of the Research Laboratories of the Royal College of Physicians and Surgeons, London.

"The effect of continually dosing with this drug is too apparent wherever it is used, benumbing the senses, and rendering more difficult every natural function. Alcohol never sustains the powers of life. It sometimes changes the symptoms of disease, but at the expense of the vitality of the body. What is called its supporting action, is a fever induced by the poison, which finally prostrates the patient. The secret of its action is found in the laws of vitality. The man who takes alcohol to help digest his food, must first throw off the alcohol, before his stomach can act healthfully.

"There is one encouraging fact to be noted in this connection, that the use of alcohol in medicine has very much diminished during the past twenty-five years, and the present tendency is constantly in that direction. Right here is an important point which I wish to make: When the physician ceases to prescribe alcohol as a medicine, the drink problem will have reached the final stage of its solution. Mankind will eventually learn that safety lies not so much in skillful doctors, or in some wonderful 'new remedy,' as in daily obedience to the laws of health. A small amount of prevention is of more worth than all the power of cure."--DR. C. H. SHEPARD, Brooklyn, N. Y.

"My observation has been that there is a decided tendency among educated physicians to give less alcohol than formerly in the treatment of disease. Of late years I have given but very little alcohol in my own practice. The tendency is due, in my opinion, to the study of the physiological action of drugs, and to the better understanding of the causation of disease and pathological processes. Modern investigators now know that we have therapeutic agents that meet the requirements of disease processes with more scientific accuracy than is obtained by the exhibition of alcohol."--DR. DONNELLY, Secretary of Minnesota State Medical Society, St. Paul, Minn.

"Dr. Pearce Gould recently made a speech to the National Temperance League on alcohol and the advantage of doing without it, both in health and in the treatment of disease. It takes a strong man to say the strong things which Mr. Gould said on the subject, especially if he happens to be a medical man. No doubt, as Dr. Gould says, the use of alcohol in medical practice is nothing now compared to what it was twenty years ago, much more forty years ago, when Dr. Todd's influence, and the reaction from the so-called antiphlogistic treatment were at their height. Public opinion has been enlightened by the evidence of leaders in medicine, such as Dr. Parkes, Sir William Gull, Dr. Gairdner, Dr. Sanderson, and others, and medical men have dared to treat disease without alcohol, or with only small quantities of it. There are physicians and surgeons of reputation and success, who are so strong in their convictions that alcohol is of little use in the treatment of disease, that it destroys tissues, lessens the resistance to microbes, deranges functions, spoils temper, and shortens life, that they are ready to testify to this effect in public, in company with redoubtable champions of the temperance cause like the Archbishop of Canterbury, Sir William White (chief constructor of the navy), and the Bishop of Derry, who have as much prejudice to contend against in their spheres as the medical man has in his. We recognize with pleasure the good done by such testimony as Dr. Gould's. Men whose record and authority in the profession are such as his have the courage of their opinions, and their honest testimony will be respected even by those who do not go quite so far in discarding alcohol as an element of diet, or as a medicine."--The Lancet, London, May 14, 1898.

"The light of exact investigation has shown that the therapeutic value of alcohol rests on an insecure basis, and it is constantly being made clearer that after all alcohol is a sort of poison to be handled with the same care and circumspection as other agents capable of producing noxious and deadly effect upon the organism. It has been shown by Abbott and others that alcoholic animals are more susceptible to infections than normal animals. And Laitinen, after having studied the influence of alcohol upon infections with anthrax, tubercle and diphtheria bacilli in dogs, rabbits, guinea-pigs and pigeons, reaches the same general results with certainty and directness. Under all circumstances alcohol causes a marked increase in susceptibility no matter whether given before or after infections, no matter whether the doses were few and massive or numerous and small, and no matter whether the infection was acute or chronic. The alcoholic animals either die while the controls remain alive, or in case both die, death is earlier in the alcoholic. The facts brought out by the researches of Abbott and Laitinen and others do not furnish the slightest support for the use of alcohol in the treatment of infectious diseases in man."--Journal American Medical Association, Editorial, September 8, 1900.

"Step by step the progress of science has nullified every theory on which the physician administers alcohol. Every position taken has been disapproved. Alcohol is not a food and does not nourish, but impairs nutrition. It is not a stimulant in the proper acceptation of the term; on the contrary it is a depressant. Hence its former universal use in cases of shock was, to say the least, a grave mistake. It has been proved by recent experiments that alcohol retards, perverts, and is destructive either in large or small doses to normal cell growth and development."--NATHAN S. DAVIS, SR., M.D., former Dean of Northwestern University Medical School, Chicago, Illinois. (Deceased.)

"It seems to me that the field of usefulness of alcohol in therapeutics is extremely limited and possibly does not exist at all. Probably every supposed indication for its use can be met better and more safely by other drugs. The recent work on the so-called food value of alcohol is the subject of much misunderstanding. While it is true that under some circumstances, for example, after a person has acquired a certain degree of tolerance to its poisonous effects, alcohol seems to act as a food in the sense that fats and carbohydrates do, I believe this to be at present a matter of little more than theoretical importance."--DR. REID HUNT, Chief of the Department of Pharmacology, Public Health and Marine Hospital Service, Washington, D.C.

"The physician should have blazoned before him, 'If you can do no good, do no harm.' If this rule is adhered to, in ninety-nine cases out of one hundred the physician will give no alcohol. In the medical wards of the Pennsylvania Hospital I have found that in acute as well as chronic disease we can do without alcohol. It does harm rather than good. Alcohol masks the symptoms of disease, so that we cannot know the patient's real condition."--J. H. MUSSER, M. D., Philadelphia, Pa., Ex-President American Medical Association.

"It is time alcohol was banished from the medical armamentarium; whisky has killed thousands where it cured one."--J. H. MCCORMACK, M. D., Secretary Kentucky Board of Health, and Organizer for the American Medical Association.

"I very rarely use alcohol in my practice. I think that its use is never essential. Physicians are using it less and less in the treatment of disease owing to the recognition that it is a narcotic, not a stimulant, and that other narcotics are usually better when a narcotic is required."--RICHARD C. CABOT, M. D., Professor of Clinical Medicine, Harvard Medical School, Boston, Mass.

"My position has been that alcohol should be prescribed with as much care as to indications and circumspection as to dose and method as in the use of any other drug that in health would prove harmful, as morphine, belladonna, aconite, quinine, etc. I believe strongly that in pneumonia, typhoid fever, and tuberculosis especially, the indiscriminate use of alcohol in the past has caused an incalculable amount of distress and needless disaster to suffering humanity."--HOWARD S. ANDERS, M. D., Professor of Physical Diagnosis, Medico-Chirurgical College, Philadelphia, Pa.

"I do not think alcohol of any value in the treatment of disease; formerly it was used a great deal in the hospital wards, and 'liquor slips' were daily signed. Now, I never order liquor in any quantity, and at times for weeks I have not signed a single slip ordering liquor."--HENRY JACKSON, M. D., Professor in Harvard Medical School.

"In the overwhelming majority of cases I am in entire sympathy with the movement to abolish the routine use of alcoholics from medicine, and I rarely advise such in my practice."--EDWARD R. BALDWIN, M. D., Saranac Lake Sanitarium, New York.

"I seldom prescribe alcohol."--GEORGE BLUMER, M. D., Yale Medical School, New Haven, Conn.

"WHEREAS, The study of alcohol from a scientific standpoint has demonstrated that its action is deceptive, and that it does not have the medical properties that we once claimed for it; now, therefore, be it

"Resolved, By the West Virginia State Medical Association, That we deplore the fact that our profession has been quoted so long as claiming for it virtues which it does not possess, and that we earnestly pledge ourselves to discourage the use of it, both in and out of the sick room."--Resolution passed at annual meeting May, 1908.

"I have been actively engaged in the practice of medicine for nearly twenty-five years, in the early portion of which I prescribed alcoholics moderately but yet with considerable frequency. For the past ten years I have been finding professionally less place for alcoholics of any sort in my practise, and for perhaps three years I have scarcely ever prescribed them. I am satisfied that my cases of pneumonia and typhoid come through in better condition without anything alcoholic, even wines, and I no longer prescribe these at all in cases of tuberculosis. I have noted also that among my professional associates of the thinking rather than of the automatic type, the medicinal use of alcohol is rapidly lessening."--C. G. HICKEY, M. D., Lecturer on Medicine, Denver and Gross College of Medicine, Denver, Colorado.

"In the thirteen years I have taught in Michigan I have not used alcohol in the treatment of disease in a routine way. Even alcoholic preparations, such as tinctures, have been used in very rare instances. I have occasion to speak on this subject every year to about two hundred students. My reasons for taking this stand are chiefly medical, though I am heartily in sympathy with the ethical and moral phases of the temperance movement."--DR. GEORGE DOCK, formerly Professor of Medicine, University of Michigan Medical College, now of Tulane University, New Orleans.

"Alcohol is distinctly a poison, and the limitation of its use should be as strict as that of any other kind of poison. It is not an appetizer, and even in small quantities it hinders digestion. The use of alcohol is emphatically diminishing in hospital practise."--SIR FREDERICK TREVES, Surgeon to King Edward.

"If during the last quarter of a century I have prescribed almost no alcohol in the treatment of disease, it is because I have found very little reason for its use, and it seemed to me that my patients got on better without it."--SIR JAMES BARR, Dean of the Medical School of Liverpool University.

"With the increase of medical knowledge and with the increase of medical observation, it is shown every year that the value of alcohol as a drug has been enormously overestimated. It is a very poor agent, and only in common use because it is so easily obtained. The medical profession is using it less and less, because they appreciate it now at its true value. Personally I never order it, because I believe patients recover better without it."--SIR VICTOR HORSLEY, Surgeon to London Hospital.

"The same care and discrimination should be given to the prescribing of alcohol as to the most deadly drug with which we have to deal. In looking at the report of Radcliffe Infirmary for the past month I see that in dealing with twenty-five cases I ordered alcohol costing exactly 1-3/4 pence."--DR. WILLIAM COLLIER, President British Medical Association, 1904.

"In England at present the use of large doses of alcohol seems to have greatly gone out of hospital practise, and opinion is certainly growing that not even small doses are required. Diseases of the stomach, liver, heart, and kidneys have appeared to me, in my practise, to be much more satisfactorily treated without beer, wines, or spirits."--DR. C. R. DRYSDALE, Consulting Physician to the Metropolitan Hospital, London.

"Alcohol is a functional and tissue poison, and there is no proper or necessary use for it as medicine."--DR. FRANK PAYNE, Vice-President London Pathological Society.

"Of scarlet fever I have treated some 2,000 cases. I have never seen a case in which, in my opinion, alcohol was necessary; no case in which its administration was beneficial; but I have seen more than one case in which its action was directly injurious. * * * Alcohol in no case averts a fatal issue where such is impending. * * * The facts are dead against alcohol. In hospitals there has been an increase of 300 per cent. in the use of milk, and a decline of 47 per cent. in the use of alcohol. Progress in treatment of disease has gone hand in hand with disuse of alcohol. The use of alcohol formerly was the outcome of ignorance, a confession of weakness and defeat; to-day it is the expression of inability to discard the fetters of an outworn routine."-- DR. C. KNOX BOND, in Medical Times.

"For many years I have dispensed almost entirely with alcohol as an aid in surgical treatment. As a student I saw it used, almost as a matter of routine, for every kind of surgical malady except head injuries, and in my early years I naturally followed the practise of my teachers; but as soon as I made trial for myself of the effect of withholding alcohol, I found how entirely overrated its value was, and how gravely mistaken had been the teaching. It is commonly held, I believe, that alcoholic stimulants are of especial value in all forms of septic inflammation, such as erysipelas, py 鎚 ia, septic 鎚 ia, and hectic fever. I believe that this belief is founded solely upon tradition unsupported by any trustworthy evidence, and untested by experiment or experience."--DR. A. PEARCE GOULD, F. R. C. S., Surgeon to the Middlesex Hospital, London.

"I have not prescribed alcohol to my patients for more than ten years, and can affirm positively that they have fared well under this change of treatment. Since I formerly followed the universal practice, I am competent to make comparisons, and these speak unconditionally in favor of treatment without alcohol. As a preventive of waste I use among fever patients nothing but real foods; in addition to milk, particularly sugar, which can be administered to any fever patient in ample quantity in the form of fruit juices, stewed fruit, sweet lemonade, fruit ices, sugared tea, etc., concerning which hundreds of investigations have demonstrated positively that it prevents the waste of both albumen and fat. As a stimulant I employ, besides hydriatic methods, which at the same time abstract heat, almost nothing but camphor, and I can affirm that it is unconditionally preferable to alcohol for its prompt results and the absence of disagreeable after-effects (intoxication, benumbing). Pneumonia, especially, subsides without alcohol to perfect satisfaction, and I rejoice to agree in this respect with Aufrecht, one of the best authorities on this disease, who in his monograph in Nothnagle's manual, acknowledges himself hostile to the use of alcohol in the treatment of pneumonia, and hopes that its use may be speedily abolished. For the reasons previously specified, I should like to see that extended to all use of alcohol in therapeutics. However, that can come to pass only when all thinking physicians clearly appreciate the fact that no substance is able to undertake the double role of a food and a poison, and, also, that for alcohol no nutritive, but only toxic properties can be claimed."--MAX KASSOWITZ, M. D., Professor in the University of Vienna, Austria.

"Besides its deleterious influence on the nervous system and other important parts of our body, alcohol has a harmful action on the phagocytes, the agents of natural defense against infective microbes."--PROF. METCHNIKOFF, Pasteur Institute, Paris, France.

"Alcoholic liquors are, to my mind, not only not valuable, but distinctly disadvantageous, in the treatment of disease, except in rare instances, as for example in the initial chill of some acute infectious disease. However, I have almost given up the use of alcohol in the treatment of disease."--DR. D. L. EDSALL, Professor of Therapeutics in the University of Pennsylvania Medical School.

"As a rule which might well be regarded as universal in the practice of medicine, alcohol in the treatment of disease is an evil. In ordinary doses and in continuous use the sum of its reactions increases exhaustion, which may terminate fatally."--DR. JOHN VAN DUYN, Professor of Medicine in Syracuse, N. Y., University Medical School.

"In sixteen years of active practice I have not used alcoholics at all. I am medical director of the Scranton Sanitarium, and I have considerable trouble in trying to cure those who use alcohol, and to undo some of the work my fellow practitioners have unwittingly made."--D. WEBSTER EVANS, M. D., Scranton, Pa.

"I am opposed to the use of alcoholic liquors as a beverage, and with rare exceptions, to their use in the treatment of diseases."--DR. EUGENE KERR, Physician to Phipps Dispensary, Johns Hopkins Hospital, Baltimore, Md.

"In my professional work I do not advise or permit the use of alcohol as a beverage or medicine in any form whatever. No alcohol is used medicinally in my hospital wards. Beer or wine is not permitted to convalescents. Children are never given tinctures. Cases of delirium tremens receive no alcohol. The hypodermic use of alcohol is not permitted in cases of shock. There are other much more effective and less depressing diffusable stimulants.

"Among my colleagues the employment of alcohol as a medicine has diminished at least seventy-five per cent. in the past fifteen years.

"I have cast it out entirely."--J. P. WARBASSE, M. D., Chief Surgeon German Hospital, Brooklyn, N. Y.

"The habitual use of alcohol in any disease is worse than harmful."--ROBERT B. PREBLE, M. D., Chicago, Ill.

"The last few years I find I have used less and less alcohol in prescribing for my patients until at the present time I use very little. I think my typhoid cases do better without alcohol than with it."--H. H. HEALY, M. D., former Sec'y North Dakota Board of Health.

"Alcohol is a poison. It is claimed by some that alcohol is a food. If so, it is a poisoned food."--FREDERICK PETERSON, M. D., Professor of Psychiatry, Columbia University, N. Y.

"Few physicians now credit alcohol as a food (that is, as a tissue builder) or as having any valuable medicinal qualities. In fact, it is considered by many to have a destructive rather than a constructive quality. I believe it should never be put into the human body."--EUGENE HUBBELL, M. D., St. Paul, Minn.

"The medical profession is learning that alcohol has been much abused in the treatment of the sick, and is largely discarding it. I hardly find occasion to prescribe it once a year."--W. A. PLECKER, M. D., Sec'y State Board of Health, Hampton, Va.

"The use of alcohol as a beverage or therapeutically, is in either case a habit of the user. The stimulation is but temporary, the reaction leaving the nerve cells of the individual with less resisting power than before the ingestion of alcohol. * * * Never permit a verbal or written prescription of yours to give rise to the use of a habit forming drug."--From a lecture to students in Omaha Medical College by J. M. Aiken, M. D., Clinical Instructor and Lecturer upon Nervous and Mental Diseases.

"The use of spirits as a stimulant in diseases, except in a very limited circle, is a mere empiricism for which no good reasons can be given. The teachings of medical men are no more to be followed blindly and without question. The tests of alcohol as a tonic, as a food, as a stimulant, as a retarder of waste, are all negative. There is no reliable evidence to support these claims, but a constant accumulation of facts to indicate the danger from the use of spirits. To give alcohol or any other drug without some rational theory in accord with the scientific researches of to-day is unpardonable."--DR. T. D. CROTHERS, Hartford, Conn., Editor of the Journal of Inebriety.

"Many physicians prescribe alcohol only because it is the desire of the patient, and because patients refuse medicine which the physicians would rather use."--EVERETT HOOPER, M. D. Boston, Mass.

"You are right in indicting alcohol for its insidious wrongs to humanity. It is an old and sly offender and very much the 'mocker' in medical practise that it has been pronounced in holy writ. It exhausts the latent energy of the organism often when that power is most needed to conserve the failing strength of the body in the battle with disease."--DR. C. H. HUGHES, St. Louis, Missouri.

"The best class of thinkers, men of the best intellectual gauge, are those who are doing away with this miserable, unscientific practise of giving liquor."--DR. BOYNTON, Clifton Springs, N. Y.

"I believe that in the scientific light of the present era alcohol should be classed among the anæsthetics and poisons, and that the human family would be benefited by its entire exclusion from the field of remedial agents."--DR. J. S. CAIN, Dean of the Faculty, Medical Department, University of the South, Sewanee, Tenn.

"Let me cite my experience in surgery for the last three years in proof of the uselessness of alcohol, and the benefit of abstinence from its administration. During that time I have performed more than one thousand operations, a large portion upon cases of railroad injuries, one hundred for appendicitis, and in none of these was alcohol administered in any form, either before, during, or after operations. I defy any one who still adheres to alcohol to show as good results. Equally gratifying results have been obtained with my medical cases, and I fail to understand how any observing and thinking physician can still cling to so prejudicial a drug as alcohol, when he has within his reach a multitude of valuable, exact, and reliable methods for combating, governing, and controlling disease."--DR. EVAN C. KANE, Surgeon Pennsylvania Railroad, Kane, Pa.

"In my neurological practice I emphatically forbid my patients the use of alcohol. This poison has a special predilection for the nervous system which it influences sometimes to an alarming extent."--ALFRED GORDON, M. D., Jefferson Medical College, Philadelphia, Pa.

"Alcohol finds no place in my remedial list. It has been banished, not from sentiment, but from knowledge secured by scientific investigation."--T. ALEXANDER MACNICHOLL, M. D., New York City, one of the founders of the Red Cross Hospital, New York.

"No sound, scientific argument can be offered for the medical use of alcohol, either internally or externally. It is a toxic substance which ought to be retired from the materia medica, and placed in the catalog of obsolete drugs along with tobacco, lobelia, and like useless but highly toxic drug substances."--DR. J. H. KELLOGG, Superintendent Battle Creek Sanitarium,

Battle Creek, Michigan.

"The majority of medical men, without making any searching investigation into the abundant recent literature upon the subject of alcohol, are disposed to regard it with less and less favor as the years go by, while those who have closely followed the thorough investigations into the physiological action of alcohol recently made by scientists, have repudiated it altogether. * * * It is a lack of information upon this subject--together with the fact that alcohol has been used as a therapeutic agent for hundreds of years, during which it has formed the basis of all tonic or stimulating treatment--that gives alcohol its present hold upon a part of the medical profession."--JOHN MADDEN, M. D., Portland, Oregon, formerly professor in Milwaukee Medical College.

"Alcohol may fill an emergency when better means are not at hand, but, apart from this, I know of no use in the practise of medicine and surgery for which we have not better weapons at our command. There is but one reason for the continued use of alcohol--men use it because they love it." DR. W. F. WAUGH, Chicago, Editor Journal of Clinical Medicine.

"If alcohol had become a candidate for recognition years ago instead of centuries ago it is safe to say that its application in medicine would have been very much more limited than we find it at the present time. Its wide therapeutic use is to be attributed in part to fallacies and misconception regarding its pharmacology, and in part to a disinclination on the part of the average practitioner of medicine to depart from old and well-beaten lines."-- WINFIELD S. HALL, M. D., Professor of Physiology, Northwestern University Medical School, Chicago.

"In its relation to the human system, alcohol is never constructive and always destructive."--PROF. FRANK WOODBURY, M. D., Philadelphia, Pa.

"The clinicians who decide for the deleterious action of alcohol in infectious conditions have what evidence of an experimental nature we possess at the present time to support their impressions. The advocates of the continuous use of the drug have this evidence against them."--HENRY F. HEWES, M. D., Harvard Medical School, Boston, Mass.

"I am very glad that you are undertaking so important a work as this in connection with the terrible problem of alcoholism. Physicians need awakening in this matter; they need reform. The evil results of alcohol are unfortunately brought to my notice each day of my life as I pursue my vocation and my public duties as Health Officer, and a reform in prescribing so as to eliminate alcohol would undoubtedly have far-reaching beneficent effects."--EDWARD VON ADELUNG, M. D., Health Officer, Oakland, Cal.

"I am forwarding you a report of 303 cases of typhoid fever treated without alcohol, and my reasons for not using it. I believe the results will not suffer by comparison with those obtained in other hospitals where alcohol is used. Wishing you lasting success in your war upon the greatest evil of the times."--J. H. LANDIS, M. D., Cincinnati, O.

"Only precise evidence that it (alcohol) is able to protect albumen from destruction can warrant its employment and establish its value as a food in the sick diet. And this evidence which is of determinative importance must be looked upon as having failed, according to the recent investigations of Stammreich and Miura (who both worked under von Noorden's direction), as well as by Schmidt, Sch 鍊 eseiffen and Roseman. The uniform result of all these experiments, arrived at by altogether different methods, is that alcohol does not possess albumen sparing power; that it even brings about an undoubted breaking down of albumen, and consequently it is entirely unequal to carbohydrates and fat."--DR. JULIAN MARCUSE, a contributing editor of Die Heilkunde, a German medical magazine. See issue of July, 1900.

"Thirty years ago the general principle of practice was stimulation. Alcohol was supposed to rouse up and support vital forces in disease. Twenty-three years ago the first practical denial was put into a permanent position in a public hospital in London, where alcohol was seldom or never used. * * * Doctor Richardson's researches showing the an 鎧 thetic nature of alcohol have had a great influence in changing medical practice in England. * * * On the Continent a number of scientific workers have published researches confirming Doctor Richardson's conclusions, and bringing out other facts as to the action of alcohol on the brain and nervous system. These papers and the discussions which followed have been slowly working their way into the laboratory and hospital, and have been tested and found correct, materially changing current opinions, and creating great doubts of the value of alcohol.

"In 1896, the prosecution of Doctor Hirschfeld, a Magdeburg physician, in the German courts, for not using alcohol in a case of septicemia, seemed to be the central point for a new demonstration of the danger of the use of alcohol in medicine. Doctor Hirschfeld was acquitted on the testimony of a large number of leading physicians from the large hospitals and universities of Europe. It was proved that alcohol was not a remedy which was specifically required in any disease; also that its value was most seriously questioned as a general remedy by many able men, and its substitution was practical and literal in most cases. Statistics were presented proving that alcohol was dangerous, and never a safe remedy, and laboratory investigations confirming and explaining its action were given. Since then a sharp reaction has been going on in Europe, and alcohol is rapidly declining and passing away as a common remedy.

"Doctor Frick, an eminent teacher of medicine in Zurich, Switzerland, and Doctor von Speyer, of the University of Berne, have made statistical studies of cases treated with and without alcohol, and have analyzed the effects of spirits as medicinal agents to check and antagonize disease, and assert very positively, that alcohol is a dangerous and exceedingly doubtful remedy. Doctor Meyer, of the University of Gottenburg, Doctor M 鰱 ius, of Leipsic, and Doctor Wehberg, of Dusseldorf, are equally prominent physicians who have taken the same position, and are equally emphatic in their denunciations of the current beliefs concerning alcohol in medicine."-- Journal A. M. A., January 6, 1900.

Dr. H. D. Didama, Dean of the Medical College of Syracuse University, Syracuse, N. Y., said in January, 1898, in the Voice:--

"For many years after my graduation at Albany, in 1846, I prescribed alcohol, and for twenty years, while occupying the chair of professor of the science and art of medicine in the College of Medicine of Syracuse University. I followed in my lectures--often reluctantly and usually afar off, but still I followed--the almost unanimous teaching of authors, ancient and modern, and the professors in the medical schools.

"Convinced that a great number of the diseases I was called to treat owed their existence or aggravation to the use, in alleged moderation, of alcoholic beverages, and that not in a few instances this use was commenced and even continued by the advice of the medical attendants; convinced also by the published experiments of many acute observers at home and abroad, and by my own observations, that almost all diseases could be managed as well if not better by the non-use of alcohol, and satisfied from the communications of some brother practitioners that the fatality in certain specified diseases was not delayed, to say the least, by the employment of increasing and enormous doses of wine, whisky and brandy, and influenced also, I must admit--overwhelmed, indeed--by what I know and what I read daily of the pauperism, domestic wretchedness, crime, insanity and incurable maladies transmitted to innocent offspring, I abandoned entirely, more than three years ago, the use of alcoholic remedies.

"I have endeavored by personal example and earnest council to dissuade my patients from the use of intoxicating beverages and medicines.

"The outcome of this practice, medically and morally, has been satisfactory to myself, and, I have reason to believe, to my patients also.

"Whatever regrets I may feel for my former teaching and practice, I have no apology to offer for my inconsistency except that once given by Gerrit

Smith:--'I know more to-day than I did yesterday; the only persons who never change their minds are God and a fool.'

"Permit me to add that while there may be an honest difference of opinion regarding the efficacy of legislative enactments in overcoming or restraining the drink habit, there should be little doubt that a whole-hearted, persistent, precept-and-example effort of the medical profession exerted as individuals on their patients and the families of their patients, and as associations on the community at large, would do immeasurable good.

"And the newspapers might aid materially in this beneficent work if, while they continue to spread before our households every day the details of the brawls and fights of drunken men and the horrible murders which they commit, they would discontinue advertising, without warning or dissent, side by side with the atrocities, the 'innocuous beers,' the pure malt whiskies, the genuine brandies, guaranteed to prevent and cure all manner of diseases."

The following testimony from an English physician is significant:--

"Although I know beforehand that their united testimony must be in favor of the practice of total abstinence from all intoxicating drinks, being most conducive to health and longevity of their patients, but very inimical to the pocket interests of themselves, my own experience is, that my teetotal patients are seldom ill, and that they get well very soon again, if they are attacked by disease. A higher principle than that of gain must influence a medical man's mind, or he will never advocate the doctrine of total abstinence."--J. J. RITCHIE, M. R. C. S., Leek.

"One of the most dangerous phases of the use of alcohol is the production of a feeling of well being in weakly, dyspeptic, irritable, nervous or an鎚ic patients. In consequence of the temporary relief so obtained, the patient develops a craving for alcohol, which in many cases can end only in one way, and, as I felt compelled to tell an assembly of ladies a short time ago, the very symptoms for the alleviation of which alcohol is usually taken are those, the presence of which renders it exceedingly desirable that alcohol should not be taken."--DR. G. SIMS WOODHEAD, of London.

In an address upon the London Temperance Hospital delivered shortly before his death, Sir B. W. Richardson gave a brief review of the influences which led him to abandon the medical use of alcohol. The following is taken from that address as reported in the Medical Pioneer:--

"I was a member of the Vestry of St. Marylebone, and we had in our parish a very serious outbreak of small-pox, attended with a considerable mortality. In his report to us Dr. Whitmore stated that in his treatment of earlier cases of the confluent and hemorrhagic, and malignant forms of disease, stimulants of wine and brandy were freely administered without any apparent benefit; and, that after consultation with Mr. Cross, the resident surgeon, they resolved to substitute simple nutriments, such as milk, eggs and beef-tea, at frequent intervals, with discontinuance of stimulants altogether. The result of the change was most satisfactory, and many bad cases did well, which under the stimulant plan they believed would have terminated fatally. Again I was struck very much by a report made by Mr. Cadbury, in which that gentleman showed the course that was going on in various hospitals. The amount of alcohol in twelve hospitals in London, taken by the inpatients, varied in ounces from 37,531 in one establishment to 300,094 in another during the year 1878. I also found, from the same author, that the whole cost in St. George's Union Infirmary for the year 1878 was ?. 3s. 6d., amongst 2,496 patients, while the cost of the same number at the average of the twelve hospitals was ?24. About this same time I also remarked that in many of the public institutions of England there was a reduction something similar in kind, if not to the same extent, and that the number of persons who suffered seemed to make better recoveries than those who were taking the free amount of stimulant. The effect of these observations chimed in very remarkably with the physiological experiments it had been my duty to carry out, and which tended to show in a most striking manner that the action of alcohol in the body very much differed from the ordinary opinion that had been held upon it, and thereupon, in my own practice, I abandoned the use of alcohol, and began to give instead small quantities of simple, nourishing, dietic food, a course I pursued up to the present time with the most satisfactory results, results I have never felt any occasion to regret. By these steps, learned in the first place from the study of alcohol in its action on man, I was led to become a believer that alcohol is of no more service in disease than it is in health, and a lengthened experience in this matter has really confirmed the correctness of the idea."

In his last report as physician to the Temperance Hospital Dr. Richardson made some remarkable statements upon the fallacy of the general ideas of stimulation. So interesting are his views that they are incorporated here:--

"Sir B. W. Richardson, M. D., who was unable to be present, communicated (through the secretary) his annual report as physician to the hospital. After twelve months further trial of the treatment of all kinds of disease in this institution without the assistance of alcohol, either as a diet or a medicine, he (Sir B. W. Richardson) was fully sustained in the belief that the plan pursued had been attended with every possible advantage. About 500 cases had come under his observation and treatment as in previous years, and these cases had been of the most varied kind, including all patients who were not directly suffering from contagious disease. In not one instance had alcohol been administered, nor had anything like it been used in the way of a substitute, and there had not been a single case in which he could conceive that it was ever called for, while the success which had attended the treatment generally had been superior to anything he had ever seen following upon the administration of alcoholic stimulants. One great truth which had forced itself upon him had reference to the doctrine of stimulation generally. It had been one of the grand ideas in medicine that there came times when sick people were benefited by being stimulated. It was argued that they were low, and in order that they might be raised and brought nearer to the natural life they required something like alcohol to quicken the circulation, quicken the secretion, and help to preserve the vitality. But the experience which was learned here tended to show in the most distinct manner that that very old and apparently rational idea was fallacious. Such stimulation only tended ultimately to wear out the powers of the body, as well as change the physical conditions under which the body worked. True lowness meant practical over-fatigue, and when the body was spurred on, or stimulated, over-fatigue was simply intensified and increased. What, therefore, was wanted was not stimulation, but repose. The sufferer was placed in the best position to gain entire rest, and all the surroundings or environments were employed which tended to prevent waste. The air was kept at the proper temperature, the body of the patient kept warm, and the simplest and most easily digested foods were used; the patient's condition then swung round to a natural state, and he began to get well. In other cases where the sick were brought under observation suffering already from excitable condition of the senses, with congestions here and there of the circulatory or nervous systems, with imperfect condition of the brain, and with the elements of what was usually denominated inflammatory or febrile state--the stimulant was already present (was, indeed the cause of the symptoms) and did not want in any degree to be enforced further by the acts of treatment. Here, therefore, they were on the safest grounds as regarded methods of administration, for they calmed as well as they possibly could both mind and body and left nature to do the rest, which she did with the best and most tranquilizing effect. On both sides, therefore, in the treatment of disease, they did good, and that was the reason, he believed, why their returns were so satisfactory. It often happened in an institution where some particular plan was carried out that the old ideas in which they had been bred were without intention refined or suppressed. For example, he had been taught, and believed for a number of years, that some medicament of a particular kind was needful for some particular train of symptoms, be the surrounding conditions what they might. There was no doubt that this same feeling had given rise to the persistent use of alcohol; but, greatly to his own surprise, he discovered that when the surroundings were all good, the rule that applied to alcohol constantly applied to other substances that were called remedies, with the result that recovery was often just as good without the particular remedies as with them, so that a revision came quite simply with regard to stimulating agents and their properties, and also with regard to every medicine that might at earlier times have been employed. He had seen many cases in this hospital recover without any other aid than that of the environments, which cases he would have said could not possibly have gone on well, or towards complete recovery, unless some special recipe had been followed. He believed the day would come when others, learning this same truth as he had been obliged to learn it, would act on such simple principles that the books of remedies would have to be vastly curtailed. It would be seen that there was such a tendency of disease to get well of itself, or by virtue of natural processes, of which people had at present but a very poor idea, that the art of physic would pass into directions how to live rather than into dogmatic assertions that particular means must be employed in addition to the common details of life for the process of cure. If therefore they learned in this hospital by their reduced death-rates the true lesson, the institution would have performed a double duty, and become one of the test objects in medicine, and in the field of disease. They made no attempt by selection, or by any side action, to exaggerate their results. The cases were taken indiscriminately, except that they gave admission to the worst cases first; that was to say, they never caused patients to come under their treatment if they saw they were only slightly affected, and were bound to get well."--Medical Pioneer.

Dr. Landmann, of Boppard-on-the-Rhine, Germany, says:--

"The members of the Association of Abstaining Physicians, reject the use of spirituous liquors in every form, and particularly declare the use of alcohol at the sick-bed a scientific error of the saddest kind. In order to war against this abuse, they earnestly appeal to the officers having charge of funds for the sick, henceforth, under no circumstances, any longer to permit the prescription of wine, whisky and brandy for sick members; but to resist to the utmost, according to the right given them by the laws insuring the sick, the taking of spirituous liquors, under the false pretext that they have a curative and strengthening effect."

Dr. Bleuler, Rheineau, Switzerland, says:--

"The treatment of chronic diseases with alcohol is contrary to our knowledge of the physiological effects of alcohol. There is no probability that its use will be beneficial, certainly its benefits have not been established. Often an injurious result is proved.

"It is not implied that there may not be some benefit in the use of alcohol in cases of sudden weakness with or without fever. But even in such cases the benefit is not demonstrated. At any rate, other remedies can with advantage be substituted for alcohol.

"The essential thing in the treatment of all alcoholic diseases, delirium tremens included, is total abstinence.

"The physiological effect of alcohol is that of a poison, whose use is to be limited to the utmost. Even the moderate use as now practiced is injurious.

"The customary beneficial results unquestionably depend chiefly on suggestion, and by making the patient believe falsely that the momentary subjective better feeling means actual improvement.

"Physicians share the blame of the present flood of alcoholism. They are, therefore, morally bound to remedy the evil. Only by means of personal abstinence can this be done."

Dr. A. Frick, professor in Zurich, is a careful student and an influential writer on alcohol. His statements are weighty. This is his testimony:--

"In larger doses, alcohol is absolutely injurious in the treatment of acute fevers, especially in case of pneumonia, typhus and erysipelas. They first of all injure the general state of the patient, they cause delirium, or increase it if already existing, and, secondly, they injure most seriously the organs of digestion and interfere with proper nourishment; thus they have a weakening effect, instead of preventing weakness, which they are usually supposed to do. In case no alcohol is used, the convalescence is much more rapid. In no case has the benefit of treatment with alcohol been established. According to the view of the most eminent pharmacologists, the stimulating effect of alcohol consists simply in a local irritation of the mucous membrane of the stomach, similar to that produced by a mustard plaster."

The following selection from the excellent address of Dr. Harvey, president of the Virginia State Medical Society, at a recent meeting, is a most timely caution:--

"Our prisons, asylums and homes are filled with the victims of the careless and indiscriminate use by the medical profession of those twin demons, alcohol and opium, which, save tuberculosis, are doing more to debase and destroy the human race than all the other diseases together. I most earnestly beseech you, young men, who are just starting out in life, to stay your hand in the use of these agents in your own persons, and in your daily work, and to beware of the seductive needle, and the cup that inebriates. Make it an invariable rule, never to prescribe alcohol, nor one of the solinaceus or narcotic drugs, if you can possibly avoid it. The use of alcohol and opium debases the minds and morals of habitu 閼, predisposes especially to Bright's disease and insanity, and lays the foundation in the offspring for the majority of the neuroses and degenerations of modern civilized life. The physical fatigue of long working hours, loss of sleep, mental strain, worry and hunger, invite the tired physician, especially, to their seductive use. To totally abstain from them is always business, and very often character, and even life itself. I feel free to speak to you on this subject very earnestly, my younger brothers, for, having prescribed alcohol for over thirty years, I am familiar with its tendencies and its dangers."

Dr. T. D. Crothers of Hartford, Conn., in an article upon "The Decline of Alcohol as a Medicine," says:--

"Thoughtful observers recognize that alcohol as a medicine is rapidly becoming a thing of the past. Ten years ago leading medical men and text-books spoke of stimulants as essentials of many diseases, and defended their use with warmth and positiveness. To-day this is changed. Medical men seldom refer to spirits as remedies, and when they do, express great conservatism and caution. The text-books show the same changes, although some dogmatic authors refuse to recognize the change of practice, and still cling to the idea of the food value of spirits.

"Druggists who supply spirits to the profession recognize a tremendous dropping off in the demand. A distiller who, ten years ago, sold many thousand gallons of choice whiskies, almost exclusively to medical men, has lost his trade altogether, and gone out of business. Wine men, too, recognize this change, and are making every effort to have wine used in the place of spirits in the sick-room. Proprietary medicine dealers are putting all sorts of compounds of wine with iron, bark, etc., on the market with the same idea. It is doubtful if any of these will be able to secure any permanent place in therapeutics.

"The fact is, alcohol is passing out of practical therapeutics because its real action is becoming known. Facts are accumulating in the laboratory, in the autopsy room, at the bedside, and in the work of experimental psychologists, which show that alcohol is a depressant and a narcotic; that it cannot build up tissue, but always acts as a degenerative power; and that its apparent effects of raising the heart's action and quickening functional activities are misleading and erroneous.

"French and German specialists have denounced spirits both as a beverage and a medicine, and shown by actual demonstration that alcohol is a poison and a depressant, and that any therapeutic action it is assumed to have is open to question.

"All this is not the result of agitation and wild condemnation by persons who feel deeply the sad consequences of the abuse of spirits. It is simply the outcome of the gradual accumulation of facts that have been proven within the observation of every thoughtful person. The exact or approximate facts relating to alcohol can now be tested by instruments of precision. We can weigh and measure the effects, and it is not essential to theorize or speculate; we can test and prove with reasonable certainty what was before a matter of doubt.

"Medical men who doubt the value of spirits are no more considered fanatics or extremists, but as leaders along new and wider lines of research. Alcohol in medicine, except as a narcotic and an æs thetic, is rapidly falling into disfavor, and will soon be put aside and forgotten."

CHAPTER XVI.

RECENT RESEARCHES UPON ALCOHOL.

In the year 1900 Prof. Taav Laitinen, of the University of Helsingfors, Finland, published an account of experiments made upon 342 animals--dogs, rabbits, guinea pigs, fowls and pigeons--to determine the effects of alcohol upon the resistance of the body to infectious diseases. He used as infecting agents, anthrax bacilli, tubercle bacilli, and diphtheria bacilli. The doses of alcohol given varied with the animal. For his "small dose" experiments he used the quantity of alcohol given as a food or as a medicine, or both, in a neighboring sanitorium. The alcohol employed was, as a rule, a 25 per cent. solution of ethyl alcohol in water. It was given either by esophageal catheter, or by dropping it into the mouth from a pipette. It was administered in several ways, and for varying times; sometimes in single large doses, at others in gradually increasing doses for months at a time, in order to produce here an acute, and there a chronic poisoning; in fact, he produced the conditions consequent upon steady, moderate drinking.

His first conclusion from these experiments, most carefully carried out, is that alcohol, however given, induces in the animal body a markedly increased susceptibility to infectious diseases; and he maintains that his experiments indicate that the use of alcohol, at least in the treatment of anthrax, tuberculosis, and diphtheria, is not only useless but probably injurious. From a number of other experiments carried out with scrupulous care he comes to the same conclusion as Abbott, Welch, and others that the predisposing to disease of alcohol must be explained by its action in producing abnormal conditions--pathological changes in the alimentary canal, liver, kidneys, heart, and nervous system. He found that the alkalinity of the blood was slightly diminished, and the number of leucocytes somewhat decreased. He also draws attention to the fact that his experiments prove that pregnant animals and their offspring are markedly affected by the continued use of small doses of alcohol. He shows, too, that the temporary lowering of the body temperature by alcohol produces the most favorable condition for the invasion of disease germs.

Since the publication of these experiments, and of others similar to them, the use of alcohol in diphtheria and tuberculosis has very largely ceased. Boards of health and charity organizations unite in warning against indulgence in alcoholic drinks as conducive to tuberculosis.

At the International Congress on Alcoholism, held in London in July, 1909, Professor Laitinen delivered two lectures. The first was upon "The Influence of Alcohol on Immunity." The following is taken from this lecture:--

"Modern researches have done much to explain the extent and nature of the protective powers by which the organism endeavors to defend itself against the attacks of all kinds of injurious agencies, and especially against invasion by the germs of infective diseases. It is now a well-established fact that alcohol weakens the normal resisting power of the body against the above-named disease-producing influences. In the hope of contributing something to the explanation of the way in which alcohol weakens the organism, I have made a number of experiments bearing upon the question of the influence of alcohol on immunity.

"Early in this century careful experiments went to show that alcohol certainly had some influence upon immunity. Two Americans, Abbott and Bergey, were the first to discover that this agent produces a diminution of the h 鎚 olytic complement in the blood-serum of certain animals which were tested. They showed also that the formation of specific h 鎚 olytic receptors (immune bodies) may be retarded by the action of alcohol.

"The extent of the evil effects upon the human body resulting from the consumption of alcoholic liquors is as yet far from being fully known, and stands in need of scientific verification. Many other injurious influences such as unsanitary dwellings, bad feeding, excessive toil, and toxic agents like nicotine, etc., may produce somewhat similar morbid effects. It is therefore necessary, in the scientific study of the question, to take these possibilities into consideration. In my investigations, the results of which I am now to lay before you, I have endeavored to select as subjects for my experiments both abstainers from alcohol, and those who indulge more or less in its use, in such a way that their conditions of life and their habits in other respects should be as nearly as possible the same. All persons, for instance, suffering from any acute or chronic disease were rejected, and very few of the persons selected were smokers. The subject of this research has been human blood, and especially its two principal components, namely, red blood-corpuscles and blood-serum, both of which up to the present time have been very little studied in relation to the question under discussion. I have gone into these matters chiefly because the modern theoretical study of immunity during the last few years has, in general, attracted greater attention to the blood, and shown the important role which the different parts, properties, and capacities of the blood play in defending the organism against internal and external injurious agencies. Further, the subtle methods employed in the study of immunity (such as organic reactions, and reactions between greatly attenuated organic liquids) would also seem to be available for our purpose, as they allow of the detection of the minutest differences which alcohol may produce in any part of the organism in question.

"During the course of this research, which has lasted over a period of three years, I sought to investigate the action of alcohol on the resistive power of human red blood-corpuscles. I wished to ascertain whether the resistivity of the red blood-corpuscles in a healthy man could be lowered by the consumption of alcohol. * * *

"It may be well for me here to explain that in this lecture I mean by the term 'drinker' a person who has taken alcohol in any quantity whatever. Many of these 'drinkers,' therefore, were in fact most moderate consumers of alcohol. By the term 'abstainer' I mean a person who has never taken alcohol in any quantity worth mentioning. In the course of my investigations I have examined blood from two hundred and twenty-three persons. They were of different classes and ages. There were professors of medicine and other physicians, University fellows, students of both sexes, hospital nurses, school-teachers, waiters, and other men and women belonging to the working-classes."

The rest of the lecture as given here is an abstract made by Professor Laitinen:--

"My studies have been directed to an investigation of the following points:

"1. I sought to ascertain whether the resistance of human red blood-corpuscles against a heterogeneous normal serum, or an immune serum, can be diminished by the use of alcohol.

"2. I have studied the action of alcohol in drinking and abstaining persons on the h鎚olytic power of blood-serum over heterogeneous red blood-corpuscles (rabbits). I have studied not only the h鎚olytic power of the human blood-serum, but also its power of precipitation in the presence of rabbit-serum, with a view to ascertain if the reaction between a known dilution of rabbit-serum and a certain dilution of serum of alcohol-users and non-drinking persons is different or not, and if the reaction is more apparent with the former or with the latter.

"3. The resisting power of serum obtained both from alcohol-drinking and from non-drinking persons was further tested by human blood, with the object of discovering whether any difference in reaction existed between the same immune serum and the two kinds of human sera above mentioned.

"4. I have studied the problem as to whether the h鎚olytic complement in the blood-serum of alcohol-drinking and non-drinking persons is altered in any way by alcohol.

"5. The bactericidal power of blood-serum from both alcohol-drinking and non-drinking persons was determined by some experiments.

"The above experiments have given the following results:

"1. The normal resistance of human red blood-corpuscles appears to be somewhat diminished against a heterogeneous normal serum or an immune serum by the consumption of alcohol, provided that tolerably large equal, or nearly equal, numbers of drinkers and abstainers of both sexes be examined, and the average of resistance be taken on both sides: this last-named precaution being necessary because the resistance of red blood-corpuscles from different human beings varies largely. The difference is often greater when using weaker solutions than when using stronger dilutions of lysin.

"2. These experiments have shown the normal h鎚olytic power of human blood-serum to be less in the case of alcohol-drinkers than in that of abstainers.

"3. The precipitating reaction between a solution of 1 per cent. human blood-serum and different dilutions of immune serum was greater in the case of drinkers than in that of abstainers.

"4. These experiments have also shown that the bactericidal power of blood-serum against typhoid bacteria was less in the case of drinkers than in that of abstainers.

"It seems clear, therefore, that alcohol, even in comparatively small doses, exercises a prejudicial effect on the protective mechanism of the human body."

The lecturer made his points clear by a carefully prepared series of charts. At its close Sir Victor Horsley, Professor Sims Woodhead, A. Pearce Gould, and several other distinguished physicians spoke in high terms of the painstaking care exhibited in the experiments.

Professor Laitinen's second lecture was upon "The Influence of Alcohol Upon Human Offspring." He sent out 15,000 circulars to his countrymen, asking many questions relative to themselves and their infant children, and received 5,845 replies relative to 20,008 children. He also studied personally a large number of drinking and abstaining families. From these studies he shows by careful tables that the drinking of alcohol by parents, even in small quantities, has an injurious influence upon human offspring. His studies in former years showed the same unfavorable influence upon the offspring of animals. One of his tables gives percentages of deaths of children in the homes of abstaining parents, moderate drinkers, and harder drinkers. Children of abstainers dying in the first year, 13.45 per cent.; of moderates, 23.17 per cent.; of harder drinkers, 32.02 per cent. Other tables show that abstainers' children gain in weight more steadily in the first year than drinkers' children, and have their teeth earlier, as a rule.

At the International Medical Congress of 1909, held in Budapest, Professor Laitinen lectured again upon his researches, and summarized his conclusions thus:--

"1. The importance of alcohol as an article of food is rendered very questionable by recent researches. 2. These researches prove that alcohol diminishes the natural power of the tissues to resist injury, promotes degeneration, and has a disastrous effect on future generations. 3. The questions of relation of alcoholic liquor to crime and of the manufacture and sale of such beverages deserve the serious consideration of the legislature. 4. It is the duty of medical men to direct more attention than formerly to the alcohol question, and by careful study to decide whether recent researches are justified or not in regarding alcohol and alcoholic beverages as a poison and one of the principal causes of degeneration in the human family; they ought also to consider whether it would not be advisable in medical practice, and especially in hospitals, either to banish it altogether or at least to prescribe it with the same care as other poisonous drugs. In this matter the attitude taken by medical men as representatives of public hygiene was of quite exceptional importance."

Metchnikoff, the illustrious Russian scientist, who has for some years been connected with the Pasteur Institute in Paris, was the discoverer of the work assigned by nature to the white corpuscles of the blood. These blood-cells are the "guardian-cells" of the body, and their duty is to destroy disease germs which may gain an entrance. They actually devour disease germs. Metchnikoff has been studying the effect of alcohol upon these protective cells, and he asserts that alcohol, even in small doses, has a harmful action on these agents of defence against disease. Alcohol seems to paralyze them more or less so that they are unable to do their full duty in destroying the infective microbes. Thus disease germs can multiply more rapidly when alcohol is in the blood. In his book called "The New Hygiene," Metchnikoff suggests that the administration of alcoholic liquors in infectious disease appears to be attended with danger to the patient.

The researches of Kraepelin, Ach, Aschaffenberg and other German scientists have become so well known through the articles by Henry Smith Williams in McClure's Magazine that only brief reference need be made to them here. Kraepelin used very small doses of alcohol for some of his experiments. He found that after 1/4 to 1/2 ounce of alcohol had been taken the time occupied in making response to a signal was slightly shortened, but in a few minutes, in most cases, this quickening action passed and a slowing process began, and continued until the body was free from the influence of the alcohol, which was sometimes four or five hours.

The ability to add figures was tested, and this decreased very rapidly under minute doses of alcohol. Memory tests showed that only 60 figures could be remembered from numbers written in columns after alcohol had been taken, while 100 figures could be remembered correctly when the mind was free from the alcoholic influence. Type-setters were tested, and the average number of errors they made and the amount of work they did in a given time was carefully recorded. After a small dose of alcohol none of the men could in the same time do as much work, or as accurate work. Yet every one of the men experimented upon thought he was doing better work after his drink. This proves the narcotic effect of alcohol.

The economic loss to a people from beer and wine drinking is worthy of serious consideration since a bottle of wine or its equivalent in beer could diminish by ten to fifteen per cent. the amount of work done by these type-setters experimented upon by Professor Aschaffenberg.

Professor Kraepelin says:--

"I must admit that my experiments, extending over more than ten years, have made me an opponent of alcohol."

He says again:--

"The laborer who wins his livelihood by the working power of his arm strikes at the very foundation of his power by the use of alcohol."

Professor Aschaffenberg says of moderate doses:--

"Any quantity of alcohol must be regarded as considerable which causes a disturbance, even if only transitory, of bodily and mental efficiency."

Dr. Reid Hunt, chief of the Division of Pharmacology, Hygienic Laboratory, United States Public Health and Marine Hospital Service, made some very interesting experiments to determine the physiological changes upon animals which would result from the strictly moderate use of alcohol. These are described in Bulletin No. 33 of the Hygienic Laboratory, published in 1907. Mice and guinea-pigs were used. The food, usually oats, was soaked in diluted alcohol, at first of five per cent. strength, then gradually increased to forty or fifty per cent. By carefully observing the weight of the mice, and not increasing the strength of the alcohol too rapidly, it was possible to keep the animals for months on this diet without any material loss of weight. After the lapse of weeks, in some cases, and months in other cases, these alcohol fed animals were given small doses of a poison known as acetonitrile. Other mice to whom no alcohol was fed were given similar doses of this poison. In the first series the mice which had received alcohol died from about one-half the quantity of acetonitrile required to kill those which had not received alcohol. In the second series with a somewhat stronger dilution the alcohol mice succumbed to one-half to one-third the dose necessary to kill the non-alcoholized animals. In no case was enough alcohol given for any symptoms of intoxication to appear, nor was there any outward indication of any injury being done by the alcohol. In another experiment a mouse was kept for four months on a diet of oats soaked in water, then 0.5 milligram of acetonitrile per gram body weight was injected. The mouse recovered. It was then fed on oats soaked in an alcoholic solution which was gradually increased to 45 per cent. After a little more than a month of this diet 0.2 milligram acetonitrile per gram body weight proved fatal. The weight of the mouse had remained about the same throughout.

Alcohol increased the susceptibility of the guinea pigs also.

Dr. Hunt says on page 33 of the bulletin:--

"These experiments with alcohol and acetonitrile are of interest in another connection. The greatest advance in recent years in our knowledge of the physiological action of alcohol has been the clear demonstration that alcohol is oxidized in the body, and may replace fats and carbohydrates and to a certain extent, the proteids of an ordinary diet. So clear has been this demonstration that the view that alcohol, in moderate amounts, should be regarded as a food is almost universally accepted by physiologists, and the drift of opinion is certainly toward the view that it is in all respects strictly analogous to sugar and fats, provided always that the amount used does not exceed that easily oxidized by the body. Under these premises it would be expected that alcohol in a diet would have the same effect upon an animal's susceptibility to acetonitrile as has dextrose, for example. This is by no means the case, however; on the contrary, the action of these substances in this regard is entirely different. Mice fed upon oats soaked in a solution of dextrose or upon cakes containing considerable dextrose, or upon rice, show a very distinct increase in their resistance to acetonitrile; such mice may recover from two or three times the dose fatal to controls. (Controls are the animals fed in the ordinary way without alcohol or in this case dextrose.-- Ed.) While these facts are not sufficient to justify the conclusion that in many cases alcohol has not a true food value, yet they are sufficient to indicate caution in applying, without further consideration, the brilliant and very exact results on the proteid sparing power of alcohol to practical dietaries."

Various other experiments were made, but there is not room here for a record of them.

In the summary Dr. Hunt says:--

"It is believed that these experiments afford clear experimental evidence for the view that extremely moderate amounts of alcohol may cause distinct changes in certain physiological functions, and that these changes may, under certain circumstances, be injurious to the body. The results also afford further evidence that in some respects the action of alcohol as a food is different from that of carbohydrates, and finally that in all probability certain physiological processes in 'moderate drinkers' are distinctly different from those in abstainers."

Professor Chittenden, of Yale University, has made extensive researches upon alcohol and digestion. A full report of these may be found in the "Physiological Aspects of the Liquor Problem." In the Medical News, vol. 86, page 721, Professor Chittenden says of the theory that alcohol is a food similar to sugar and fats:--

"It is, I think, quite plain that while alcohol in moderate amounts can be burned in the body, thus serving as food in the sense that it may be a source of energy, it is quite misleading to attempt a classification or even comparison of alcohol with carbohydrates and fats, since, unlike the latter, alcohol has a most disturbing effect upon the metabolism or oxidation of the purin compounds of our daily food. Alcohol, therefore, presents a dangerous side wholly wanting in carbohydrates and fats. The latter are simply burned up to carbonic acid and water, or are transformed into glycogen and fat, but alcohol, though more easily oxidizable, is at all times liable to obstruct, in some measure at least, the oxidative processes of the liver, and probably of other tissues also, thereby throwing into the circulation bodies such as uric acid, which are inimical to health; a fact which at once tends to draw a distinct line of demarcation between alcohol and the two non-nitrogeneous foods--fat and carbohydrate."

Dr. S. P. Beebe, now of the Cornell Medical College Laboratory, New York City, has made some very valuable experiments with alcohol. It is well known that impairment of the functions of certain organs results in the appearance in the urine of nitrogeneous compounds which do not normally occur there. In certain diseases of the liver the same quantity of nitrogen may be excreted as in health, but a portion of it is in the form of acids never found in the urine during health. Dr. Beebe, with this knowledge in mind, sought to discover the effects of alcohol upon the excretion of uric acid in man. Most of the experiments were made on the same person, a young man in good health, of regular habits, unaccustomed to the use of alcohol in any form. Absolute alcohol, diluted with water, whisky, ale, and port wine were used at different times. Dr. Beebe reported his experiments in the American Journal of Physiology, vol. 12, No. 1. His conclusions are given as follows:-
-

"After a consideration of these experiments, it hardly seems possible to doubt that alcohol, even in what is considered by the most conservative as a moderate amount, causes an increase in the excretion of uric acid, and this effect is seen almost immediately after taking the alcohol. The following points indicate that the effect is due to a toxic effect on the liver, thereby interfering with the oxidation of the uric acid derived from its precursors in the food: Alcohol taken without food causes no increase. The maximum increase occurs at the same time after a meal as it does when purin food but no alcohol is taken. Alcohol is rapidly absorbed and passes at once to the liver, the organ which has most to do with the metabolism of proteid cleavage products.

"There is no evidence that the alcohol has merely hastened the excretion of urates normally present in the blood; the increased excretion means that a larger quantity has been in circulation, and although it is classed by Van Noorden among the substances easily excreted, still most physiologists would consider the presence in the blood of this larger quantity as undesirable. Certainly in pathological conditions it might be harmful.

"If we accept the origin of the increased quantity of uric acid to be in the impaired oxidative powers of the liver, the results of these experiments will have greater significance than can be attributed to uric acid alone. For the impaired function would affect other processes which are normally accomplished by that organ, and the possibilities for entrance into the general circulation of toxic substances, of intestinal putrefaction, for instance, would be increased. The liver performs a large number of oxidations and syntheses designed to keep toxic substances from reaching the body tissues, and if alcohol, in the moderate quantity which caused the increase in uric acid excretion, impairs its power in this respect, the prevalent ideas regarding the harmlessness of moderate drinking need revision."

Dr. Winfield S. Hall, professor of physiology at the Northwestern University Medical School, Chicago, has interpreted these researches of Beebe and Hunt in a very striking way. He says that they prove that the oxidation of alcohol in the body is a protective oxidation, the same as the oxidation of any other poisonous substance by the liver. His views have such an important bearing upon the commonly accepted theory that alcohol is in some sense a food that they are given here, somewhat abbreviated, as a fitting finish to this chapter. Dr. Hall says:--

"The fact that alcohol is oxidized in the body has been generally misunderstood. The first impression naturally was: 'Foods are Oxidized; Alcohol is Oxidized; therefore alcohol is a food.' But many difficulties appeared. A real food promotes muscular, glandular and nerve activity, and its oxidation maintains body temperature. But alcohol disturbs muscular, glandular, and nervous activity, and its oxidation does not maintain body temperature. When one eats a real food it is assimilated largely by muscle tissue and is oxidized for the purpose of liberating the life energy. When one ingests alcohol it is carried by the blood to the tissues, mostly to the liver, where it is oxidized, as any toxine would be, for the purpose of making it harmless. Its oxidation liberates heat energy but this energy cannot be utilized by the body even for the maintenance of body temperature. If a food is defined as a substance which, taken into the body, is assimilated and used either to build or repair body structure, or to be oxidized in the tissues to liberate the energy used by the tissue in its normal activity, then alcohol is not a real food.

"But, if alcohol is not a real food, what is the significance of its oxidation? It has been long known that the liver produces oxidases and that it is the site of active oxidation of mid-products of katabolism of toxins and of other toxic substances. Alcohol, usually formed as an excretion of the yeast plant, is also found as a mid-product of tissue katabolism. On a priori grounds we should expect alcohol to be oxidized in the liver along with leucin, tyrosin, uric acid, xanthin bodies, and various amido bodies. There have recently appeared two most important papers based upon extended researches upon man and lower animals. These researches practically clear up this knotty question."

Dr. Hall then reviews the work of Dr. Reid Hunt and Dr. S. P. Beebe, and continues:--

"The value of this work can hardly be over-estimated. In the first place the rapid oxidation of the alcohol in the liver is explained. Alcohol itself being one of the toxic substances which reach the liver from the alimentary canal is at once attacked by the liver, and if the oncoming tide of alcohol is not too great it will practically all be oxidized.

"But the liver oxidation of other toxic substances is impaired in the meantime so that they get past the liver to the tissues, where they may do injury. Some of these toxins are excreted unoxidized by the kidneys. There are three ways of accounting for this condition: (1.) The oxidation capacity of the liver is limited. The physiological limit of alcohol ingestion is that amount which taxes the oxidation capacity of the liver to its limit. When thus taxed all other toxic substances including uric acid and the xanthin bodies pass through the liver unoxidized to appear in the urine. (2.) The presence of alcohol in the blood, through its toxic action upon the liver cells, impairs the hepatic oxidation capacity and thus permits toxic substances to pass unoxidized. (3.) A combination of these conditions may represent the real situation. It is hardly conceivable that the relation of alcohol to the liver activity is not covered in the hypotheses above formulated.

"We may therefore accept it as practically demonstrated by the researches of Beebe, Hunt, and others that the oxidation of alcohol in the liver is simply one of the defensive activities of that organ, i. e., it is a protective oxidation and belongs strictly in the same category with the oxidation of uric acid, xanthin bodies, leucin, tyrosins, and the amido acids.

"The next question which arises is, why does the liver select alcohol first and oxidize that substance to the exclusion of other toxic substances up to the oxidation capacity? The answer is probably to be found in the chemical composition of alcohol.

"It oxidizes very easily, much more so than any of the other toxic substances which gain access to the liver. Its early oxidation may be due to this fact alone, or in part to an actual selection on the part of the liver. Another question of importance: Is the energy liberated in the oxidation of alcohol in the liver available for the use of the muscles, nervous system, or glands?

"If this question is answered affirmatively, then alcohol is a food. If negatively then alcohol is not a food. Let us reason together. All body oxidations may be classified in two groups: (1.) Active oxidations which take place in the active tissues--muscles, nervous system, or glands--and take place incident to action. It is under the perfect control of the nervous system and is proportional to normal activity. (2.) Protective oxidations which take place in the liver. This class of oxidation processes is wholly independent of the usual tissue activity and is proportional to the ingestion of toxic substances and quite independent of muscle action, brain action, or gland action, other than liver action.

"If the oxidation of alcohol in the liver belongs to class 1, the following consequences should be found: (1.) The ingestion of alcohol would lead to an increase in muscular power and in the working capacity of the brain or glands. (2.) The ingestion of alcohol would serve to maintain body temperature in the healthy individual subjected to low external temperature. (3.) The accession of muscle, brain, or gland activity would be proportional to the amount of alcohol ingested, but laboratory observations and general experience show that none of these things are true; i. e., the ingestion of alcohol decreases muscle, brain, and gland work, and depresses body temperature when external temperature is low.

"In the nature of the case there can be no proportional relation. The oxidation of alcohol does not therefore belong to class 1. If the oxidation of alcohol in the liver belongs to class 2, the following consequences would be found: (1.) The ingestion of alcohol would be followed by its early oxidation in the organs in question. (2.) If the oxidation capacity of the liver is limited this capacity may be overloaded by exceeding the physiological limit of alcohol. (3.) If the oxidation capacity of the liver is taxed nearly to its limit in the oxidation of uric acid, xanthins, and other toxic substances, the introduction of alcohol may seriously interfere with this protective oxidation by overtaxing the capacity. (4.) If the oxidation capacity is overtaxed, an excess of uric acid, xanthin bodies, and other toxic substances will get by this portal and reach the active tissues or the kidneys. Now all of these things take place, so we are forced to the conclusion that the oxidation of alcohol is a protective oxidation. In the light of this presentation the significance of Dr. Hunt's work becomes very clear. The alcohol given to the animals taxed the oxidation capacity of the liver to the limit and left the organism defenseless against bacterial or other toxic substances."

CHAPTER XVII.

MISCELLANEOUS.

ALCOHOL BATHS:--The action of alcohol upon the surface of the body is that of a refrigerant. Alcohol baths for debility, weakness, and states of exhaustion are opposed by non-alcoholic physicians. The old custom of bathing a new-born babe with whisky was simply a superstition, and a dangerous one, because the infant should not have a refrigerant applied to its body so soon after leaving the warm nest where it had been sheltered so long. Warm water is the proper liquid for a baby's bath until it becomes hardy. There is nothing of strength imparted by an alcohol rub; the 'rub' is good, but vinegar, or water, or olive oil can be used according to what is desired. Alcohol is not necessary internally nor externally. Its proper use is for mechanical purposes and to give light and heat.

WILHELMINA LEMONADE:--Take four or five rough-skinned oranges (according to size) and two pounds of sugar, in big lumps. After having cleaned the oranges, rub the sugar with them, till the oranges are quite white--the sugar yellow. Place the sugar in a big earthernware pan or jar, and add three pints of cold water. Then cover it up and let it stand two days, stirring it occasionally to help the melting. Now take two ounces of citric acid, dissolved in a little boiling water, and add it to the syrup, stirring the whole.

Then strain the whole through a fine sieve, covered with muslin, so that it becomes perfectly clear. In well-corked bottles it will keep for more than a year. Mix one-third of the lemonade with two-thirds water. [Instead of the oranges five or six lemons may be used.]

BEVERAGES FOR THE SICK:--Unfermented Grapejuice. Hot milk. Egg cream, made as follows: Beat the white and yolk separately, add milk and sugar, and stir well, flavor to suit taste. Egg lemonade--beat yolk and sugar thoroughly, add lemon and water, shake well, then add white, beaten stiff. Barley water, made by boiling pearl barley five or six hours, and straining the water from it; add milk or cream if wished. These are used in the National Temperance Hospital of Chicago.

BATHS:--"If all people understood the value of water to cool, cleanse, invigorate and sustain life, and how to use it, and would use it, one-half of all the afflictions from disease would be removed; and the other half might be banished if all the people understood how and what to eat, how to breathe, and the necessity of daily vigorous exercise. A daily towel bath will do more to counteract disease, and restore the body to its normal health condition, than any other method or remedy yet discovered. After the bath, the body should be thoroughly rubbed with a crash or Turkish towel. Rub until a warm glow is produced. This bath is a fine tonic if taken upon rising in the morning."

HOT WATER AS A MEDICINE:--"One is never," says a physician, "far from a pretty good medicine chest with hot water at hand. It is a most useful assistant to the mother of a family of small children, who is frightened often to find herself confronted by a sudden illness of one of her flock, without her usual dependence--the family doctor. If the baby has croup, fold a strip of flannel or a soft napkin lengthwise, dip into very hot water, and apply to the child's throat. Repeat and continue the application till relief is had, which will be almost at once. For toothache, or colic, or a threatened lung congestion, the hot-water treatment will be found promptly efficacious if resorted to. Nature needs only a little assistance at the first sign of trouble to rally quickly in the average healthy child, and often hot water is all that is wanted."

ALCOHOL INJURIOUS TO THE INSANE:--Dr. Richard Maurice Bucke, whose valuable paper on "The Evolution of the Mind" appeared in the December number of the Journal of Hygiene, in a recent report of the Asylum for the Insane in London, Canada, makes the following statement concerning the use of alcohol in the institution over which he presides:--

"As we have given up the use of alcohol, we have needed and used less opium and chloral; and as we have discontinued the use of alcohol, opium and chloral, we have needed and used less seclusion and restraint. I have, during the year just closed, carefully watched the effect of the alcohol given, and the progress of cases where, in former years, it would have been given, and I am morally certain that the alcohol used during the past year did no good. With humiliation I am forced to admit that in the recent past my noble profession has been to an alarming extent, and is still too much so, guilty of producing many drunkards in the land, directly or indirectly, by the reckless and wholesale manner in which so many of its members have prescribed alcoholic stimulants in their daily practice for all the aches and pains, coughs and colds, inflammations and consumptions, fevers and chills, at the hour of birth and at the time of death, and all intermediate points of life, to induce sleep and to promote wakefulness, and for all real or imaginary ills."

TOBACCO AND THE EYESIGHT:--"Prof. Craddock says that tobacco has a bad effect upon the sight, and a distinct disease of the eye is attributed to its immoderate use. Many cases in which complete loss of sight has occurred, and which were formerly regarded as hopeless, are now known to be curable by making the patient abstain from tobacco. These patients almost invariably at first have color blindness, taking red to be brown or black, and green to be light blue or orange. In nearly every case, the pupils are much contracted, in some cases to such an extent that the patient is unable to move about without assistance. One such man admitted that he had usually smoked from twenty to thirty cigars a day. He consented to give up smoking altogether, and his sight was fully restored in three and a half months. It has been found that chewing is much worse than smoking in its effects upon the eyesight, probably for the simple reason that more of the poison is thereby absorbed. The condition found in the eye in the early stages is that of extreme congestion only; but this, unless remedied at once, leads to gradually increasing disease of the optic nerve, and then, of course, blindness is absolute and beyond remedy. It is, therefore, evident that, to be of any value, the treatment of disease of the eye due to excessive smoking must be immediate, or it will probably be useless."--Journal of Inebriety.

"Dr. Isaac Fellows was for many years a prominent physician in Los Angeles. A temperance man, he was persuaded by an old physician whom he loved to try for a year substituting alcohol in drop doses in water for such patients as demanded alcoholic stimulants. He was delighted with the result. When his patients found they could not have wine, beer or brandy under the guise of medicine, but must take it in drop doses in water, as they did their other medicines, they speedily learned to do without 'a stimulant.'"--Pacific Ensign.

ADVERTISED "CURES" FOR DRUNKENNESS.

"Poudre Coza, an English product, is sold at $3.00 for thirty powders. On analysis these powders were found to contain an impure form of sodium bicarbonate, together with a little aromatic vegetable matter. Gloria Tonic was examined by the Massachusetts Board of Health, and found to consist of sugar of milk and cornstarch, with a small quantity of ground leaves resembling those of senna. White Ribbon Remedy was found to be made of milk sugar and ammonium chloride. Of course such things are clearly frauds, as they can have no power to destroy a craving for liquor. The Infallible Drink Cure was 98 per cent. sugar and 2 per cent. common table salt. Another 'cure' was made of chlorate of potash and sugar. Cases of poisoning by chlorate of potash are on record. Another 'cure' contained tartar emetic, a dangerous poison. Most of the liquid 'cures' for drunkenness sold prior to the passage of the National Pure Food Law contained large quantities of cheap alcohol. It is safe to say that practically all of the secret cures for drunkenness are fraudulent, and some are dangerous.

"If a man wants to quit drinking, he can be helped by a proper diet, and by frequent use of the Turkish bath, or even of the ordinary hot bath at home, with a quick cold sponge or shower bath each morning as a tonic. The hot bath is to draw out impurities from the system. The diet should consist of plenty of fruit, nuts, grains and vegetables. It is better to eat no meat. It has been fully demonstrated in Lady Henry Somerset's work with women drunkards that a vegetarian diet is a great help in allaying the alcohol crave. The Salvation Army, in England, have also found by experience that a meat-free diet is a great aid in overcoming the drink habit.

"Dr. T. D. Crothers, who has for years conducted a large sanitarium for the cure of inebriety, at Hartford, Connecticut, says that a valuable remedy to break up the impulsive craze for spirits is a strong infusion of quassia given in two-ounce doses every hour. As desire for liquor abates the quassia can be given less frequently, until it is no longer needed.

"Dr. Alexander Lambert, of Bellevue Hospital, New York, has been treating drunkards and other drug habitues successfully of late. A description of his treatment may be found in Success for November, 1909."

MEDICAL PUFFS OF WHISKY AND OTHER ALCOHOLICS:--"Every medical man knows how he is pestered with advertising circulars of so-and-so's genuine whisky, and what-do-you-call-em's extra stout, to say nothing of the tempting offers of wines and spirits on sale with special discounts to medical men. Other enterprising firms send samples or offer to send them with the implied understanding that a testimonial is to be given, or that at least the wares in question will be recommended to patients. Even our medical papers have not always been incorruptible. We have little expectation ourselves of being favored with an offer of full-page advertisements of extraordinary wines and spirits. We are not prepared to recommend them except as vermin killers. Nor are we prepared to remain silent as to their alleged virtues. The whole system of testimonials is a huge imposture. Granted that the sample is all that it is described as being, who can guarantee that what is served to the public in the face of severe competition will be up to the sample?

"But there is another and a sadder view of the case. We cannot believe that all the eulogies of all the medical trumpeters of the wines and the spirits are wilfully false or even exaggerated. It is a lamentable fact that a vast number of doctors have a genuine faith in the value and virtue of these pernicious drinks. It is not simply a question of medicinal use, though even on that we should join issue. These things are vaunted as valuable for the promotion of health in spite of all the accumulating evidence to the contrary. We wish that these doctors would carefully study this evidence. The pity of it is that the very worst offenders are the least likely to study it. We suppose they must die out, and be replaced by men less prejudiced and bound by the chain of alcoholic habit. We can only regret that they should be doing so much harm in fastening the fetters of drink on other people, and hindering their emancipation from the evil customs which play havoc amongst us."-- Medical Pioneer.

ALCOHOL AND CHILDREN:--"Parents often labor under the delusion that alcoholic drinks are good for children and act as tonics. Mothers will put drops of brandy into the milk with which their children are fed, increasing the quantity with the age of the recipient. In the illness of children the same is given to meet disturbances of the stomach or to increase growth and development, without taking the advice of any medical man as to the wisdom of the practice. This is all erroneous. The excitement of the central nervous system under alcohol, excitement which seems to be a relief to weariness and to give strength, is nothing more than temporary at best, and injurious, causing in fact symptoms of alcoholic poisoning, abnormal excitement, ending, in extreme cases, in convulsions succeeded by exhaustion of body and mind, and inducing a kind of paralysis. Many cases of stomach and gastric catarrh in children followed by emaciation and debility are due to the early administration of alcoholic drinks; and impediment of growth from the same cause is thereby produced. The most serious derangement is that of the nervous system, and the development in the young, under the influence of alcohol, of what is known as nervousness, to which is added the moral paralysis with which the habit of alcoholic drinking smites its victims in the very spring-time of life."--PROF. DEMME, of Berne, Switzerland.

"The action of the New York Board of Health, in recommending to tenement house parents, that on the hottest days of summer a few drops of whisky be added to the water or food of their infants, has received a strong protest and rebuke in a meeting at Prohibition Park, where the opinions of eminent physicians, collected by the Voice, were read, condemning such a course. A resolution of protest was also adopted."--Sel.

"For nineteen years we lived with a physician whose success may be estimated from this one item: He had between 1,600 and 1,700 labor cases, and never once lost the mother, and only twice the child, and what seems still more remarkable never used instruments. When other physicians, as often happened, would come to him to know how he did it, he always answered, 'A woman will do anything if you only encourage her.' Nor was obstetrics his specialty--he had none.

"In a fifteen years' practice in Chicago and New York, where these diseases are so very fatal, and he was much sought after to treat them, he did not lose a case of scarlet fever, diphtheria or cholera infantum which he managed himself, and saved many a one where he was called in consultation, or after some other physician. Now when such a man after an experience more than fifty years long and as wide as the continent, gives it as his unqualified opinion that wines, beers, liquors of every kind, alcohol itself, are not medicines and should never be used as such, for SCIENTIFIC reasons, not to mention moral, is not his opinion entitled to a hearing? Isn't it probable it weighs more than the doctor's you were just quoting? Is it too great a risk to act upon it?"--Pacific Ensign.

"A lady, Mrs. A., tenderly nurtured, refined, cultured, moving in an influential position, belonged to a family in whom the tendency to intemperance existed. Realizing the danger, she, for seven years of her married life, adhered to total abstinence. Illness came, and the doctor ordered wine; and her husband, deaf to her arguments, insisted on her taking it. She fell into habits of intemperance. Her husband died, and for a time she pulled up and trained as a hospital nurse; but temptation prevailed, and she fell from bad to worse. Loving hands received her time after time, and at last placed her in an Inebriate Home. For a short time she did well, but soon became unmanageable. After another desperate period she entered a second home, but after leaving she yielded again, was twice in prison, and fell into the lowest degradation and utter ruin, surely deserving our deepest pity. Her doctor and her husband had persisted in working her fall in spite of her own strongest convictions."--Selected.

THEY DID NOT DIE.--"Dr. Lord of Pasadena suffered from rheumatism of the heart for more than half of a long lifetime. No doctor ever felt his pulse (which intermitted) without exclaiming, 'Why, doctor, you have no business to be alive with such a pulse,'--or something similar. For nineteen years his wife never retired without having at least one medicine she could put her hand on in the dark, the ammonia bottle within reach, the electric battery ready to start like a fire-engine, and preparations for heating water in less than no time. His acute attacks usually came in the night--an uninterrupted night's sleep was something unknown to either the doctor or his wife in all these years.

"They lived in sight of an open grave, and seldom a week passed when it did not seem as if death had actually occurred. If ever a case called for alcoholic stimulants this one did. But none were ever administered, none were ever kept in the house. The doctor's standing orders were: 'If all the doctors in the country order you to give me liquor, and say my life depends upon it, don't do it. Tell them I know more about it than they do. It won't save my life; it will only lessen what little chance I have.' All who knew about this case, and hundreds did, were driven to the conclusion that if these two people, one in this condition and the other feeble, could live all alone as they did, miles from a doctor, and neighbors not near, and could get along without alcoholics of any kind, everybody can do the same everywhere. And the doctor finally wore out his heart trouble and died of another disease."-- Pacific Ensign.

An English weekly journal is responsible for the following anecdote:--

"A Birmingham physician has had an amusing experience. The other day a somewhat distracted mother brought her daughter to see him. The girl was suffering from what is known among people as 'general lowness.' There was nothing much the matter with her, but she was pale and listless and did not care about eating or doing anything. The doctor, after due consultation, prescribed for her a glass of claret three times a day with her meals. The mother was somewhat deaf, but apparently heard all he said and bore off her daughter, determined to carry out the prescription to the very letter. In ten days' time they were back again, and the girl looked a different creature. She was rosy-cheeked, smiling and the picture of health. The doctor congratulated himself on his diagnosis of the case. 'I am glad to see that your daughter is so much better,' he said. 'Yes,' exclaimed the excited and grateful mother. 'Thanks to you, doctor! She has had just what you ordered. She has eaten carrots three times a day since we were here, and sometimes oftener-- and once or twice uncooked--and now look at her!'"

THE REST CURE:--"After all, the veneer of civilization is quite thin. Scratch most people, and very near the surface you come on the savage. This is specially true when they are sick. They at once want charms and miracles to restore them to health, and come to the doctor or 'medicine man,' as they look upon him--with this demand: 'I want something, doctor, to fix me up.' But he, unhappy man, has not wherewith to satisfy them, unless he is a quack.

"He knows that in most cases all he can do is to give advice as to how best Nature may be allowed to effect a cure; for Nature is the great physician, and the doctor's main duty is to stand by and see that she gets fair play. Nature's chief cure, in a large number of the diseases to which flesh is heir, is rest. The tired man needs rest. The tired brain, the tired stomach, the tired liver and kidneys, need the same rest.

"So, when the patient turns up with an overworked and exhausted organ of some sort within him--be it what it may--heart, brain or stomach--the true physician prescribes, first and chiefly, not drugs, but rest.

"Now, this is generally the advice the patient doesn't want. His desire is for a bottle of something, no matter how nasty it may be, which shall 'fix him up,' and let him go on doing what he has been doing previously. Common-sense is always at a discount, and never more so than in this case. The tired brain-worker doesn't want to stop. Give him something to whip up his brain and his body, something to drive the spurs into them. 'What I want,' he says, 'is a really strong tonic'; though, if he knew that before, what was the use of coming to the doctor? Or he would like to be told to take a glass of whisky-and-water when he is tired, which is the maddest and most disastrous advice that could be given.

"The man who has been ill-treating his stomach, eating too much or too well, also demands a tonic--something to give him an appetite so that he may eat more. And his poor overwrought stomach is all the time crying out for rest.

"So it is all along the line. The possessor of an inflamed and swollen knee prays for a liniment to rub into it which will cure it straight away, and is highly disgusted when told that he will have to lie up for a week or two.

"Again, for the tired stomach the cure is starvation. Let the person live on his own fat, and a little milk-and-water for a few days, and his stomach will take courage again and return to work with renewed zest. But it is the most difficult thing in the world to persuade the patient or his kind relatives of the truth of this. There are many diseases in which, for a short time at least, the less food the sick person has the better. But the relatives are always much wiser than the doctor. They insist 'that the strength must be kept up,' and would like to force the patient to eat more than he does when well. 'You will let his strength down, doctor,' is a common complaint, and one of the difficulties hospital authorities have to face is to prevent kind friends from smuggling in food to the inmates, who, in their opinion, are being brutally starved.

"I myself have cured people by making them rest--lie in bed and starve. But the next time they were sick, I wasn't the doctor."--"PHYSICIAN" in Our Federation.

"The blessings of sunlight and fresh air should be more appreciated. The sun is the godfather of us all. The source of all light, heat, electricity and energy, what wonder that it was once worshipped as the Creator. The future will recognize it not only as the best disinfectant, an all powerful preventive of disease, but also as a wonderful healer of disease. The more people can be taught to live in pure air out of doors, and bask in the rays of the sun, the less of disease there will be to prevent."--DR. C. H. SHEPARD, Brooklyn, N. Y.

ALCOHOL TESTED.

"Some years ago Dr. Beddoes, a physician of eminence, was very anxious to put to the test the disputed question as to the power of alcoholic liquors to give strength to the system. He discovered that those who had most calls upon their physical endurance were the smiths who were engaged in forging ship's anchors, for at one moment they would be exposed to a heat so fierce that one marveled that any human organization could endure exposure to it, and then their work would call them away to a temperature that was chilly and cold, added to which all the time their work lasted they were bathed in a profuse perspiration, the demands upon their physical energy were so great. To counteract this perpetual drain upon their system they were in the habit of drinking unlimited quantities of beer, which their masters provided for them as a matter of course, and a sine qua non. One day, as they were resting from their work at midday, Dr. Beddoes made his appearance amongst some of these men who were employed in a certain foundry, and submitted a formal proposition to them, to this effect, that twelve of their number, the strongest and stanchest, should be selected for an experiment, and they should work for a week, six of them drinking only water, and the other six taking their beer as usual. His proposition was laughed to scorn. The men would not hear of it. 'Look here, mate,' said their spokesman, 'do you want us to be all dead men; you don't know what our work is, and how it takes all a man's strength to weld an anchor. Why, if we did not have our beer and plenty of it, it would be all up with us in a brace of shakes.'

"The doctor said: 'I should be very sorry for any harm to come to you. You know I am a doctor, and I will be constantly at hand to see if any of you are going wrong, and I promise that if I see any of you breaking down I will at once stop my experiment.' And then taking out of his pocket ten crisp five-pound notes, he displayed them to the anchor smiths. 'I will put down these notes, ?0 in all; six of you shall try water for one week honestly and fairly; if you pull through without giving in, the ?0 shall be yours; if not, I'll take the ?0 back again. Is it a bargain?'

"This clenched the matter, and very soon the doctor's offer was accepted, and a gang of six men volunteered to begin their work on the Monday without beer. The beer drinkers did their best to chaff the water drinkers, and aggravated them by taking good care to show them how very nice it was to have recourse to unlimited beer. The water drinkers kept firm, and the first day, to their astonishment, found that they could do just as much work as the rest of their mates. On Tuesday the water drinkers began to crow over the beer drinkers, for they found that, while the latter complained and grumbled at the heat, they were enabled to take the work in a philosophical kind of way. Wednesday, Thursday and Friday wore away, and the teetotal band became more and more triumphant, the laugh was all on their side, for not only did they feel more comfortable than their beer-loving companions, but the ?0 came nearer and nearer, and at last, on Saturday, when the time for finishing work came, they threw down their tools and their hammers, and crowded up to the doctor to claim the prize, and to give a faithful record of their experiences; and one and all declared that they had done their hard work with more ease and comfort to themselves than ever it had been done before, and, instead of feeling tired and jaded, as they often did on the Saturday afternoon, they were quite ready to begin work again, and if the doctor had another ?0 to dispose of, they would most gladly give him a chance of protracting his experiment for another week. The doctor expressed himself perfectly satisfied with the trial which had already taken place, and left the place amidst three hearty cheers, while the men proceeded to discuss the ins and outs of the matter among themselves."--National Advocate.

BEER-DRINKING INJURES HEALTH.

"I think there is no doubt that beer-drinking is deleterious to health, and personally I have never seen any case of disease where I thought it useful. I believe it is more deleterious to health than the stronger spirits, and this opinion is derived from the report of the actuaries' investigations for our insurance companies a few years ago."--DR. JOHN M. DODSON, Dean of the Medical Department of the University of Chicago.

"My connection with large medical institutions for many years past has given me, I think, an excellent opportunity to observe the effect of beer-drinking and the use of other alcoholic liquors in many cases. I can say as a result of my own observation that beer-drinking has a very pernicious effect upon nearly every organ of the body. It produces disease of the stomach and digestive tract, of the heart and circulating system, of the kidneys and liver, and of the nervous system. In addition to this it lessens the vigor and vital resistance of the whole body, makes the beer drinker very much more susceptible to infection such as pneumonia, and other acute infections, and also lessens his ability to recover from illnesses of any kind. An untold amount of misery and disease would be avoided if the use of beer and other intoxicating liquors could be wiped off the face of the earth."--DR. W. H. RILEY, Battle Creek Sanitarium, Battle Creek, Mich.

In the report of Bellevue Hospital, New York City, for 1904, Dr. Alexander Lambert, in speaking of delirium tremens, says: "The delirium tremens from beer does not come on so readily as that from whisky, but is slower in clearing up." Page 138 of report.

"Apart from its toxic effect it is seldom realized how harmful beer may be by promoting obesity, and, in susceptible persons, favoring dilatation of the stomach."--DR. E. P. JOSLIN, Professor in Harvard Medical School.

"It is not the concentrated alcoholic liquors alone that cause heart and kidney trouble but pre-eminently the continued immoderate use of beer. Nothing is more false than the belief that the progressive dislodgement of other alcoholic drinks by beer will diminish the destructive influences of alcoholism. * * * It has been conclusively established by thousandfold experiments that soldiers in all climates, in heat, cold and rain, endure best the most fatiguing marches when they are absolutely deprived of alcoholic drinks."--PROF. G. VON BUNGE, M. D., Basle, Switzerland.

"Beer, wine and spirits furnish no element capable of entering into the composition of blood, muscular fibre, or anything which is the seat of vital principle. If a man drinks daily 8 or 10 quarts of the best Bavarian beer in a year he will have taken into his system as much nourishment as is contained in a five-pound loaf of bread."--Liebig, the great German chemist.

"Beer-drinker's heart is a term well-known to the physicians of our large hospitals, and indicates a special condition of unhealthy enlargement of the heart due to dilatation, accompanied by some increase of tissue and of fat. Doctors Bauer and Bollinger found that in Munich one in every sixteen of the hospital patients died from this disorder. It is common in Germany--the land of beer-drinking--and proves incontestably that the habit of drinking even such a mild alcoholic beverage as lager-beer is one that is undesirable and unwise."--From "Alcohol and the Human Body," by Sir Victor Horsley, M. D., London.

"Nothing is more erroneous from the physician's standpoint, than to think of diminishing the destructive effects of alcoholism by substituting beer for other alcoholic drinks, or that the victims of drink are found only in those countries where whisky helps the people of a low grade of culture to forget their poverty and misery."--PROF. STRUMPEL, Breslau, Germany.

"The result of extolling beer as the mightiest enemy of whisky and brandy has been that the consumption of the distilled liquors has changed very little, while to these liquors has been added beer, the use of which has led to a great and still increasing beer alcoholism. * * *

"The beer drinker who is not at all a drunkard in the popular sense, is very frequently the victim of chronic inflammation of the kidneys. * * * An enlarged and fatty condition of the liver, marked by a dull pain in the region of the organ, often follows from the habitual use of beer. The death-rate from liver diseases among brewers of beer in England is more than double that in all other occupations. * * * Beer-drinkers have a marked tendency to enlargement of the stomach, and to chronic diarrhoea. Beer causes also inflammation of the nerves. This is often announced by 'rheumatic' pains in the legs. * * * Beer alcoholism, as well as alcoholism in general, lowers the resistance of the body to all diseases by injuring most of the organs. And herein lies the chief danger in the general wide-spread use of beer. The drinker is especially open to attacks of infectious disease. * * * The brutalizing effect of beer-alcoholism is shown most clearly by the fact that in Germany crimes of personal violence, particularly dangerous bodily injuries, occur most frequently in Bavaria where there is the highest consumption of beer."--DR. HUGO HOPPE, Nerve Specialist, Konigsberg, Germany.

"The life insurance companies make a business of estimating men's lives, and can only make money by making correct estimates of whatever influences life. Now they expect a man otherwise healthy, who is addicted to beer-drinking, will have his life shortened from 40 to 60 per cent. For instance if he is twenty years old and does not drink beer he may reasonably expect to live until he is 61. If he is a beer-drinker he will probably not live to be over 35. If he is 30 years old when he begins to drink beer he will probably drop off somewhere between 40 and 45 instead of living to 64 as he should. There is no sentiment, prejudice or assertion about these figures. They are simply cold-blooded business facts, derived from experience, and the companies invest their money on them just the same as a man pays so many dollars for so many feet of ground or bushels of wheat."--DR. S. S. THORN, Toledo, Ohio, in U. S. Senate Document, published in 1901.

"Fatty degeneration of various organs is frequently witnessed in beer-drinkers. Diabetes mellitus is frequently due to beer-drinking, and is made much worse by its continuance. In Germany more than half of the cases in the inebriate asylums enter from beer-drinking. In Bavaria, the women are not able properly to suckle their children because of the universal consumption of their favorite national drink. Indeed, so grave are the evils caused by beer-drinking that the fight against beer should now be conducted as strenuously as that against stronger liquors."--DR. LEGRAIN, Paris, France.

DRUG DRINKS.

In the report of the President's Homes Commission, Senate Document 644, may be found a list of soft drinks examined by the Bureau of Chemistry. The report says:--

"Attention is directed to the danger of soft drinks containing caffeine, and extract of coca leaf, the active principle of the latter being cocaine. * * * We have seen how the opium habit may be acquired by the use of the various proprietary or secret preparations, and so the cocaine habit may be developed by the use of these much lauded soft drinks. * * * No wonder that insanity and diseases of the nervous system are on the increase."

The following is a list of drinks examined by the Bureau of Chemistry. Investigation showed that these contained both caffeine and extract of coca leaf:

Afri Cola, Ala Cola, Cafe Coca, Carre Cola, Celery Cola, Chan Ola, Chera Cola, Coca Beta, Coca Cola, Pilsbury's Coke, Cola Coke, Cream Cola, Dope, Four Kola, Hayo Kola, Heck's Cola, Kaye Ola, Koca Nola, Koke, Kola Ade, Kola Kola, Kola Phos, Koloko, Kos Kola, Lime Cola, Lima Ola, Mellow Nip, Nerv Ola, Revive Ola, Rocola, Rye Ola, Standard Cola, Toka Tona, Tokola, Vim-O, French Wine of Coca, Wise Ola.

The manufacturers of some of those listed claim that their coca extract is prepared from a decocainized coca leaf, the refuse product discarded in the manufacture of cocaine. The Coca Cola company claims that their coca extract is now without cocaine, and most of the recent analyses show this to be true, yet the Pure Food Commissioner of North Dakota says in his report for 1907 that Coca Cola as examined by him, "Gave a reaction for cocaine." It is easy to see that so long as even refuse coca leaves are used some cocaine may at times be in the product.

As cocaine is the most destructive drug known to humanity its presence in any of the so-called temperance drinks is a frightful evil calling for speedy legislation. It is practically impossible to cure a person of the cocaine habit. This drug causes insomnia, dyspepsia, chronic palpitations, and complete paralysis of will-power, with a tendency to criminal acts. When a person becomes habituated to its use he suffers torments when not under its influence. The real cocaine fiend will rob or kill to get the drug. What can be thought of men, who knowing the deadly nature of this drug, will hide it away in a drink sold as harmless to children and women who would never touch beer or wines? It is placed in the drink to form a craving for that drink and thus create a demand that will enrich the conscienceless manufacturers.

The following preparations were found to contain caffeine, but there was no evidence to the effect that coca leaf in any form had been used in their manufacture:

Calcycine, Celery Cocoa, Citro Cola, Deep Rock Ginger Ale, Fosko,

Heck's Star Pepsin, Koke, Koke Ola, Kalafra, Kumfort, Lime Juice and Kola, Lon Kola, Meg-O, Mexicola, Pau Pau Cola, Pedro, Pepsi Cola, Speed Ball, To-Ko, Vril.

The report says that the following list were not examined but from their names, and from the evidence submitted, they contain either caffeine or coca leaf extract, or both: Charcola, Cherry Kola, Cola Soda, Cola Ginger, Field's Coca, Imported French Cola, Jacob's Kola, Koko Ale, Kola Cream, Kola Pepsin Celery Wine Tonic, Kola Vena, Loco Kola, Mintola, Mate, Pikmeup, Ro-Cola, Schelhorn's Coca, Vine Cola, Viz.

Dr. Harvey W. Wiley, chief of the Bureau of Chemistry, says that the sale of all such drinks should be prohibited.

Caffeine is a drug much used in headache remedies. It is derived from the kola nut, and from tea and coffee. It is also made artificially from uric acid occurring in the guano or bird manure deposits of South America. This bird manure product is said to be used in some of the drinks while in others caffeine obtained from refuse tea sweepings is used. The sales-manager of the Coca Cola Company says the caffeine in their product is made from tea. It is claimed by the manufacturers of caffeine drinks that they are as harmless as tea or coffee. But physicians advise against the use of tea and coffee for children and for delicate, nervous people, and every intelligent person knows that these drinks should not be indulged in immoderately. The secret caffeine drinks at the soda-fountain are not warned against because few people know of what they are made. So it frequently happens that children whose parents do not permit them to drink tea and coffee are taking caffeine in a much more injurious form at the drug stores.

Dr. Harvey W. Wiley, Chief of the Bureau of Chemistry, says: "When caffeine is separated from tea and coffee, and used as a separate drug, it exerts a much more specific action upon the system than when in natural combination. Its general effect is to induce that unhappy state described as nervousness, with deranged digestion and impaired health." Dr. H. H. Rusby,

Dean of the College of Pharmacy, of Columbia University, New York City, a high authority, says: "Caffeine is a genuine poison, both acute and chronic. Taken in the form of a beverage it tends to the formation of a drug habit, quite as characteristic, though not so effective, as ordinary narcotics. Permanent disorders of the cardiac function, and of the cerebral circulation, result from its continued use."

The Druggists Circular, for May, 1908, contained a query from a druggist as to a good formula for a kola nut soda syrup. The answer was in part as follows: "There are two kinds of druggists. One kind puts any and every kind of stuff into stock, and passes it out to his customers, young and old, ignorant or learned, foolish or wise, his only desire being to get a profit. The other kind of druggist refuses to stock some things at all. Kola drinks owe their vogue to the caffeine which they contain. Caffeine is a poison which is cumulative in its effects, and an excess of which has not infrequently caused death. We believe you would better be on record as discouraging rather than encouraging the growth of the caffeine habit, especially among young people, who constitute a large part of the soda-water trade."

The London Lancet of January 25, 1908, reports the results of experiments made in Paris with kola given to horses to determine its action in relieving fatigue. It apparently diminished fatigue, but the horses receiving it lost more weight than those to whom it was not given. The experimenter said this showed that kola (caffeine) like alcohol, can give the tissues a lash with a whip, but that such energy, artificially produced, is at the expense of the organism. So, when people see the alluring advertisements of caffeine drinks which "relieve fatigue," let them beware of the relief which carries with it injury to the body.

Of the most widely advertised of these caffeine drinks the government report says: "The prevalence of the 'Coca Cola fiend' is becoming a matter of great importance and concern." (See volume on Social Betterment of Senate Document 644, page 268.) M. M. A.

SPECIAL MEDICAL DIRECTIONS FOR WOMEN.

"In the treatment of diseases of women, alcohol has been considered a very important remedy. Because it affords relief from pain, many resort to its use during painful menstruation. Each month either whisky, or some medicine containing a liberal supply of alcohol, is considered a necessity.

"The alcohol habit is not infrequently formed in this way. I have in my mind several cases of inebriety which were traceable to the habit of taking something to relieve pain at these periods. A woman whose husband held a high official position, thus acquired a craving for alcohol and became a confirmed drinker. He was finally compelled to place her in an institution for treatment.

"Alcohol affords relief, not by lessening the internal congestion which causes the pain, but by paralyzing or benumbing the nervous system. In fact, alcohol, instead of relieving, aggravates the internal congestion. It is a deceiver, for it makes the patient believe she is benefited when in fact the condition is made worse. The uterus has become more congested by its use, and when the paralyzing effect of the alcohol has worn off the pain will be found more severe, and the demand for alcohol increased correspondingly. The only safe and wise plan when suffering from pain due to internal congestion is to remove the cause. If uterine misplacement exists suitable treatment must be taken to correct this. Almost immediate relief from pain due to congestion of the pelvic organs may be obtained by taking a hot full bath. A hot foot or leg bath is also a good treatment since the warming of the extremities quickens the circulation in the limbs and relieves congestion in the pelvic region.

"There are various forms of dysmenorrhea or painful menstruation and each form has a treatment by itself. The congestive type which is due to taking cold is better relieved by a hot sitz bath before the date expected, the temperature of the water should be 101?103?with the feet in water a degree or two hotter. If at the time of the period the pain still continues, an enema or vaginal douche will usually give the necessary relief unless the patient should be exposed to cold by allowing the hands, arms, feet or legs to become chilled.

"Many women do not dress their limbs warmly enough at any time. Just before the menstrual period the tendency is for the pelvic organs to become congested; there is a greater tendency to cold feet then, than at any other time. I would therefore advise warmer clothing on the limbs at such times. The drinking of hot pepper tea, ginger tea, etc., is a pernicious practice, for these irritants inflame the mucous membrane of the stomach and intestines. Hot lemonade or hot water will afford the same relief without leaving an inflamed surface behind to be irritated by the next meal.

"There are some cases of great constriction of the uterine canal which have reflex irritability in the stomach. Those having the stomach affected cannot take food, the least thing is rejected. It is best for such to remain quiet in bed, applying heat to the stomach and abdomen and to the feet until relief is experienced. Those suffering from headache should also remain quiet in bed. Some resort to anodynes and form the habit of using codeine, morphine. All these are bad and should be avoided. I have never found it necessary to give one dose of either to relieve pain at such times. Hot applications with the enema, vaginal douche, or foot bath, has usually been all that was required.

"I recall many cases of severe pain where the extremities were cold and clammy and the entire body was in a hysterical contraction that were immediately relieved by a hot vaginal douche. The muscles relaxed, the patient warmed up and recovered nicely.

"For securing sleep in insomnia, a hot toddy is often used, but a quicker and better effect can be gained by a hot, or neutral bath. The latter given at 99?or 100?for twenty minutes will produce sleep and refreshment, as it equalizes the circulation by bringing the blood to the surface.

"It is safer under all circumstances to do without alcohol or other dangerous drugs in treatment of these diseases."--DR. LAURETTA E. KRESS, Washington, D. C.

NOTE--An experienced nurse says that prompt relief in painful menstruation may often be found by sitting upon a toilet water-jar half full or more of hot water. The steam rises and the heat relieves.

TOTAL ABSTINENCE AND LIFE INSURANCE.

Nothing shows more clearly and convincingly that alcoholic liquors have a tendency to shorten life than the figures published by life insurance companies. A most interesting and valuable paper upon this theme was read before the Actuarial Society of America, in 1904, by Mr. Joel G. Van Cise, actuary of the Equitable Life Assurance Society of the United States. In it he gives the experience of different life insurance companies which have separate sections for total abstainers and non-abstainers. The Mutual Life Insurance Company of New York, one of the large companies, showed after a few years' experience with the two sections a death-rate 23 per cent. higher among the drinkers than among the abstainers. The Sceptre Life for the years from 1884 to 1903, inclusive, gave the following: Expected deaths of abstainers, 1,440; actual deaths, 792, being 55 per cent. of the expected. Expected deaths of non-abstainers, 2,730; actual deaths, 1,880, or 79 per cent. of the expected. The Scottish Temperance Life from 1883 to 1902 gave the following: Abstainers, expected deaths, 936; actual deaths, 420, or 45 per cent. of the expected. Non-abstainers, expected deaths, 319; actual deaths, 225, or 71 per cent. of the expected.

Mr. Van Cise goes on to show that the statistics which have been published from time to time, giving the percentages of mortality in the various occupations of life, invariably show a higher death-rate among those engaged in the liquor business than among those engaged in other lines of work, except such as are specially hazardous. He says: 'The higher death-rate among liquor dealers is so universally recognized by life assurance companies that a number of them will not issue policies, even on the lives of the richest brewers, upon any terms, and not one of the companies, to my knowledge, admits liquor dealers upon as advantageous terms as those engaged in other ordinary occupations.' He then quotes from a circular sent to the agency force of a prominent United States company, in which attention is called to a rule which forbids the taking of any risks on bartenders: 'Saloonkeepers, generally, not taken, but best of this class may be accepted on 10 or 15 year endowments only.' Others connected more remotely with the liquor business might be taken with a charge of $5.00 per thousand extra. The circular of instructions adds that the limitations of liquor dealers are made necessary 'by the very excessive rate of mortality found to exist among persons so employed.'

Mr. Van Cise closed his address before the Actuaries' Society by saying: 'I contend that the facts given in this paper show conclusively that the effect of total abstinence is to lower the death-rate, and increase the average duration of human life.'

The Equitable Company had a section for total abstainers for a few years which was discontinued on account of the new insurance laws which came into effect in 1907. The actuary writes in response to inquiry: 'We are very careful in our selection of risks, and only those who drink in moderation will be accepted. I think it safe to say that, other things being equal, all American life insurance companies would consider a total abstainer a more desirable risk than a moderate drinker.'

The United Kingdom Temperance and General Provident Institution, of London, is a large and successful company which was organized in 1840, expressly for total abstainers, because at that time larger premiums were asked from abstainers than from drinkers, the common opinion then being that alcoholic liquors were necessary to health. In 1846, this company added a general section, in which carefully selected moderate drinkers were accepted, but each section was kept entirely separate from the other. This separation has continued to the present time, both classes paying the same premiums, but sharing in profits according to the earnings of the section to which the members belong. From 1866 to 1900, for every 100 deaths in the temperance section there were 137 deaths in the moderate drinking section, based on a corresponding number of lives at risk. The dividends for a recent five years average $20 to the temperance members, and $17 to the drinking members.

The actuary of this English company, Mr. Roderick Mackenzie Moore, read a paper before the Institute of Actuaries, in 1903, in which he reviewed the work of this company during its history of sixty years' experience with abstainers and over fifty with non-abstainers. He showed that there has been no marked difference in the number of policies in force in the two sections, and the average amount of the policies in each section has been about the same, so that the comparison is as fair as could possibly be made. He gives these figures: 'Non-abstainers, male, expected deaths, 8,911; actual deaths, 8,947; per cent. of actual to expected, 100.4. Abstainers, male, expected deaths, 6,899; actual deaths, 5,124; per cent. of actual to expected, 74.3.' This shows a difference of 26.1 per cent. between the actual and expected deaths of abstainers and moderate drinkers, and the full figures show the death rate among the drinkers to be 35 per cent. higher than among the abstainers.

The American Temperance Life Insurance Association was organized in 1887. It gives a lower premium rate to members of the abstainers' section than to those in the general section. The circulars sent out by this company state that the average life of moderate drinkers is thirty-five and a half years; tipplers, fifty-one years; total abstainers, sixty-four and one-fifth years.

Very interesting is the result of an inquiry made of various insurance companies not long ago as to whether they consider the habitual user of intoxicating beverages as good an insurance risk as the total abstainer; 'if not, why not?' All but two out of forty-one companies answered, 'No.' The two answered, 'Depends on quantity used.' In answer to the 'Why not?' the Etna said, 'Drink diseases the system and shortens life'; Hartford Life, 'Moderate use lays foundation for disease'; Knights of the Maccabees, 'Drink tends to destroy life'; Knights Templar and Masons' Life Indemnity, 'Drink lessens ability to overcome disease'; Sun Life, 'Drink injures constitution. Habit apt to grow'; Massachusetts Mutual Life, 'Drink causes organic changes. Reduces expectation of life nearly two-thirds.' The rest of the answers are much the same as these.--M. M. A.

###